A GUIDEBOOK TO HUMAN
SERVICE PROFESSIONS

Second Edition

A GUIDEBOOK TO HUMAN SERVICE PROFESSIONS

Helping College Students Explore Opportunities in the Human Services Field

Edited by

WILLIAM G. EMENER, PH.D.

MICHAEL A. RICHARD, PH.D.

JOHN J. BOSWORTH, M.A.

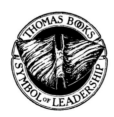

CHARLES C THOMAS • PUBLISHER, LTD.
Springfield • Illinois • U.S.A.

Published and Distributed Throughout the World by

CHARLES C THOMAS • PUBLISHER, LTD.
2600 South First Street
Springfield, Illinois 62704

©2009 by CHARLES C THOMAS • PUBLISHER, LTD.

ISBN 978-0-398-07851-5

Library of Congress Catalog Card Number: 2008041517

With THOMAS BOOKS *careful attention is given to all details of man-*
ufacturing and design. It is the Publisher's desire to present books that are sat-
isfactory as to their physical qualities and artistic possibilities and appropri-
ate for their particular use. THOMAS BOOKS *will be true to those laws*
of quality that assure a good name and good will.

Printed in the United States of America
CR-R-3

Library of Congress Cataloging-in-Publication Data

A guidebook to human service professions : helping college stu-
dents explore opportunities in the human services field / edited by
William G. Emener, Michael A. Richard, John J. Bosworth. -- 2nd ed.
    p. cm.
ISBN 978-0-398-07851-5 (pbk.)
  Rev. ed. of: I'm a people person. c2003.
  Includes bibliographical references.
  1. Human services--Vocational guidance. 2. Social service--
Vocational guidance. 3. Educational counseling--Vocational guidance.
4. Mental health services--Vocational guidance. 5. Rehabilitation
counseling--Vocational guidance. 6. Health counseling--Vocational
guidance. 7. Employees--Counseling of--Vocational guidance. I.
Emener, William G. (William George) II. Richard, Michael A. III.
Bosworth, John J. IV. I'm a people person.

  HV10.5.I4 2009
  361.973023--dc22

                                        2008041517

CONTRIBUTORS

Michael V. Angrosino, Ph.D., is Professor Emeritus of Anthropology at the University of South Florida. He specializes in the cultural dimensions of mental health policy and service delivery and has served as Editor of *Human Organization,* the journal of the Society for Applied Anthropology. His most recent publications include: *Naturalistic Observation; Doing Ethnographic and Observational Research*; and the forthcoming *Oral History: A Window on the Past.*

Michael B. Brown, Ph.D., is Professor of Psychology and a member of the school psychology faculty at East Carolina University in Greenville, NC. He has a Ph.D. in school psychology from Virginia Tech and is both a licensed psychologist and a National Certified School Psychologist. His research interests include school psychologists' job satisfaction, childhood cancer, and school-based health centers.

Robynanne Cash-Howard, M.A., is currently in private practice and provides Vocational Expert testimony in many arenas. She has worked in a wide variety of rehabilitation settings since 1985 and has taught as an Adjunct Professor at the University of South Florida. She also holds the following national certifications: Certified Rehabilitation Counselor, Certified Vocational Evaluator, Certified Case Manager, Certified Life Care Planner and Social Security Vocational Expert.

John L. Daly, Ph.D., is an Associate Professor and Director of Public Administration at the University of South Florida. He also serves as President of Creative Insights Corporation, a consulting firm located in Lutz, Florida. John is a past U.S. Fulbright Scholar to Swaziland (1998–99 & 2005–06). His research has appeared in numerous national and international public administration and human resource management journals. His most recent book, *Training in Developing Nations* (M.E. Sharpe) was published in 2005.

Peggy A. Dupey, Ph.D., is Assistant Dean of Students at the University of Nevada, School of Medicine and Adjunct Assistant Professor in the Department of Counseling & Educational Psychology at the University of Nevada.

Colleen A. Etzbach, Rh.D., is an Associate Professor at Emporia State University teaching in the undergraduate and graduate rehabilitation programs. She received her B.S. and M.S. from Mankato State University and doctorate from Southern Illinois University. She is a licensed clinical professional counselor and certified rehabilitation counselor. She has extensive experience working in the public and private rehabilitation sectors.

Gary G. Gintner, Ph.D., is an Associate Professor and Division Leader of the Leadership and Counseling Programs at Louisiana State University. He served as the 2007–2008 president of the American Mental Health Counselors Association, and has published and presented extensively in areas such as the DSM, practice guidelines and substance abuse. His 30 years of clinical experience include inpatient care and outpatient mental health, and he currently serves as the clinical director of a Louisiana-based employee assistance program.

Arthur M. Guilford, Ph.D., is a Vice President of the University of South Florida and is the Campus Executive Officer of the USF Sarasota-Manatee Campus. His doctorate in speech-language-hearing sciences is from the University of Michigan. A former Chair of the Department of Communication Sciences and Disorders for 14 years, his research interests are in pediatrics, neurogenics and educational issues and his scholarly publications are extensive and include another new book published in 2007.

William E. Haley, Ph.D., is a Professor in the School of Aging Studies at the University of South Florida. Dr. Haley has a professional background in clinical psychology and has conducted extensive research and published widely on family caregiving, stress and coping, and end-of-life care for older adults.

Kathryn Hyer, Ph.D., MPP, is Associate Professor and Director of the Training Academy on Aging at the School of Aging Studies, University of South Florida. Before embarking on her academic career, Dr. Hyer worked as a policy analyst for Governor Babbitt, administrator for home care programs, and foundation consultant.

Scott Johnson, Ph.D., directs the Family Therapy Ph.D. Program at Virginia Tech and is Associate Director of Tech's Office of Recovery and Support. He holds degrees in English, Music, Poetry, and Family Therapy, and has written many scholarly and popular articles. He was president of the American Association for Marriage and Family Therapy, and is on the editorial boards of the *Journal of Marital and Family Therapy and the Journal of Feminist Family Therapy.*

Thomas S. Krieshok, Ph.D., is a Professor in the Department of Psychology and Research in Education at the University of Kansas, where he focuses on career decision making.

William A. Lambos, Ph.D., is President of Cognitive Neuro Sciences, Inc. in Tampa, Florida. He possesses a postdoctoral certification in Neuropsychology from Fielding Graduate University, is a Licensed Neuropsychologist and certified as a family mediator by the Supreme Court of the State of Florida. Dr. Lambos has mediated a wide variety of family issues and finds the practice of mediation a source of joy and a synergistic complement to his practice as a neuro/clinical psychologist.

Brent Mallinckrodt, Ph.D., received his doctoral degree in Counseling Psychology from the University of Maryland. He currently serves as Director of the Counseling Psychology program at the University of Tennessee and as Editor of the *Journal of Counseling Psychology.* He is was a recipient of the APA Division 17 (Counseling Psychology) Scientist-Practitioner Award and the University of Missouri Graduate Mentor of the Year Award. His research interests include adult attachment, psychotherapy processes, and social support.

Mary Finn Maples, Ph.D., is Professor and Coordinator of Higher Education Student Development at the University of Nevada, Reno. She is a former president of the American Counseling Association (then APGA) and the Association for Spiritual, Ethical & Religious Values in Counseling (ASERVIC).

Donna M. Massey-Anderson, Ph.D., is an assistant professor in the Department of Sociology, Anthropology, Social Work, and Criminal Justice at The University of Tennessee at Martin. Her primary research interests include the transfer of juveniles to the adult criminal court system, Weed and Seed program evaluations, and an examination of the inmate social system. She holds a B.S. in Criminal Justice and a M.A. in Sociology from East Tennessee State University, and a Ph.D. in Criminology and Criminal Justice from The Florida State University.

Gail Mears, Psy.D., is an Associate Professor of Counselor Education and Chair of the Counselor Education and School Psychology Programs at Plymouth State University. She has held leadership positions in multiple professional counseling organizations and is a past president of the American Mental Health Counselors Association. Her interests in counseling supervision and clinical training are informed by 25 years of experience as a clinical mental health counselor in community mental health, private practice, and college counseling.

Bruce M. Menchetti, Ph.D., is an Associate Professor in the School of Teacher Education at Florida State University. His research interests include transition of students with disabilities from school to adult life, supported employment, and the community inclusion of individuals with severe disabilities. Dr. Menchetti has directed federal grants to prepare personnel to work effectively with individuals with disabilities as well as grants to demonstrate best practices in supported employment and transition systems change.

Mary F. Mushel, M.A., is retired after serving for many years as an Adjunct Professor and Undergraduate Advisor in the School of Aging Studies, University of South Florida. She has extensive experience in gerontology, medical technology, and health care administration, as well as in teaching and advising students.

Karen R. Nicholas, Ph.D., is an Assistant Professor in the College of Education at Southeastern University in Lakeland, Florida. Dr. Nicholas is a national educational consultant to local districts and state departments of education regarding their accountability to NCLB and IDEA guidelines. Her research interests include developing writing strategy programs for students with learning disabilities and inclusive practices for teacher preparation programs. Dr. Nicholas received her Ph.D. in Special Education from Florida State University.

Vincent E. Parr, Ph.D., is the founder and president of the Institute for Advanced Study in Tampa and the president of the Center for Rational Living and the Rational Living Foundation also in Tampa. He is a licensed Clinical Psychologist specializing in Rational Emotive Behavior Therapy and Cognitive Behavior Therapy, a Rational Emotive Behavior Supervisor, and was hand picked by Dr. Albert Ellis to be on the Board "in Waiting" to carry on his work and teachings after his death.

Dennis Pelsma, Ph.D., is a Professor at Emporia State University. He has worked as a classroom teacher, counselor (K–12), and counselor educator in Kansas, Missouri, and Illinois.

John D. Rasch, Ph.D., is a Professor and former Chair of the Department of Rehabilitation and Mental Health Counseling at the University of South Florida. He publishes several electronic resources for rehabilitation counselors and individuals with disabilities, including a website that is a review guide for the national certification examination in rehabilitation counseling at: http://luna.cas.usf.edu/~rasch/index.html.

Paul E. Spector, Ph.D., is a Distinguished Professor and Director of the Industrial/Organizational Psychology Doctoral Program at the University of South Florida. He is also director of the NIOSH funded Sunshine Education and Research Center's Occupational Health Psychology program. His research focuses on employee behavior, health, and well-being in organizational settings. A 1991 ISI Web of Science study listed him as one of the 50 highest impact contemporary researchers (out of over 102,000) in psychology worldwide.

Destin N. Stewart, M.S., received her B.S. in psychology with a minor in world religion from Florida State University and her Master's of Science degree in clinical psychology from Mississippi State University. She is currently working to complete her Ph.D. in counseling psychology at the University of Tennessee, where she teaches general psychology, sees clients at the University Counseling Center as a practicum student and pursues her research interests in social issues and psychotherapy effectiveness.

Lori Foster Thompson, Ph.D., is an Associate Professor in the Industrial/ Organizational Psychology program at North Carolina State University. Her research, teaching, and consulting pertain to employee reactions to emerging technologies, organizational surveys, and 360-degree feedback. She also studies careers. She has coauthored a book, some chapters, and various articles on these topics and currently serves on the editorial board of *The Industrial-Organizational Psychologist* (TIP), the *Journal of Organizational Behavior, and Ergometrika*, where she is Associate Editor.

Gerry Tierney, Ph.D., is Professor of Anthropology in the Behavioral and Social Sciences Department at Webster University, where she teaches courses in cultural anthropology, applied anthropology, and criminal justice. She has also taught anthropology in Austria, Japan, Thailand, and England and has conducted field research in Alaska and Japan.

Paul S. Trivette, Ph.D., is a school psychologist in the Winston-Salem/Forsyth County North Carolina Schools. He has a Ph.D. in counseling and school psychology from Virginia Tech. He taught for five years in the Counselor Education program at Bowling Green State University in Ohio. He is a National Certified School Psychologist and a Licensed Professional Counselor in North Carolina and remains active in the supervision of school psychology interns and practicum students in his school district.

Susan Craft Vickerstaff, Ph.D., worked as a health care and psychiatric social worker for 20 years before going into academics. She earned a Master of Social Work degree and a Ph.D. in Social Work from the University of Alabama and a Master of Public Health degree from the University of Alabama in Birmingham. She retired from the University of Tennessee at Martin in 2006 and currently teaches part-time at the University of Alabama.

Courtney A. Waid, M.S., is an assistant professor in the Department of Criminal Justice and Political Science at North Dakota State University. Her primary research interests include the effectiveness of inmate treatment programs on female recidivism, the reform of juvenile detention practices, and factors impacting the fear of crime/victimization. She holds a B.A. in psychology, an M.S. in criminal justice, and is currently a doctoral candidate in the College of Criminology and Criminal Justice at the Florida State University.

We dedicate this book to seven special, successful, and loving professionals whose "people skills" and current and prospective successful career journeys bring us great pride, and from whom we learn so much about life. Our seven young and adult children:

Michael A. Richard, Jr. (Food Services/Management)

&

Meighan J. Richard (Elementary Education)

and

Karen R. Nicholas (Special Education)
Barbara J. Karasek Emener (Business/Sports Marketing)

&

Scott W. Emener (Business/Technology Communications)

and

Brooke E. Bosworth and Lindsay R. Bosworth
(Future careers undetermined yet bound for Success)

PREFACE

While the nineteenth century in the United States was considered the agrarian age for employment, the twentieth century revolved around the machine and industrial age–giving birth to the technological era in the eighties and nineties. During the first decade of the current millennium, we appear committed to advancing communications technology. What better time in history than during such change, is it to focus on a most important arena in the world of work–human services.

As our libraries reveal, volumes have been written in the past about human service careers–most focusing on specific fields such as medicine, law, education, social work, counseling and psychology, among others. And except for a 1991 text by William G. Emener and Margaret A. Darrow, *Career Explorations in Human Services*, and the 2003, first edition of this current book by Michael A. Richard and William G. Emener, *I'm A People Person: A Guide to Human Service Professions*, few have introduced a variety of different careers designed for those persons undecided about their future, beyond "a desire to work with people."

One of the greatest challenges of our new millennium will be in the social science, human service, and interpersonal communications fields. With the increasing emphasis on technology for human interaction–cell phones, e-mails, pagers, the Internet, fax machines, ipods, and voice mail, it is possible for an employee to spend eight hours a day at work, in full productivity without speaking face-to-face with even one individual.

Perhaps one of the most compelling persuasions for this text is the nature of the people who will be reading it–the Next Great Generation. As university professors, we have experienced today's college students to be bright, energetic, and caring individuals who are turning back toward traditionalism, but with a twist–they are comfortable with a fresh application of older values, which includes the value for the human element. These new millennium students, many of whom are children of the baby-boomers, are being viewed as being conventional, confident, sheltered, idealistic, achieving, and team-oriented. And it is not uncommon to find that behind the green hair and body piercing is an individual who came to college with a determination to find meaning in life and graduate with the skills and abilities to make a difference in the world and be in positions that will make the world "a better place for people to live." All the more reason so many college students are choosing human service as a vocation which they see as more than a way of earning a living or a career–for many it is a calling.

Furthermore, graduate programs in human services are experiencing a burgeoning influx in applications for admission from persons who are in midlife and wanting to opt out of the "data and things world" and into the "people world." Also significantly impacting peoples' choices of human service careers are the increasing variety and diversity of opportunities available in what can be described as "new careers." Gerontology and counseling, communication sciences and disorders, case management, applied anthropology, and student development in higher education were relative infants in the woods less than a generation ago. Yet, it is evident that the more technological advances occur in our society, the more society will need "people helping people."

Life in the twenty-first century is uncertain at best. This book, nonetheless, presents helpful information pertinent to many professional career opportunities and facilitatively challenges the young and not-so-young persons seeking to make the world a better place. Beyond the traditional academic and knowledge qualifications for many human service professions–all that is necessary for the readers of this text who choose careers in human service–this book also embraces and reflects its editors' and authors' desire to kindle the flames for a new generation who have a real passion for helping people.

This book is divided into four parts.

Part I, containing one important chapter, assumes that you have made a decision or are seriously inclined to invest yourself into a journey that would end up with you being an employed professional, working with and helping people–a people person. Furthermore, it assumes that you would like to know what you now should do with your occupational leanings, interests, and/or commitments. But you then ask, "Now what do I do?" Following a discussion of some of the tangible and intrinsic reasons why people want to be human service professionals, the chapter defines and discusses career choice and human services, as well as the concepts of career, job, and professionalism. It then concludes with a statement of the overall objective of this book–to explore the professions comprising the human services–and offers specific recommendations regarding how to best use it.

Part II includes 18 contributed chapters–each authored and coauthored by a total of 30 very busy professionals who all have graduate degrees (mostly Ph.D.s), have many years of service delivery experience, are accomplished scholars, and hold or have held numerous leadership positions in, and have taught many graduate courses in, their respective professional disciplines. And this just scratches the surface. Thus, they clearly constitute an All-Star team in professional human services. Moreover, each of these chapters address 10 specific aspects of the 18 specific human service professionals: (1) the state of the art of the profession; (2) its history and development; (3) its mission(s) and objectives; (4) the predominate profile(s) of the clients it typically serves; (5) its philosophical assumptions and pre-eminent theory(-ies); (6) an appreciation of its real world application(s) and salary indices; (7) professional preparation and development; (8) work settings; (9) its professional organizations; and, (10) its future outlook.

Part III provides those who may be unable, unwilling, or unqualified to attend graduate school alternatives within human services. It is not uncommon for an individual to not have the financial resources to attend graduate school. Many have the passion to work with people who are hurting, but not the means. And if this is your situation, this chapter is written for you.

Others, may have the passion or may not have the resources, but find life circumstances currently prevent them from pursuing their dreams. Or they need to work but long to work in a job that involves helping others. And if this is your situation, this chapter is written for you.

Less than 10 percent of the public ever attend and/or completes graduate school; some are through with their education and want a job. The authors have known many people who want to attend graduate school but lack the necessary skills or abilities. Many of these people have a burning passion but do not try or are denied attendance in human service graduate programs. Again, if this is your situation, this chapter is written for you.

This chapter presents a brief overview of five major occupational areas where individuals with nongraduate degrees frequently find employment working with people. Within each area, specific jobs are described, and salary and outlook information is given. The five areas where persons with degrees in human services or an interest in working with people frequently work are: (1) Behavioral and Mental Health; (2) Human Resources; (3) Education; (4) Police and Public Safety; and (5) Leisure and Recreation. This is not meant to be all inclusive but rather a taste of the possibilities that are available to those who want to work with people but do not have a graduate degree. For all of you who have the passion to work with people but the opportunity to attend graduate school is now nonexistent, dim, difficult or uncertain—this chapter is for you.

Part IV offers an in-depth discussion of professionalism in human services and defines and addresses the big four human service regulatory mechanisms: certification, licensure, registration, and accreditation. Following discussions of autonomy and professional behavior, professionals' codes of ethics, the roles of knowledge in professional decision-making, and professionals' ultimate decisions, the reader is then invited to think about his or her "professional self-concept."

This last Part also concludes the book with an intriguing challenge: be sure that when you eventually become a human service professional—caring for and helping vulnerable individuals (who also may be hurting, in trouble and/or uninformed and unable to meaningfully help themselves)—that you have a professional obligation to offer them the best help and assistance available.

As we say and infer throughout: if you invest yourself while reading this book, the included thoughtful, knowledgeable, and practical approaches will provide a valuable point of embarkation on your journey to a personally and professionally rewarding career as a human service professional.

We sincerely hope you benefit from reading and studying the material herein and find it helpful in your personal decision-making . . . and also that you enjoy the journey.

WGE, MAR & JJB

ACKNOWLEDGMENTS

First and foremost, we extend a hearty "Thank-you!" to the 30 authors of the book's 18 contributed chapters (2–19). As we delineate and then say in the Preface, they clearly constitute an All-Star team in professional human services and we are grateful to each of them for meaningfully contributing to this endeavor.

In view of our repeated experiences during this endeavor, we want to thank all the "behind the scenes" persons who made this text possible. It would have been much more difficult without you. And on an individually deserved note, John graciously acknowledges Linda M. Wright for her unerring enthusiasm, patience, and persistence in teaching him sophisticated ways of using his computer and working with e-mails and the Internet.

Our respective families—wives, children, grandchildren, and loved ones—have been respectfully caring and compassionate when over the past few months we replied to many of their requests with, "Okay, as soon as I finish editing this chapter." Their unerring love did not go unnoticed and to all of them we extend our sincerest appreciation.

Bill, Mike and John

CONTENTS

Part III. Professional Human Service Occupations

Part IV. Ethics and Professionalism

A GUIDEBOOK TO HUMAN SERVICE PROFESSIONS

Part I

THE ROAD TO BECOMING A HUMAN SERVICE PROFESSIONAL

Chapter 1

OKAY, YOU WANT TO WORK WITH AND HELP PEOPLE . . . NOW WHAT DO YOU DO?

WILLIAM G. EMENER, MICHAEL A. RICHARD & JOHN J. BOSWORTH

*It is one of life's greatest compensations that we cannot sincerely try
to help someone else without helping ourselves.*

–Ralph Waldo Emerson

Although Mr. Emerson coined the above pearl of wisdom approximately 150 years ago, it still is poignant today and indeed pertinent to the essence of this book. The befitting "if-then" follow-up scenario would be:

IF you agree with and embrace Emerson's philosophical tenet,
IF you are a "people-person" person, and
IF you can identify and invest yourself in a human service professional career,
THEN at the end of the day you will have won the ultimate trifecta:
You will be helping others,
You will be helping yourself, and
You will be getting paid for it.

And a bonus payoff would be that you would feel good about yourself, you would feel good about your life, and you would feel good about the way you would be living it.

In our collective roles as vocational evaluators, rehabilitation counselors, mental health counselors, psychologists, professors, and undergraduate/graduate advisors, we often have heard people ask, "I am a people person, but now what do I do?" Among other things, these words have served as seeds of inspiration for this book. Furthermore, the origin for this book has grown from both the positive and the negative events we have experienced in our professional careers. For the most part, we are pleased to say, our experiences have been positive as related to our students' and clients' concerns regarding their career choices in human service occupations. Nonetheless, because of the negative experiences we indeed realized and deeply appreciated that there was a need for a book such as this one.

In our roles as editors of this book, we want to offer the following experiences from our individual professional careers as a prelude to the essence of this book's existence.

Dr. William G. Emener:

While I have enjoyed many opportunities of

witnessing students and clients make positive and meaningful career choices, I also have experienced the unfortunate side of graduate school choice being made on inadequate information. Fittingly, I would like to share a story from my recent experiences that are illustrative examples of the need for adequate information when making graduate school choices and the power of that information.

My story has a less satisfactory ending (other than to accentuate and emphasize the need for this book). As an advisor to graduate students, I often visit with them regarding the sequencing and scheduling of their courses, progress toward graduation and plans after graduate school. One very intelligent, skilled, and emotionally healthy student was visiting with me near the end of her last Practicum course. She was approaching graduation, needing only to complete her Internship.

During our conversation she appeared somewhat despondent, describing her Practicum experiences as less than satisfactory. Although she liked her supervisors, clients and co-workers, she related ". . . it was the situation, the experience and the future career opportunities" that contributed to her dissatisfaction.

The crux of her story was that as she had progressed in her graduate studies, had gained more and better information and more practical experience, and now was clearly aware that she had probably entered the wrong program of study. Her dilemma, being that she was almost at the end of her program and after a two-year investment in school, was that she felt dissatisfied with the career commitment she had made two years ago. Our Mental Health Counseling Program (at the University of South Florida) was not in concert with her philosophical and professional goals. She had gained more information about the role of various human service professionals, and it became increasingly evident that for her a Clinical Psychology Program would have been more meaningful and professionally rewarding. Unfortunately she per-

ceived no other choice than to complete her degree due to family obligations and needs. She completed our master's degree program and is a successful Licensed Mental Health Counselor. To this day, however, she believes she would have been happier as a Clinical Psychologist. (She has told me, nonetheless, that once her children are grown she may go back to school to obtain a degree in Clinical Psychology.)

Dr. Michael A. Richard:

While working as a Vocational Evaluator and Rehabilitation Counselor, I discovered that many of my clients would express interest in pursuing a career in human services. The vast majority indicated they wanted to pursue degrees in Nursing or Rehabilitation Counseling. Upon questioning, many clients disclosed that the foundation of their desire to enter these fields began as a result of their personal experiences with professionals specifically in these careers. For these individuals, the most recent and/or common contacts with human service professionals were with their rehabilitation counselor and/or nurse.

In an attempt to broaden their choices, part of their time was spent in career exploration. For most persons interested in, and qualified to enter, undergraduate Nursing and Rehabilitation Counseling careers, I provided information intended to expand their career options. This information essentially consisted of data describing other majors and occupations comprising the field of human services. In those early years of professional development, the information provided them was limited due to my own lack of knowledge. Thus, it primarily consisted of information about degrees and occupations in Psychology, Sociology, Rehabilitation Counseling, Nursing and Education. Although admittedly limited, this information was intended to help them make more informed choices when developing long-ranged career goals.

Generally, my professional experience has

plainly indicated that with adequate and relevant information and self-knowledge, clients typically are able to make more satisfying and meaningful career and educational choices. I also have found that this proposition holds true for persons wanting to enter one of the human services.

In view of the fact that long-range career goals in human services often require a commitment to graduate school, I would also address this with my clients. Basically, as an undergraduate and graduate Student Advisor I became aware that students need more detailed information on postgraduation options. The more I worked in higher education I increasingly became aware of the range and availability of human service career options that might be available to undergraduates. I also became progressively more appreciative of the richness and variety of career options available to students—he key of course being that people have adequate information on which to make their choice. I would like to present the following story to illustrate my positive experience with this belief.

Near the end of a semester, a former colleague of mine, Perry Kaly, on the St. Petersburg Campus, referred a very bright and intelligent psychology major to me for career counseling. The student stated he was majoring in psychology, and had some misgivings about entering graduate school and then working in the area of clinical psychology. In addition, he said he did not want to continue on for a doctoral degree immediately after completing his master's degree. His academic advisor had wisely encouraged him to seek career counseling. During our interview, it was quickly revealed he had limited knowledge of other graduate programs available to him. The extent of his knowledge was limited to the fields of social work, sociology, and psychology. He had some vague ideas as to what persons working in these professions did, but knew little more. He also could identify only a few other "human service professions" by name, yet

he had no idea what these professions actually involved. It was evident that he had insufficient knowledge and awareness of what career options he could consider. Fortunately, this student was eager to gain knowledge and to educate himself as to other options. Furthermore, regarding his self-knowledge, he had an in-depth and accurate sense of self-awareness. In this instance, all I needed to do was to provide him with sufficient information, and help him organize and synthesize the information once he obtained it. Ultimately, he decided to enter a Mental Health Counseling program and he was extremely pleased with his choice. He related that his program of choice, compared to clinical psychology, placed a greater emphasis on counseling application rather than theory and research, which better suited his personality, temperament and professional goals.

Mr. John J. Bosworth:

As an adjunct faculty member teaching mostly undergraduate students, I am granted the challenging yet highly rewarding position of having an enormous influence on students, as they contemplate and pursue graduate education and career path decisions. In one course that I teach, "A Survey of Human Service Professions," I usually start each semester engaged in an informal dialogue with students as to why they even considered enrolling in the course. Some say they want to go to graduate school in psychology, social work, or rehabilitation counseling and others have no idea, they're just not sure of which direction they should travel, or even if they want to pursue a career in human services. The most prominent feeling or attitude that permeates the first few weeks of class following this discussion is a vague sense of indecision, uncertainty, and skeptical curiosity. Good! They are in the right place.

As each semester progresses, I am continually reminded of the lack of knowledge most students have in forming an accurate representation of what being in the human service profes-

sions is all about. I am not surprised though, as I was once an undergraduate student, and faced the same insecurities, indecision, and lack of direction. As we listen to guest speakers, representing many of the professions outlined in this book, and compare and contrast theory and practice, students start to get a better feel for the many opportunities available. Most of my students report, at the end of the semester or through the early stages of their graduate programs, that the class and the previous edition of this textbook were integral in their career decision-making process.

The early questions such as "What is the difference between a counseling psychologist and a clinical psychologist?", "How long does it take to become a rehabilitation counselor?", "Can a mental health counselor have a private practice or testify in court?", "What about nurses ?", or "Do social workers conduct therapy?", seem to get answered as we progress. I consider it my duty and priority as an educator to provide a comprehensive, objective, accurate, and enthusiastic portrayal of the human service professions. My reward comes often, in the form of phone calls or e-mails, thanking me for taking time to listen, writing letters of recommendation, and providing a virtual laboratory for career and vocational guidance and exploration.

These are but three stories that exemplify the many others from our professional experiences. Other stories include, for example, one about a nurse who discovered that public administration is actually more appealing, a rehabilitation counselor who would rather be working in gerontology, and a school teacher who would rather be employed in the criminal justice system.

Fortunately, life often gives us second chances and choices that can be extremely rewarding. For example, Dr. Emener is not the college basketball coach he once dreamed of being, Dr. Richard is not the applied anthropologist in a university setting he once fancied, and Mr. Bosworth is not persuading indecisive juries as a prominent trial attorney. Nonetheless, all three of us now happily work as professionals in the health care field—as counselors doing counseling and psychotherapy with people in need of help, *and* as university professors—educating and training counselors and therapists. In these roles, like many of the authors contributing chapters to this book, we have found great satisfaction in helping troubled people; furthermore, we also are able to write professional journal articles, publish books and work with many distinguished professionals, occasionally including basketball coaches, applied anthropologists, and forensic or legal experts.

CAREER CHOICE

Authors in the professional literature have debated how to organize and structure the development and choice of careers (Brown & Brooks, 1987; Isaacson & Brown, 1997; Jepsen & Dilley, 1974; Richard & Emener, 2003). A further debate continues over the philosophical assumptions, definitions, and differences between careers, occupations and jobs (Brown & Brooks, 1987; Isaacson & Brown, 1997; Savickas & Lent, 1994). For the purpose of this book, nonetheless, we will be working from the following assumptions of career choice.

From an *a priori* perspective, the basis for this book accepts the proposition that career development is a process of growth, culminating in a person gravitating toward and choosing an occupation related to their personality (Brown & Brooks, 1987; Holland, 1985; Super, 1980). It also is assumed that satisfaction with career choice is related to the extent to which an individual is able to implement and utilize abilities, interests, personality traits, and values (Brown & Crace, 1996; Super, 1980).

Furthermore, people search for and are able to identify environments that will let them fulfill their attitudes and values and take on compatible roles (Holland, 1985). If people are provided with accessible, accurate, and relevant career information, it will enhance the process of developing a wide range of alternatives. This, in turn, will facilitate the development of better career plans, focus preparation, and increase satisfactory employment (Isaacson & Brown, 1997; Mitchell & Krumboltz, 1987; Richard & Emener, 2003; Schein, 1982).

HUMAN SERVICES DEFINED

As with the general term "careers," *human services* have been variously defined. Typically these professions involve a professional providing a service that is perceived as helpful by the individual who has sought assistance (Bernstein, 1996; Corey, Corey & Callanan, 1988; Egan, 2002). The most efficient definition describes the players in this process as "helper" and "helpee" (Egan, 2002; Emener, 1991).

For the purpose of this book, *human services will be defined as unique, useful and purposeful activity by a specialized professional designed to assist a consumer with their personalized issues*. Furthermore, *the services provided are clearly defined, and require specialized training to obtain the requite skills* (Crouch, 1997; Egan, 2002; Emener & Darrow, 1991; Perry, 1996; Richard & Emener, 2003).

CAREERS AND JOBS DEFINED

The differences between jobs and careers have essentially been described as differences in the level of dedication over time to one's work (Emener & Darrow, 1991; Cullen, 1978; Perry, 1986; Richard & Emener, 2003). A career is essential a lifelong enterprise that encompasses a purposeful process of planning, perseverance, and lifelong development (Crouch, 1997; Holland, 1985; Super, 1980). Persons who work in the human services as described in this book general meet these criteria. Each of these professions involves an individual developing a plan to acquire an advanced degree. Once implemented, the degree program will necessitate that the person perseveres until the minimum education is completed. The educational requirements, when met, usually will involve a lifelong process of professional development and commitment to that occupation (Bernstein, 1996; Emener, & Darrow, 1991; Hollis & Wantz, 1993; Richard & Emener, 2003).

This latter requirement typically involves such activities as pursuing certification and/or licensure, the acquisition of continuing education and individualized professional growth (Crouch, 1997; Emener & Darrow, 1991; Perry, 1996; Richard & Emener, 2003). A career in human services often means that the person's occupation will become part of their personal self-concept (Bernstein, 1996; Nugent, 2000). For example, people are often seen in relation to their careers. How often have you heard someone being introduced in some manner similar to, "This is Katie; she is a nurse."

On the other hand, a person may hold several different jobs while pursuing a career (Emener & Darrow, 1991; Richard & Emener, 2003; Salacuse, 2000). For example a nurse, over the course of a lifetime, may work as an ER nurse, in a physician's office, and then in home health care.

PROFESSIONS DEFINED

To fully benefit from this book, the construct of "profession" needs to be clarified. There have been many models and definitions of describing what a profession is. However, we will limit our discussion to the "human service" professions. In the broad spectrum of human services, specific standards and criteria exist separating the professional from the paraprofessional (Brammer, 1993; Egan, 2002; Perry, 1986).

For most human service professions, these criteria can be found in the "Preamble" of the American Personnel and Guidance Association's 1965 *Ethical Standards Handbook*. Essentially three criteria for a trade or skill to be called a professional are addressed and they are as follows:

1. The existence of a body of "specialized knowledge, skills and attitudes."
   a. it is derived through scientific inquiry and scholarly learning;
   b. is constantly tested and extended through research and scholarly inquiry;
   c. comprises a literature of its own (even though it may, and at times must draw from other areas of knowledge); and,
   d. is known and practiced by members of the profession.
2. The exaltation of service to the individual and society above and beyond personal gain which:
   a. includes the possession of a philosophy;
   b. is translated into a code of ethics which is known and practiced by members of the profession, and
   c. the public recognizes, has confidence in, and is willing to compensate members for the provision of their service.
3. The members of the profession:
   a. have acquired the professions body of specialized knowledge, skills, and

attitudes through professional preparation (preferably on the graduate level):
   i. at a college or university
   ii. through continuous in-service training, continuing education, and personal growth after the completion of formal education;
   b. constantly examine and improve the quality of the profession's professional preparation, in-service training, and continuing education programs;
   c. constantly examine the quality of services to the individual and society;
   d. limit membership, and the practice of the profession, only to persons meeting stated standards of preparation and competencies; and,
   e. are afforded a life career and permanent membership as long as services meet professional standards.

As will be evident throughout this book, these criteria are similar to principles upon which, and serve as the basis from which, most human services are formulated and practiced. Furthermore, these principles have served, and will continue to serve, as the foundation of service provisions (Bernstein, 1996; Nugent, 2000; Richard & Emener, 2003).

OBJECTIVE

The primary objective of this book is to explore the professions comprising the human services. Although a case can and may be made for the inclusion of other professions, the editors believe the ones presented herein are a worthy representation of "human services." The areas addressed in the chapters include a formal response to the following questions about each profession:

1. What are the philosophical assumptions and major theories of the profession?
2. What is the current state of the art of the profession, its history, and what distinguishes it from other human service professions?
3. What type of persons do these professionals typically serve?
4. What is it that persons working in this profession do for the persons, groups, organizations, etc. served?
5. What are the minimal requirements to enter the profession?
6. What opportunities are available to those who work in the profession?
7. What are the primary professional organizations and governing bodies?
8. Where can someone go to find out more information about the profession?
9. What are the opportunities and what is the outlook for persons wanting to enter this profession?

RECOMMENDED UTILIZATION OF THIS BOOK

There are a variety of approaches beneficial for persons involved in the task of exploring careers in human services. Based on the work of Emener and Darrow (1991) and Richard and Emener (2003), as well as on our experiences as human service professionals and professional human service educators, the following suggestions, if followed, will augment your exploration process.

1. Visit with persons currently employed as professionals in the area(s) of interest to you.

During the visit, talk candidly to the professional and don't be afraid to ask questions. There are no "stupid" questions (as in many aspects of life, the only "stupid ques-

tions" are those not asked)– most professionals were once in your shoes. Also, talking to more than one professional in the field will give you a better indication of the professions "real world."

2. Visit several places where these professionals work and function.

It is suggested that you make several visits, and if possible "shadow" a professional and even consider volunteering some of your time at these sites. Importantly, these visits will give you a "feel" for the environments in which the professional works. These experiences also will give you a deeper understanding and appreciation of the demands these professionals face on a daily basis.

3. Think about "who you are" and "how you feel" about yourself, in the context of what it would be like working in this profession.

It is important to spend time questioning and imagining what it would be like if you were actually working in these environments, meeting the career demands, and dealing with routine circumstances. It is important that you answer these questions about yourself in the specific professional role, honestly and accurately.

4. Consider how others may perceive you as a person.

This does not mean that you "do" what others want you to do and/or become what they believe you should become. However, there are likely significant others in your life who "know" you and what you are like as a person. These persons may include family and friends who have firsthand experience with you as a person. Finally, some or all these people may be impacted by your final decision. A husband or wife, children, parents, and siblings all may have a stake in your choice. It may be that you will feel more self-assured and confident when making your career decision if you have considered how these persons may be affected.

CONCLUDING THOUGHTS

In the process of addressing issues related to these four areas, it is vital that you keep an open mind about yourself and maintain flexibility in your eventual occupational choice. In the final analysis, it is important that you attempt to identify what would be rewarding to you about a career. The four areas previously discussed, considered openly and truthfully, should give insight and reassurance into "why" your final choice would be right. One last piece of advice: your exploration does not have to strenuous or solemn. Approach it as a child would with sincere curiosity, wonder, enthusiasm, and humor.

We wish you all the best on your journey—may you find the professional niche that gives you a sense of personal and professional meaning and fulfillment. Lastly, sometime in the future, we hope that you too can occasionally smile when reminded of Emerson's pearl of wisdom and can marvel at the fact that you are getting paid to do what you are doing.

REFERENCES

American Personnel and Guidance Association. (1965). *Ethical standards casebook.* Washington, DC: Author.

Bernstein, G. (1996). *"Human services?–That must be so rewarding": A practical guide for professional development* (2nd ed). Baltimore: P.H. Brookes.

Brammer, L.M., (1993). *The helping relationship: Process and skills* (5th ed). Boston: Allyn & Bacon.

Brown, D., Brooks, L., & Associates. (1987). *Career choice and development* (4th ed.) San Francisco: Jossey-Bass.

Brown D., & Crace, R.K. (1996). Values and life role decision making: A conceptual model. *The Career Development Quarterly, 44* (3) 211–223.

Corey, G., Corey, M.S., & Callanan, P. (1988). *Issues and ethics in the helping professions* (3rd ed.) Pacific Grove, CA: Brooks/Cole.

Crouch, A. (1997). *Inside counseling: Becoming and being a professional.* Thousand Oaks, CA: Sage.

Cullen, J.B. (1978). *The structure of professionalism: A quantitative examination.* New York: Petrocelli Books.

Emener, W. G., & Darrow, M.A. (1991). *Career explorations in human services.* Springfield, IL: Charles C Thomas.

Egan, Gerald (2002). *The skilled helper: A problem-management and opportunity development approach to helping* (7th ed.). Pacific Grove, CA: Brooks/Cole.

Holland, J.L. (1985). *Making vocational choices: A theory of vocational personalities and work environments* (2nd ed.). Englewood, Cliffs, NJ: Prentice-Hall.

Hollis, J.W., & Wantz, R.A. (1993). *Counselor preparation 1993–1995: Program and personnel* (8th ed.). Muncie, IN: Accelerated Development.

Isaacson, I.E., & Brown, D. (1997). *Career information, career counseling, career development* (6th ed.). Boston: Allyn & Bacon.

Jepsen, D.A., & Dilley, J.S. (1974). Vocational decision making models: A review and comparative analysis. *Review of educational research* (Bulletin).

Mitchell, L.K., & Krumboltz, J.D. (1987). Social learning approach to career decision making: Krumboltz's Theory. In D. Brown & L. Brooks (Eds.), *Career choice and development* (4th ed.) San Francisco: Jossey-Bass.

Nugent, F.A. (2000). *Introduction to the profession of counseling.* Upper Saddle River, NJ: Merrill.

Perry, P. A. (1996). *Opportunities in mental health careers.* Lincolnwood, IL: Career Horizons.

Perry, T.D. (1986). *Professional philosophy: What it is and why it matters.* Boston: D. Reidel.

Richard, M.A., & Emener, W.G. (2003). *I'm a people person: A guide to human service professions.* Springfield, IL: Charles C Thomas.

Salacuse, J. W. (2000). *The wise advisor: What every professional should know about consulting and counseling.* Westport, CT: Prager.

Savickas, M.L., & Lent, R.W. (Eds.) (1994). *Convergence in career development theories: Implications for service and practice.* Palo Alto, CA: Consulting Psychologist Press.

Schein, E. H. (1982). Increasing organizational effectiveness through better human resource planning and development. In R. Katz (Ed.),

Career Issues in human resource management. Englewood Cliffs, NJ: Prentice-Hall.

Super, D.E. (1980). A life span, life space approach to career development. *Journal of Vocational Behavior, 16,* 282–298.

Part II

HUMAN SERVICE PROFESSIONS

Chapter 2

APPLIED ANTHROPOLOGY

Michael V. Angrosino & Gerry Tierney

Anthropology is not a human service profession but rather a liberal arts discipline that pays particular attention to applying its cross-cultural theories, methods, and substantive data to health and human services problems. Most of the larger departments of anthropology now include applied anthropology training, and several of them have training programs as part of their degree options.

Anthropology literally means the study of humankind. Anthropologists develop generalizations about the behavior of people in the more or less permanent groups that define their collective identities. They also document the extent of human diversity throughout human history and around the world. In the U.S., anthropology has traditionally been divided into four subfields. In an undergraduate curriculum, a student can expect to be introduced to all four of these sub-fields, although specialization is expected at the graduate level. The four subfields are: (1) *physical (biological) anthropology*, which studies humans as biological organisms, traces their evolution and examines biological variations within the species; (2) *cultural anthropology (ethnology)*, which studies the ways of life of living human societies; (3)

archaeology, which documents the past of human cultures through an examination of their material remains; and (4) *anthropological linguistics*, which explores the ways in which language functions as an important human trait, facilitating the many and complex forms of communication that make it possible for humans to maintain and pass on cultural knowledge.

Like many other social scientists, anthropologists are interested in testing hypotheses, or developing case studies to illustrate presumed general trends. More than most other social scientists, however, they prefer to do so in the context of fieldwork (a relatively long-term immersion either in the living society or at the site of a bygone society's material remains. Anthropologists like to work in the "natural laboratories" of human societies, gaining a kind of subjective insight into the culture or physical condition of a people even as they collect objective data about those people.

BRIEF HISTORY

Anthropology emerged as an independent discipline in the second half of the nineteenth century; it was particularly interested in the peoples of Africa, Asia, the Pacific, and Native America. Applications of anthropology began with the formation in 1879 of the Bureau of American Ethnology as part of the Smithsonian Institution. Its mandate was to collect information about the indigenous people of North America whose lives were being deeply and disastrously impacted by contact with European Americans. Franz Boas, the most influential American anthropologist of the early twentieth century, used his anthropological knowledge to formulate a powerful critique of the prevailing racism of the day. At a time when official immigration policy was harshly discriminatory against all but northern Europeans, Boas marshaled scientific evidence to show that other people were not "inferior." Anthropologists also contributed their expertise to the Bureau of Indian Affairs (BIA), an influential mediator of native policy in the U.S., and to the Bureau of Agricultural Economics (BAE), an agency of the Department of Agriculture. They also worked in the private sector, studying conditions in factories and other work sites.

By the early 1940s, there were increasing numbers of scholars applying their insights to various contemporary human problems. They joined together in 1941 to establish the Society for Applied Anthropology, now commonly referred to as SfAA. Members of the SfAA were deeply involved in the Second World War effort and conducted research on programs for emergency feeding and food rationing, the design of various kinds of military equipment, and the cultures of people and places involved in the war (which, of course, grew to include most of the world). Anthropological study of Japanese culture resulted in policies for the occupation of Japan and the development of the postwar Japanese constitution. Anthropological studies of the culture of the Pacific islands informed the postwar administration of the territories that had passed from Japan

to the U.S. under United Nations trust. The postwar period saw an expansion in the enterprise known as *development*–the effort to promote positive economic and political change in the societies of the Third World that were then emerging from colonialism. Anthropologists made development more culturally sensitive by showing that not all development must result in economic and political institutions that match those of the capitalist, industrial, urban nations.

For most of the twentieth century, applied anthropologists were primarily affiliated with universities and/or museums and conducted their applied projects as sideline consultancies. However, beginning in the 1970s, anthropologists began seeking (and obtaining) full-time employment outside the academic world. Such full-timers are now usually referred to as *practicing anthropologists* to distinguish them from traditional applied anthropologists. Working within government agencies or in the private sector, practicing anthropologists bring together the professional expertise required at the work site with the academic research skills of their discipline. These professionals, however, also run the risk of losing their identification as anthropologists because the jobs they occupy may call for anthropological skills and insights but are rarely identified as such and because their primary responsibilities are to their employers, not to the discipline itself (i.e., they are not teaching students their newly acquired professional competencies, nor are they contributing to professional journals in ways that disseminate their new insights). For this reason, the modern era has seen the proliferation of applied/practicing-oriented training programs at several universities; such programs are an important way of maintaining the link between the academic discipline and its increasingly dispersed members.

This same period has also seen the emergence of various movements of political consciousness (civil rights for minorities, women, people with disabilities, people of various sexual orientations, and so forth). Anthropologists have been more willing than ever to contribute their expertise as advocates for such movements, sometimes working for grassroots activists, sometimes in collaboration or partnership with them, sometimes as activists themselves. Modern applied and practicing anthropologists thus learn to walk a fine line between traditional scientific objectivity and commitment to one or another strategy of political or economic action.

MISSION

The 1941 charter of the Society for Applied Anthropology stated that applied anthropology has as its primary objective, the scientific investigation of "the principles controlling the relations of human beings to one another . . . and the wide application of those principles to practical problems" (see SfAA website). The Society continues to promote the idea that anthropologists demonstrate a particular capacity to help solve human problems by: building partnerships in research and social action; acknowledging the perspectives of all people involved; focusing on challenges and opportunities presented by biological variability, cultural diversity, ethnicity, gender, poverty and class; and addressing imbalances in resources, rights, and power.

The Society has identified nine major goals for the twenty-first century: (1) to improve the capacity of the Society to respond to policy issues identified by the membership as particularly important; (2) to enhance the reputation of the Society's publications and leading repositories of applied knowledge, skills, and methods; (3) to advance anthropological perspectives through public outreach and effective media coverage; (4) to promote and expand ser-

vices to various member constituencies, especially students at all levels and MA and PhD-level professionals working outside of academia; (5) to expand the readership of the Society's printed and electronic publications; (6) to strengthen its international constituency and endeavors; (7) to increase the diversity of people encompassed within its activities, especially regarding the representation of ethnically underrepresented groups; (8) to support and expand interdisciplinary networks, membership, and perspectives; (9) to advance the Society's capacity to serve its members, committees, and the discipline through contracts, grants, and cooperative agreements with organizations committed to enhancing the quality of life in local communities.

TYPICAL CONSUMER PROFILE

Client Profile

Applied anthropologists work with, for, and in host communities for whom services are being planned or among whom existing services are being evaluated. Such communities may be domestic or international, rural or urban, although anthropologists characteristically work with communities that differ from the "mainstream" and who, as a consequence, do not have ready access to the decision-making processes of the policy makers. Applied anthropologists may therefore see themselves as "brokers" between the policy establishment and the people who are the objects of policy. As noted above, there are applied anthropologists who maintain an academic affiliation, but a growing number of practicing anthropologists work within agencies or organizations (both public and private sector) that formulate and/or carry out policies. It is now common for applied anthropologists to work as members of multidisciplinary teams rather than as solo researchers.

Typical Needs of Clients

Applied and practicing anthropologists serve their host communities or agency worksites in a variety of ways. Some of them are *program administrators* and are particularly valued when the work force and/or service population of an agency is culturally diverse or somehow different from the "mainstream" population. Others are *program evaluators*, an increasingly important role given the growing emphasis on accountability in both public and private sector programs. Because anthropologists are comfortable with qualitative research methods (see below), including in-depth interviewing and unobtrusive observation, they can add a human dimension to the process of evaluation that is not possible with standardized surveys or cost-benefit accounting methods. Still others work as *needs assessors*. One of the most common problems in the field of human services is that so much planning is done in a top-down manner—"experts" project from theoretical models (or from supposedly analogous cases) in developing programs for specific communities. Sometimes a community's perception of its needs may not be the same as what the experts' models predict, leading them to underutilize—or even reject—programs supposedly designed for their benefit. Since anthropologists are trained to operate on the basis of long-term immersion in a community, they have the ability to see the world from the perspective of that community and hence to add a grass-roots dimension to the identification of needs and to the planning of services to meet those needs.

Social impact assessors deal with the estimation of consequences of programs of service or technological change. Building an oil pipeline may be a good idea from the point of view of general energy policy; but if the pipeline runs through an indigenous area and disrupts the range of plants and animals on whom the native people depend for their livelihood, the policy can turn out in such a way that its negative consequences outweigh the potential benefits. Because the human services are, by definition, programs designed to impact people, it is fundamental to have a good understanding of how particular people in particular communities, at particular times in their history will respond and to make such understanding an integral part of the cost-benefit analysis of the overall situation. Thus there is an increasing need for those who can serve as cultural diversity trainers for agencies with multicultural staffs and/or service communities. Anthropologists—whose primary disciplinary focus has always been the comparative study of human cultures—are obvious candidates for such positions.

Finally, applied anthropologists may be called on in a general way as *policy analysts*, providing a holistic view of policy. Another problem in the human services, in addition to top-down planning, is the tendency to think in terms of one-size-fits-all solutions. In fact, there are many different constituencies with different social, economic, regional, ethnic and cultural perspectives. Policies must be made and implemented with an eye to the diverse complexity of the real world.

PHILOSOPHICAL ASSUMPTIONS

Culture

Anthropology is, above all, the "science of culture," and it approaches the object of study in a comparative way. That is, anthropology is interested in all manifestations of culture throughout human history and in all parts of the world. *Culture* is a term used casually and carelessly in everyday discourse, but it has a meaning for anthropologists. *Culture* refers to a set of rules or standards shared by members of a society, which when acted upon by the members produce behavior that falls within a range of variation the members consider proper and acceptable. That set of rules forms a kind of system, which means that the component parts are integrated and mutually reinforce one another. Culture is thus studied *holistically*. For example, we might perceive a problem of unequal distribution of food resources in a certain community. But if we approach that problem solely on an economic basis, we will miss the fact that rules and customs about distribution probably reflect prevailing norms about family organization, interpersonal responsibilities, and standards of leadership and governance. They are likely to be embedded in symbolic systems (such as mythology or ritual or art) that are the vehicles for their transmission across generations. Intervention in one segment of a culture will necessarily produce a ripple effect in all the other aspects of the culture to which it is connected. Intervention that targets only one aspect of society, as if it exists in a vacuum, is likely to produce unintended consequences that must be addressed, perhaps at great cost, at a later time.

The shared standards of culture can be found at many levels. Traditional anthropologists were most concerned with small, autonomous, isolated tribal societies in which the boundaries of a culture were easy to see. In the modern world, however, such tribal isolates are hard to find and anthropologists are just as likely to study cultures in such contexts as ethnic communities in a big city, dispersed communities defined by shared interests, or even "virtual communities" as they are emerging on the Internet. In such settings, the boundaries tend to blur; in fact, most people in the modern world

belong to several distinct, overlapping cultures. The challenge to modern anthropology is to discern which group identification takes precedence in a given situation when there might be several such groups competing for attention or resources.

Perhaps the most important aspect of the culture concept is that culture is *learned* behavior. The learning process often occurs over many generations–so much so that people are often unaware of why they do certain things or how things they take for granted came to be in the first place. But it would be wrong to assume that culture can never be changed–that people are too stubborn or too set in their ways to be open to change. By definition, that which is learned can also–with patience and tact–be unlearned, or learned in a modified way.

Anthropology is, furthermore, interested in both the physical and social sides of the human experience. The *biocultural perspective* means that much of what we do is genetically patterned, but the ways in which we interpret our behavior and make choices about what we will and will not make, do, and think about are all factors of the learned behavior we call *culture*. Often, the innovations that come through the cultural learning process will have profound biological effects. For example, when humans learned to control the use of fire (between 500,000 and 1 million years ago), there was a new selective pressure–it became desirable to have people with intelligence sufficient to understand the abstract leap from out-of-control-and-dangerous natural fire to controlled-and-beneficial fire and to learn the complex steps required to make and use fire properly. It is not surprising, therefore, that there was a marked increase in the size and complexity of the human brain as those with lesser intelligence were selectively bred out of the population.

In sum, the anthropological, comparative view of culture means that we first document the specific aspects of one particular culture and do so without prejudice or preconception. But then we attempt to put that culture into a larger perspective by attempting to find patterns or trends that describe the dynamics of culture as universal human phenomena.

Cultural Relativism

Anthropology is both a scientific discipline and a basis for approaching solutions to human problems. In both of those senses, anthropology operates on the principle of *cultural relativism*, which means that each culture is a distinctive adaptation to its own particular environment; it is inappropriate to evaluate one culture in terms of the standards and values of any other culture. This principle came to the fore under the influence of Franz Boas, who was appalled at the tendency of an earlier generation of anthropologists to rank cultures according to presumed levels of development and even to equate "primitive" cultures with the behavior of children, criminals, the insane, or apes. The enduring tendency to stereotype and undervalue other cultures without carefully examining them is known as *ethnocentrism*. Boas recognized that all human groups are defined by culture and that culture is neither rational nor irrational, neither good nor bad in any absolute terms; cultures come to be because people need to solve particular problems in their own environments. It makes no sense, he pointed out, to say that western civilization is "better" than the culture of an African tribe because we have motor cars and the telegraph and it does not; after all, it has survived quite happily and successfully for many generations with the culture that suited its traditional environment.

It is important, however, not to confuse cultural relativism with moral relativism (a belief that there are no absolute standards of right and wrong). Cultural relativism is not a way of saying that anything that any group does is okay. There are clearly customs and practices that come to be entrenched in a society (or that are imposed on them by external force) that are certainly not okay. Indeed, the entire enterprise of applied anthropology is predicated on the assumption that sometimes societies encounter problems–things they want or need to change. Anthropologists, as students of culture, are in a position to help them do so. *Cultural relativism* mainly refers to a position from which the study of culture must proceed. It is a reminder that our task is to describe the diversity of the human experience and to do so without uninformed value judgments. Only then will we have an objective base from which to make decisions about change.

METHODOLOGICAL CONSIDERATIONS

These philosophical ideas are put into action by anthropological researchers, including those engaged in applied projects. The most familiar methodological manifestation of anthropological ideas is the *ethnographic method*; *ethnography* means the description of a culture as a result of long-term immersion of the researcher in the community he or she is studying (a process sometimes referred to as *participant observation*). It is based on detailed observations, structured as well as informal interviews, and other devices, both qualitative and quantitative, all with the intent of converging on a holistic picture of the community, enhanced by the subjective understandings of the researcher as he or she attempts to get at the "insider's" view of issues and problems. Any social research method can be part of an ethnographer's toolkit, as long as it can be applied in the natural setting (as opposed to the laboratory or clinic) and as long as it occurs in the context of ongoing interaction between the researcher and those being studied.

In former times, anthropologists referred to the people they studied as subjects, an academic term that in the modern world has unfortunately taken on patronizing colonialist connotations. Anthropologists now acknowledge that they owe a debt of gratitude to people who share their time and insights with them, often with little or no visible return. They no longer consider themselves to be doing research "on" or "about" some subject community but rather see the research process as a collaborative enterprise. Some applied anthropologists would even claim that their most important duty is to teach members of the community the techniques of research so that they are empowered to do it for themselves. It is not always easy for researchers, secure in their many years of advanced education, to work in a collaborative, empowering framework, but this is at least the stated ideal of contemporary practitioners.

MAJOR THEORIES

As in any scientific discipline, anthropological theories are essentially elaborated means to explain generalizations and patterns; in anthropology, those patterns are generated by the process of comparative ethnography. Three main theoretical orientations (each of which includes numerous specific theories and models) stand out as having been of particular importance to modern applied anthropologists: functionalism, conflict theory and interactionism. Functionalist theory stresses the orderly interdependence of a society and its component parts and looks toward incremental adjustments needed to restore equilibrium when dysfunction arises. *Conflict theory* emphasizes the tensions that result from exploitation and competition for natural resources. *Interactionist theory* concentrates on everyday interpersonal dynamics operating within a socially constructed perception of reality.

AREAS OF APPLICATION

Almost every conceivable area of social service has been the setting for applied anthropology in recent years. In the field of the environment and resource-based industries, anthropologists have helped farm farmers' cooperatives and aquaculture projects; fostered the participation of women in development projects; and explored the impact of government and international regulations on the management of fisheries. Anthropologists have been active in disaster and risk assessment in cases of oil spills, hurricanes, famines, nuclear waste and chemical spills. Social impact assessment relative to dam, highway, and oil pipeline projects has also benefited from input from anthropologists. Anthropologists have long studied the process of technology transfer, for instance the impact of introducing steel axes to a people previously limited to stone tools. More recently, they have studied the effect of computers, the Internet, fax machines, and other advances in communications media and transportation technology on the globalization of the workplace.

Anthropological contributions to the health field are so numerous that the field of *medical anthropology* has emerged as perhaps the single most prominent specialization among applied anthropologists. Medical anthropologists study the formation of health policy, the delivery of services, and effective methods for health education/

health promotion in multicultural settings. One area of special concern in recent years has been the AIDS epidemic. Given the fact that AIDS/ HIV infection is highly correlated with certain kinds of social behaviors, anthropologists have had a great deal to contribute to our understanding of the spread of infection within and across populations. They have made particular contributions to understanding the ways in which people of diverse cultural backgrounds define and act on their sexuality so that programs of education and prevention can be tailored to make sense to members of those populations.

Anthropologists have worked in the field of *criminal justice*, contributing, for example, to a needs assessment study of both administrators and inmates of state penal institutions, as well as to studies of community attitudes toward policing. Biological anthropologists have been in the forefront of the development of *forensic anthropology*, which involves the analysis of human remains as they are linked to criminal cases. Several popular TV shows have highlighted, and glamorized, the growing field of forensic anthropology. Anthropologists have been interested in *education* and have been active in multicultural curriculum design and program evaluation. Linguistic anthropologists have been particularly interested in studies of how people (especially children) learn. Anthropologists have worked in the private sector, helping businesses gain a better understanding of their activities and customers for purposes of marketing, as well as for research and development of new product lines. The traditional concern with *indigenous peoples* has continued into the modern world, with projects involving the administration of aboriginal, native, or tribal peoples in various parts of the world. Contemporary applied anthropologists have been active in the movement for indigenous self-government, and linguists among them have been in the forefront of efforts to preserve and dis-

seminate long-suppressed tribal languages.

Archaeological anthropologists have helped develop the field of *cultural resources management*, or the preservation of "heritage materials," both prehistoric and historic. Federal and state legislation now mandates that any construction project of a certain size submit both a report of the cultural resources that might be impacted by disturbing the earth and a plan for mitigating those impacts by retrieving and archiving those resources in an appropriate place. Now more than ever, there is an attempt to coordinate such efforts with tribal councils and other indigenous peoples' representatives to make sure that prehistoric remains are treated respectfully.

PREPARATION AND DEVELOPMENT TO WORK IN FIELD

An advanced degree is generally the prerequisite for a career as a practicing anthropologist or part-time consultant. The M.A. is the degree of choice for those working full-time outside of academe, as well as for those who opt for a career in teaching at the elementary, secondary, or community college levels. Those interested in university employment usually need a doctorate. Most of the larger departments of anthropology in the United States and Canada have at least a few survey courses in applied anthropology and some of them (e.g., University of Kentucky, University of Arizona, and the University of Florida) allow students to select applied anthropology as a specialized thesis topic. But there are as of this writing some forty institutions (most notably the University of South Florida and the University of Memphis) that have advanced degree programs specifically designed to train applied anthropologists. Some institutions have instituted "dual degree" programs that combine a traditional anthropology Ph.D. curriculum with that for a master's degree in public health, business administration, social work, criminal justice, or education. Well regarded advanced degree programs specifically in medical anthropology have been developed at the University of California–at both Berkeley and San Francisco campuses, Case Western University, and the University of Connecticut. There have been moves in recent years to develop criteria to certify training programs and licensing for applied and/or practicing anthropologists (i.e., adopting a professional model such as that in social work), but as of this writing, these efforts have not resulted in concrete action.

Admissions criteria vary from one school to another and often change from year to year. But a grade point average of 3.0 (overall, and in the major) and a Graduate Record Exam Score of 1100 are generally the minimum standards for an application to be favorably reviewed. An undergraduate major in anthropology is not necessarily a prerequisite for entering a graduate program in anthropology. Beyond the formal criteria, a clear and well written statement of career goals and positive, detailed letters of reference are important elements in a successful application.

Undergraduates have been able to find positions on applied projects directed by members of their department faculty. Such experience is very valuable and will look impressive on an application to graduate school, but it is very rare for someone with only undergraduate training to make a successful career as an applied/practicing anthropologist.

WORK SETTINGS

In addition to the academic settings noted above, applied anthropologists (especially archaeologists and physical anthropologists) may find work in museums, some of which are attached to universities, while others are government-supported or privately operated. Indigenous groups in the U.S. and elsewhere now also sponsor their own museums, and while they give preference to tribal members for permanent staff positions, they may welcome as consultants people from outside the tribe who have special skills.

Anthropologists may work directly in government agencies. Some federal agencies have a good history of employing anthropologists: the National Parks Service (usually archaeologists interested in cultural resources management, but also cultural anthropologists who can work on matters involving the social impact of land-management programs), the Bureau of Indian Affairs (most recently in the area of preparing documents for Congress to grant federal recognition to Indian tribal units), and the Centers for Disease Control (a wide variety of basic research, as well as needs assessment and program evaluation research related to various aspects of public health). Anthropologists have been hired by various states' departments of education, health, and transportation. Among nongovernment agencies (NGOs), the World Bank, the United Nations (especially its UNESCO and UNICEF agencies), and the World Health Organization have been eager to hire anthropologists, particularly for projects in international health and development.

Opportunities also exist in the private sector, although such positions will rarely be advertised under the label "anthropology." The private sector includes not only business concerns but also public interest advocacy groups. It is important for the budding practitioner interested in a private sector career to learn to market his or her skills even in the absence of a defined position title of "anthropologist."

PROFESSIONAL ORGANIZATIONS

The SfAA publishes *Human Organization*, the most widely read international journal of applied social science; indeed, its name was deliberately selected to reflect the multidisciplinary reach of those with a cultural perspective on social issues. In the 1980s, it also began publishing *Practicing Anthropology*, a more informal magazine devoted to the specific concerns of nonacademic practitioners. The SfAA also sponsors an annual meeting at which scholarly papers are presented and where members have an opportunity to network with others with similar interests.

In the 1980s, the American Anthropological Association (the largest and most influential umbrella organization representing anthropologists of all persuasions) created the National Association for the Practice of Anthropology (NAPA) in order to secure an organizational presence for applied/practicing anthropologists within the mainstream of the discipline. NAPA publishes a regular series of bulletins–collections of papers on topics of interest to its constituencies. It also produced a widely disseminated DVD documenting applied and practicing anthropologists in their work settings. Many practitioners, particularly those with no ongoing ties to a university department, have grouped themselves into Local Practitioner Organizations (LPOs), which provide peer group support and local networking. There are especially active LPOs in Washington, Memphis, Tucson, and Tampa, cities with large concentrations of anthropologists working in the community.

APPLIED ANTHROPOLOGY CAREERS

Because there is no single career track for anthropologists outside the university, it is difficult to make any generalizations about career advancement, opportunities, or salaries. Such matters are determined by the particular positions that anthropologists fill; as noted above, such positions may not have the label "anthropologist" in their titles or job descriptions. Nevertheless, there are two excellent sources for more detailed information, including sample profiles of applied/ practicing anthropologists at work. The first is the NAPA DVD noted above. Entitled *Anthropology: Real People, Real Careers*, it features anthropologists working in the US and abroad, in government, human services, manufacturing, and retail. The DVD is available from the American Anthropological Association (see the References for contact information).

The second source of note is a 2002 booklet, *Careers in Anthropology: What an Anthropology Degree Can Do for You* by W. Richard Stephens. It profiles 15 anthropologists and their jobs. It is interesting to note that most of the professionals profiled in the video and the booklet work at jobs that do not seem to have an obvious anthropological content; it is therefore instructive to read the anthropologists' complete profiles in order to understand how they make use of their anthropological skills even in jobs that seem far removed from the traditions of academic anthropology.

OUTLOOK

People with anthropological training must create their own career niches, usually beginning the job search with a "pathfinder," a process that involves researching the main issues related to a particular area (health care, criminal justice, international business, and so forth), interviewing people who have direct experience in that area, and searching out the main journals, books, and professional associations dealing with the area. The pathfinder can thus suggest any needs for further training and the upgrading of skills. An effective job search would also include: (1) developing a resume that highlights skills and experiences that even a nonanthropologist would understand and value; (2) seeking out a mentor who is already established in the area in which you want to work; (3) getting involved in networks of people in the area who know and appreciate your skills; (4) getting to know the agencies for which you might want to work; (5) being prepared to take on short-term jobs at short notice; and (6) seeking out volunteer opportunities in agencies in which you might ultimately want to work.

Close to half the people now graduating with advanced degrees in anthropology are working in nonacademic settings, and every indication is that this trend will continue. Specialized practitioner-oriented graduate programs continue to be developed. There is a growing body of empirical, methodological, and theoretical literature that is of particular interest to applied and practicing anthropologists. The first generation of non-academic practitioners is now well established in fields such as international aid, business, medicine, public administration, architecture, charitable organizations, governments, unions, advocacy, and consumer protection agencies. They are, therefore, in a position to assist newer anthropologists in identifying suitable careers and helping them achieve their goals.

SUMMARY

Anthropology is no longer the study of arcane, antique, esoteric materials. It is an academic discipline that can equip its practitioners to engage with the major social issues of the day and to find employment in the various public and private sector agencies that deal with those issues. The discipline as a whole is increasingly accommodating to those who seek to apply anthropology beyond its traditional academic confines.

Anthropologists have at their disposable a body of knowledge based on the comparative study of human cultures and the evolution of the species. They are adept at working within communities to find out people's perceptions and needs and so avoid the trap of elite, top-down planning and service delivery. The holism of anthropology encourages its practitioners to be open to a wide variety of approaches–to become, in effect, creative problem-solvers.

REFERENCES

Baba, M.L. (1994). The fifth subdiscipline: Anthropological practice and the future of anthropology. *Human Organization*, 53(2), 174–186.

Chambers, E. (1985). *Applied anthropology: A practical guide.* Englewood Cliffs, NJ: Prentice-Hall.

Ervin, A.M. (2000). *Applied anthropology: Tools and perspectives for contemporary practice.* Boston: Allyn & Bacon.

Fluehr-Lobban, C. (Ed.). (1991). *Ethics and the profession of anthropology: Dialogue for a new era.* Philadelphia: University of Pennsylvania Press.

Higgins, P.J., & Paredes, J.A. (Eds.). (1999). *Classics of practicing anthropology, 1978–1998.* Oklahoma City, OK: Society for Applied Anthropology.

Hill, C.E., & Baba, M.L. (Eds.). (2000). *The unity of theory and practice in anthropology: Rebuilding a fractured synthesis.* Washington, DC: National Association for the Practice of Anthropology.

Hyland, S., & Kirkpatrick, S. (1980). *Guide to training programs in the applications of anthropology* (3rd ed.). Memphis, TN: Society for Applied Anthropology.

Koon, A., Hackett, B., & Mason, J.P. (Eds.). (1989). *Stalking employment in the nation's capital: A guide for anthropologists.* Washington, DC: National Association for the Practice of Anthropology.

Kushner, G. (1994). Training programs for the practice of anthropology. *Human Organization, 53*(2), 186–192.

Manderson, L. (1996). Handbook and manuals in applied research. *Practicing Anthropology, 18*(3), 3–40.

McDonald, J.H. (Ed.). (2002). *The applied anthropology reader.* Boston: Allyn & Bacon.

Omohundro, J. (2002). *Careers in anthropology* (2nd ed.). Mountain View, CA: Mayfield.

Omohundro, J. (2005). Career advice for anthropology undergraduates. In J. Spradley & D. McCurdy (Eds.), *Conformity and Conflict* (11th ed.), pp. 399–410. Needhan Heights, MA: Allyn & Bacon.

Stephens, W.R. (2002). *Careers in anthropology: What an anthropology degree can do for you.* Boston: Allyn & Bacon.

Trotter, R.T. (1988). *Anthropology for tomorrow: Creating practitioner-oriented applied anthropology programs.* Washington, DC: American Anthropological Association.

van Willigen, J. (1987). *Becoming a practicing anthropologist: A guide to careers and training programs in applied anthropology.* Washington, DC: National Association of Professional Anthropologists.

van Willigen, J. (1993). *Applied anthropology: An introduction* (2nd ed.). Westport, CT: Bergin & Garvey.

van Willigen, J., Rylko-Bauer, B., & McElroy, A. (Eds.). (1989). *Making our research useful: Case studies in the utilization of anthropological knowledge.* Boulder, CO: Westview.

Weaver, T. (1985). Anthropology as a policy science: Part I, A critique. *Human Organization, 44*(2), 97-106.

Weaver, T. (1985). Anthropology as a policy science: Part II, Development and training. *Human Organization, 44*(3), 197–206.

Wulff, R.M., & Fiske, S.J. (Eds.). (1987). *Anthropological praxis: Knowledge into action.* Boulder, CO: Westview.

WEBSITES

American Anthropological Association, www.aaa net.org [see especially its link to the National Association of Practicing Anthropologists and to information about the DVD *Anthropology: Real People, Real Careers*].

Society for Applied Anthropology, www.sfaa.net [see especially its education, employment, organizations, and students links].

Chapter 3

AUDIOLOGY, SPEECH-LANGUAGE PATHOLOGY, AND SPEECH-LANGUAGE-HEARING SCIENCE

ARTHUR M. GUILFORD

It has been estimated that as many as 46 million people in the United States have some type of communication disorder (National Institute of Deafness and Other Communication Disorders, 1995). Of these, some are born with their disorder(s) such as those individuals born deaf (an inability to hear sounds) or those born with a neuromotor condition such as cerebral palsy or a craniofacial anomaly (cleft lip or palate). There are others with acquired communication disorders who have suffered their losses as a result of disease (e.g., cancer or meningitis), accident (traumatic brain injury), or vascular changes (stroke or cerebrovascular accident). There are specialists who can offer help to individuals with communication disorders and their families. These specialists are called audiologists, speech-language pathologists, and speech, language, and hearing scientists.

DISCIPLINE

A discipline is an area of study or specialization of study, while a profession is an area of practice. The discipline of communication sciences and disorders (CSD) encompasses the study of the human communication process, the science of human communication, the breakdowns in the processes of human communication (referred to as communication differences or disorders), and the efficacy of the applied disciplinary practices. The professions represented in the discipline of communication sciences and disorders are speech, language, and hearing science, audiology, and speech language pathology. Related areas of practice within the discipline are those dealing with issues of deafness and deaf education (e.g., those who develop and apply educational and rehabilitative techniques for individuals with severe and profound hearing impairments). Communication sciences and disorders is a relatively new discipline and is not offered at all colleges and universities. Currently, there are approximately 250 programs in the United States that offer graduate educational opportunities in this discipline. Of these, not all offer work in both audiology and speech-language pathology.

It has only been about 20 years that the descriptor "communication sciences and disorders" has been consistently used. However, the terms speech pathology and audi-

29

ology have been used longer. The first use of the term speech pathology occurred in the 1920s and appeared for the first time in print in the University of Iowa catalogue in the 1924–1925 academic year (Moellor, 1976). The American Speech-Language-Hearing Association (ASHA) added the term language many years later (1976), as it became apparent that communication disorders were more complex than just speech production problems.

Drs. Ray Carhart and Norton Canfield coined the word audiology during World War II. This new science focused on the aural rehabilitation of individuals who had suffered war-related hearing loss. World War II was a catalyst for both audiology and speech pathology as it served to foster a union between the two professions and it produced enormous numbers of individuals requiring audiological or speech-language pathology services due to war-related injuries. During this era, the Veteran's Administration hospitals grew in order to accommodate the war-injured, and almost all of these facilities included rehabilitation programs in audiology and speech language pathology.

Communication sciences and disorders have drawn heavily from a number of other fields. Some fields that have contributed to this discipline include psychology, medicine, physics, biology, linguistics, education, rehabilitation, anatomy and physiology, counseling, computer science, and speech communication. Because this discipline grew first through the practice of the professions and then later defined and refined itself, there has been some concern among researchers in universities and other settings that research in communication sciences and disorders has failed to keep pace with the practice demands. We have attracted many thousands into practice but have failed to attract as many graduates into research careers within the discipline. One of the most promising current employment opportunities is to work in university settings teaching and conducting research. As with many disciplines, we have suffered from the "graying of the professorate," as retirement rates exceed the numbers of those who wish to replace them. Therefore, both practicing professionals and individuals desiring research and teaching careers are in high demand in this discipline.

THE PROFESSIONS

The American Speech-Language-Hearing Association (ASHA) is the primary professional, scientific, and accrediting association for the professions of audiology and speech language pathology. ASHA considers communication science and disorders to be a single discipline with two separate professions: audiology and speech language pathology. A third entity of this discipline that should be considered is speech, language, and hearing sciences, although there is no direct service delivery with this component of the discipline. There are more than 130,600 audiologists, speech-language pathologists, and speech, language, and hearing scientists who are members or affiliates of ASHA. The mission of ASHA is to ensure that all people with speech, language, and hearing disorders have access to quality services in order to help them communicate more effectively (www.asha.org).

Audiology

Audiologists are hearing health care professionals. Audiologists specialize in the prevention, identification, and assessment of hearing disorders. Audiology is practiced in many different work settings. Audiologists test and diagnose hearing disorders in infants, children and adults, and they prescribe and dispense hearing aids and assistive listening devices while instructing people in their use. They also help prevent hearing loss through programs of hearing conservation, work with people needing aural rehabilitation through such approaches as auditory training, speech reading and sign language instruction, and conduct research into influences on hearing, new evaluation methods and rehabilitative devices such as cochlear implants (www.asha.org). The number of audiologists has grown rapidly in the past 50 years, but there remain fewer audiologists than speech-language pathologists. There are an estimated 18,000–20,000 practicing audiologists in the United States today. It has been suggested that audiology grew out of the practice of speech pathology and otology—the medical profession that deals with diseases of the ear and the peripheral hearing mechanism during World War II (Newby, 1958).

Audiologists are often employed in medical environments such as physician's offices, hospitals, and rehabilitation settings. Some audiologists work in educational settings such as universities, public or private schools, and schools for the deaf or hard of hearing. These professionals are usually referred to as educational or rehabilitative audiologists. One of the fastest growing segments of this profession is that of private practice in which the practitioner tests hearing and dispenses hearing aids when required by the patient's hearing loss. The employment site directly influences the type of activity performed by the audiologist. For those working with physicians' offices, they spend the majority of their time determining the nature and extent of the hearing loss, the likelihood of pathology in the auditory system, and the potential benefits of amplification through a hearing aid. Those employed in educational or rehabilitation settings are more likely to provide assessment and rehabilitative services but dispense few, if any, hearing aids (Powers, 2000). Some audiolo-

gists elect to belong to single professional groups such as the American Association of Audiologists (AAA) or Audiology Foundation of America (AFA) for their professional representation; however, the majority continues to join ASHA.

Recent demographics (2007) reveal that the majority of audiologists work in healthcare facilities (71.4%) and 17.2 percent work in educational settings. Audiologists serve clients of all ages from birth through the geriatric years. Many states, for example, have supported infant hearing screening which is performed on newborn infants prior to being released from the hospital. These programs are usually required through the Early Intervention Programs (EIP) in the state and may be paid for by dollars generated through Individuals with Disabilities Education Act (IDEA), part C, which specifies services for all infants and toddlers from birth to three years of age. Other audiologists provide services to older children in educational settings or to adults in physicians' offices, hospitals, rehabilitation centers or private practices. A large part of the practice in these settings is the fitting and dispensing hearing aids or other assistive listening devices.

Speech-Language Pathology

Speech-language pathologists help individuals develop their communication abilities and diagnose and treat speech, language, swallowing, and voice disorders. Their services may include prevention, identification, evaluation, treatment, and rehabilitation of communication disorders. Speech-language pathologists conduct research: (a) to develop newer and better ways to diagnose and remediate speech, language, and swallowing disorders (a major growth area); (b) to work with children who have delays in language development and to provide treatment to people who stutter and to those with voice and articulation problems; and (c) to provide assistance and service to people with foreign or regional accents who want to learn another speech style. It has been estimated there are more than 113,000 practicing speech-language pathologist in the United States today.

Speech disorders are most often associated with speech sound production or articulation, fluency, and voice. Many forms of speech disorders are developmental in nature as they reflect that the child has never learned the correct form. Language disorders are characterized by difficulties in the content, form, use and comprehension of the language system. Language disorders among children are most often developmental in nature, but among adults they are usually acquired due to trauma, disease or neurological impairment. Swallowing disorders (dysphagia) refer to difficulties in preparation of the food in the mouth to be swallowed (oral stage dysphagia); manipulation of the food (referred to as bolus) to the back of the oral cavity to be swallowed; the pharyngeal stage of actually swallowing the bolus; and the esophageal stage as the bolus passes through the esophagus to the stomach.

The history of speech-language pathology as a profession is longer than audiology's. As early as the 1920s, academic course work in speech correction was offered in some universities. The disorder of speech fluency, which is referred to as stuttering, provided some of the initial interest in the profession and produced early research as well as academic and clinical interest. This early work focused on discovering the causes of stuttering and interestingly was often conducted by researchers in universities who suffered from this condition (e.g., Charles VanRiper and Wendall Johnson). Later, research in stuttering expanded to include the provision of clinical services to assist in the remediation of this disorder.

Speech-language pathologists are often referred to by a variety of titles or names; however, ASHA has recommended the use of speech-language pathologist. In many schools, practioners are referred to as speech clinicians, speech teachers, speech therapists, or speech correctionists. In hospital and rehabilitation settings, many are called speech therapists as this term is correlated with the professions of physical and occupational therapy. This is rather misleading because physical and occupational therapists work under the direction of a physician who prescribes the therapy. The speech-language pathologist works independently to evaluate, determine eligibility of service, prescribe treatment, and deliver the service (Powers, 2000). Malone (1979) has indicated that speech-language pathologists have been identified by as many as 100 different titles dependent upon the work setting.

The work environments for speech-language pathologists are expanding. Approximately 59 percent work with children in preschools, elementary or secondary schools, while the remaining 41 percent work in other settings. These settings include, infant and early childhood programs often associated with state agencies, medical settings such as hospitals, rehabilitation centers, freestanding speech and hearing centers, nursing homes, home health care, and private practice. The fastest growing segment of employment for speech-language pathologists for the last couple of decades has been private practice (www.ASHA.org).

Salaries in speech-language pathology and audiology are competitive and, with critical shortages reported in both areas, salaries have steadily improved. A median 10-month starting salary in the school system is reported to be $52,000 and a residential/day school salary is approximately $60,000 (ASHA 2006 Schools Salary Survey at www.ASHA.org). Salaries in hospital settings would have a large range as well, but would likely be between $55,000 and $70,000 for a 12-month salary. Starting salaries for Ph.D.s have increased, and most institutions start assistant professors in these disciplines at $60,000 to $70,000 for a nine-month salary.

Speech, Language, and Hearing Sciences

Speech, language, and hearing scientists do not usually deliver direct services to people with communication disorders unless they are also certified or licensed audiologists or speech-language pathologists. There are, however, many audiologists and speech-language pathologists who conduct clinical research and have greatly contributed to the applied and theoretical knowledge base of the discipline. In its strict sense, speech, language and hearing science is concerned with anatomical, physiological, perceptual, and linguistic aspects of the human communication process because these processes may contribute to the production and comprehension of the speech and language systems.

Speech, language, and hearing scientists often come from a variety of backgrounds that may include medicine, acoustics, psychology, biology, linguistics, physics, and of course, communication sciences and disorders. Due to this diversity, it may be somewhat difficult to define the limits of the speech, language and hearing scientists, as they will often have broad research backgrounds and interests. The majority of these scientists hold advanced degrees such as the Doctor of Philosophy (Ph.D.) and have extensive research training and education.

The majority of speech, language, and hearing scientists are employed in university settings. However, some work for governmental agencies or in independent public or private laboratories. Some are engaged in research that deals only with the normal process of human communication, while others are involved with both normal and disordered communication. Because of the need for research, speech, language, and hearing scientists are important to the growth of the knowledge base of the professions of audiology and speech-language pathology.

ACADEMIC PREPARATION IN SPEECH-LANGUAGE PATHOLOGY AND AUDIOLOGY

The official policy of the American Speech Language-Hearing Association (ASHA) is that the minimum requirement for the practice of the profession of audiology will become a doctoral degree by the year 2012. Specifically, many universities have developed a clinical doctorate or Doctor of Audiology (Au.D.) degree to meet this challenge. Prior to this policy change, the master's degree was the minimum requirement for the profession. It has long been ASHA's policy that a master's degree should be the minimum qualification for those working in speech-language pathology. ASHA provides a Certificate of Clinical Competence (CCC) to audiologists and speech-language pathologists who meet the strict requirements of their profession. In speech-language pathology and in masters-level audiology programs, the CCC is awarded to individuals after the completion of a clinical fellowship experience and the successfully passing the National Examination in Speech-Language Pathology or Audiology. For students enrolled in Doctor of Audiology programs, the CCC is often earned in the fourth and final year of the program rather than after the program has been completed. In addition, many states now have licensure laws for the professions of audiology and speech-language pathology. In 1969, Florida was the first state to establish professional licensure for these professions and since then a steady increase in the number of states requiring licensure has followed. Some states have teacher certification for speech-language pathology, but few have it for audiology. In some states, it is possible to work in an educational setting in which fees are not charged without holding the CCC, these practitioners work under a state's professional license or teacher certification program. Laws, rules, and regulations vary by state and should always be investigated prior to obtaining employment.

ASHA also accredits graduate educational programs that meet its standards. When investigating programs, one should remember it is easier to obtain the certificate of clinical competency when one has graduated from an accredited institution. In addition, if one wishes to become a certified audiologist or speech-language pathologist, he or she will have to abide by the ASHA Code of Ethics, which sets the highest standards for professional conduct and performance (www .asha.org). A copy of the Statement of Practices and Procedures of the Board of Ethics (last revised 1998) may be found and reviewed in print in Asha, 40 (Suppl.18) or online at www.asha.org. Anyone interested in working as either a speech-language pathologist or audiologist should carefully review this material prior to pursuing a career in these professions.

HUMAN COMMUNICATION AND ITS DISORDERS

Generally speaking, communication is an exchange of ideas between the sender(s) and the receiver(s). You say something, and I respond. I say something, and you respond. A message is sent, and a message is received. In order to communicate, we must have someone with whom to talk. We also must have something to say, a reason to say it, and some means through which to communicate

this message (Beebe, Beebe & Redmond, 1996). Communication is a social process, so we must have someone with whom to speak. Who that person is will affect topics of conversation and how topics are presented or discussed. We don't speak to our parents in the same way that we speak to friends. Nor do we talk with people at first meeting in the same manner as we talk with them after having been friends with them for several months. There are topics that we might feel comfortable in discussing with our same sex friends that we would be less likely to discuss with someone of the opposite sex. If we were speaking to a young child we would alter our speech in one way, but if we were speaking to one of our professors we would change our speech in another way. There are three rules to effective communication.

1. *We must have something to say.* Most of us, at one time or another, have found ourselves in a situation in which there is a high expectation for conversation, and yet we can think of nothing to say. Typically, the situation itself is the cueing mechanism that provides the common bond between speaker and listener and assures an opening topic for conversation.

2. *We must have a reason to communicate.* In some situations, we may want to inform others or request information from them. We may want to exert some control over others either directly (e.g., "Close the window") or indirectly (e.g., "Don't you think its cold in here?"). In either case, the reason is basically the same (i.e., regulatory).

3. *We need to have a way to send our message.* We need to use an efficient system that will convey our ideas to a wide range of people as simply as possible. Grammar helps us do just that. We need a way to transmit our message. In most situations, we use speech for com-

munication. It is the most expedient form of communication, and it is understood by nearly everyone we are likely to encounter in our local communities.

Speakers and listeners cue and respond to each other while creating conversations. Each conversation begins with the speaker formulating a message that is transmitted to the listener who then formulates his interpretation of the message. Formulation, transmission, and interpretation comprise the first step in the conversational process.

Formulating a Message

Before a conversation can be developed, a message must be formulated. The idea is then translated into the appropriate lexical items or words, with careful consideration of the rules for selecting and sequencing speech sounds (phonemes). After the appropriate lexical items have been selected, it is necessary to order them according to the conventions of the speech community. For example, Americans say "The white house," but the French say "La maison blanc." These conventions are realized through rules of grammar, which add structure to messages so the listener receives the intended meaning. The utterance, "The boy hit the girl" clearly does not convey the same meaning as "The girl hit the boy."

Once the message has been formulated according to content, lexicon, and grammar, it is ready to be transmitted from the brain of the speaker to the brain of the listener. This second step may be referred to as transmitting a message.

Transmitting a Message

Through transmission, a message is sent from the brain of the speaker to his speech mechanism—specifically to his lips, tongue, jaw, pharynx, larynx, velum, and lungs. The speech mechanism acts as a unit to articulate the message, setting air molecules in vibration according to patterns that have been programmed by the cortex of the brain. The message travels through the air to the listener where the ear acts as a receiver. His or her eardrums are set in vibration. This, in turn, impinges on the tiny bones of the middle ear that amplify the sound and send the message on to the inner ear (the ossicular chain). Here, tiny hair cells are set in vibration. Their action modifies neural activity along the auditory nerve, sending the message to the brain where the process of interpretation takes place.

Interpreting the Message

The message is received in the temporal region of the brain where it is analyzed according to its grammatical and lexical features. On the basis of this decoding process, the listener organizes an interpretation of the message sent by the speaker.

The total process of formulating, transmitting, and interpreting messages in interpersonal exchanges is referred to as the speech chain (Denes & Pinson, 1973). Two additions to the chain must be considered to derive a description of a basic model of communication. First, the listener's response must be considered; without it, there is no way to determine if the message has been received or if it has been interpreted correctly. Second, the model must be expanded to show the conversational nature of communication. For a conversational model, we would have to link a series of speaker-listener units in such a way that the respective roles of speaker and listener alternate. This process of conversational turn-taking continues until it reaches some natural conclusion or until turn-taking has ended.

CULTURAL DIVERSITY

There are several variables that affect communication and its success or failure. Age, gender, ethnic background, and education affect communication. Furthermore, each of us is a member of a language community because our own culture will influence what words we select, our speech patterns, how closely we stand together, how intently we look at each other, and all of the direct and indirect aspects of our language use. Speakers and listeners must share competence in a common language if they are to communicate fully and easily (Owens, Metz & Haas, 2000). We also have to respect the diversity within our community and create opportunities to learn and incorporate aspects of other cultures into our own for effective cross-cultural communication. Speech-language pathologists must be particularly sensitive to cultural differences, as understanding these variations may greatly influence the diagnosis and treatment of communication and swallowing disorders. Culture and diversity play a role in all diagnostic and treatment plans (Rosa-Lugo & Champion, 2007).

COMMUNICATION DISORDERS

Communication is our most human characteristic. It is essential to learning, working, and enjoying social relationships. ASHA has estimated that one in ten Americans has a communication disorder due to stroke, undetected hearing loss, stuttering problem, head injury, language disorder, or some other disorder that interferes with speech, language or hearing (www.asha.org). Communication disorders may be manifested in many different ways. The significant defin-

ing feature is that the disorder impedes the formulation, transmission, or interpretation of a message. It is important to identify at least three distinct aspects of communication that may be affected by a disorder. Language is the first aspect to consider as it involves the use of an arbitrary rule system (grammar) of the speech community in formulating messages. Second, the speech aspects of the production of the message are composed of articulation, resonance, voicing, and fluency or rhythm. The third aspect of communication includes the nonverbal cues we use as we communicate, such as facial expression, gestures, and posture.

The management process of communication or swallowing disorders is a complex one and most often begins with the identification process and ends when the individual no longer has need of the specialized services. The overall steps in the management process are outlined below.

1. Identification or diagnosis occurs as the initial aspect of the management process. This may occur as the result of an initial screening in which all individuals are subjected to the same process. Screening procedures are often used in child-find programs, in which the goal is to identify the young child who is at risk for communication disorders. Screening examinations are not diagnostic in nature but identify potential risk factors that may lead to the definitive identification of a communication or swallowing disorder. Often potential clients are referred to the speech-language pathologist or audiologist by physicians, teachers, family members, or themselves.

2. Referral to other specialists may be made at the conclusion of the screening process. Frequently this would involve referral to a speech-language pathologist, audiologist, social worker,

psychologist, or other professional for comprehensive diagnostic services. Speech-language pathologists use a wide variety and complexity of test instruments to evaluate and diagnose the communication or swallowing disorder. These evaluations are performed in a variety of settings (clinic, hospital, rehabilitation center, school, or home); however, swallowing evaluations are almost always performed with the assistance of medical personnel, in either in-patient or out-patient hospital or nursing-home settings. Audiologists require specialized equipment and a sound booth for comprehensive diagnostic assessment.

3. Team staffing is required in many settings. It is particularly valuable in educational settings or early childhood settings where professionals and family members meet to develop either a Family Support Plan (FSP; for infants and toddlers birth to 3 years) or an Individualized Educational Plan (IEP; for children 3–21 years). Development of both of these plans requires parental/ family participation as well as participation by a staffing specialist or family coordinator and any other professionals who were a part of the evaluation process. These plans will determine the intensity and frequency of treatment as well as other professionals involved in the management program for the infant, toddler, or child.

4. Clinical services are provided in a variety of settings and under various levels of intensity. For instance school systems frequently use small-group intervention or provide the service in a classroom setting utilizing a collaborative or consultative model. Clinical services with adults usually take place individually but may involve small group interaction as well. For example,

group interaction is often helpful and appropriate for stroke patients and their families or for patients who have had their larynges removed due to cancer. Many times, these individuals profit such group interaction and support. The duration of clinical services will be determined by the severity of the communication disorder, the amount of progress made in treatment, and the willingness of the client to continue participation in the rehabilitative process. Speech-language pathologists frequently repeat diagnostic testing in order to measure progress made in therapy and to recommend dismissal only when the individual stops making progress in the treatment process.

5. Dismissal from treatment may occur due to many factors. The most likely case is that the individual has made sufficient progress in treatment of the disorder and additional treatment is no longer required. It is important to realize that due to the overall condition of the individual, not every communication or swallowing disorder will be completely remediable. For example, in persons with progressive neurological disorders, the combination of behavioral treatments (speech-language clinical services) and the medical treatments may be unable to turn back the progression of the disease. In these individuals, the decision may be made that continued treatment is no longer warranted. Children may be dismissed from clinical services as they no longer require them. In these cases the teacher(s) may be asked to continue to monitor the success of treatment and refer the child back should additional needs develop. In other settings, family members will be asked to similarly monitor their child's continued progress. Evidence-based practice should

always be followed in treatment and dismissal. An excellent review of this approach may be found in Hinckley (2007).

The following section addresses several of the most frequently observed communication disorders that the audiologist and speech-language pathologist treat on a routine basis. Due to the length of this chapter, it is not possible to cover all in detail, nor is it possible to cover all etiological, evaluation, and treatment aspects to these communication disorders.

Language Disorders

Language disorders comprise the single largest group of communication disorders for children. Language disorders fall into several different categories and may not receive a specific diagnostic label due to the age of the child. The type of clinical interventions varies considerably between an infant or toddler and a school-aged child or adolescent. Language disorders generally cluster themselves around the child's ability to handle the content of language (semantic elements or word meaning), the form of language (grammatical form, phonology, and morphological markers), or the use of language (knowledge of the social aspects of language). Each of these systems is considered to be rule-governed because they are consistently applied across the language.

There are many different causes of language disorders, and sometimes the cause may not be precisely known. For a variety of reasons, children may fail to follow a typical course of development of their communication skills. When children fail to follow typical developmental patterns, it becomes a concern and early intervention may be required. It is estimated that approximately 6 to 10 percent of infants born each year do not follow the same synergistic developmental sequence that promotes communicative competency. Therefore, at any given time 630,000 to 1,050,000 infants may be experiencing social, emotional, behavioral, and preacademic difficulties (Billeaud, 1998). The number of children requiring special services to meet their communicative or other needs continues to grow. Consequently, increasing numbers of speech-language pathologists are working in early intervention programs or preschool programs for children with disabilities. The most common reason for referral of young children between the ages of two and three years is failure to learn conventional communication.

Approximately 7 percent of all school-age children experience difficulties in learning their native language, and more than one million children receive language intervention services in the schools each year (U.S. Department of Education, 1990). Many more children receive treatment in private facilities, private schools, centers, and agencies, so the numbers of children requiring services for language disorders is generally higher than reported by the federal government. Children who reach five years of age and older and are still experiencing difficulty with their language are at-risk for other problems, including learning disabilities, reading difficulties, and other academic failures. When these problems continue throughout the school-age years, language problems may persist into adulthood (Gillam & Bedore, 2000).

Language disorders are also seen in adults. The most common cause of language disorders among adults is a condition called aphasia, which results from neurological damage, most commonly cerebrovascular accident or stroke. Other causes of aphasia may include gunshot wounds, blows to the head, traumatic brain injury, or brain tumors. According to the American Academy of Neurology (www.aan.com), 700,000 people incur strokes each year resulting in 80,000 new cases of aphasia annually. The National Aphasia Association (www.aphasia.org) estimates that over one million Americans suffer from aphasia. There are a variety of language problems that may be evidenced in individuals suffering from aphasia. Some of these problems may include expressive or receptive language problems, word-finding problems, and reading and writing difficulties. These language difficulties vary in severity and are often related to the site of lesion within the brain and the extent of the overall brain damage (Chapey & Hallowell, 2001).

In addition, individuals with aphasia may also suffer from neuromotor communication disorders such as dysarthria, dysphagia, or apraxia. Dysarthria and apraxia are neurogenic speech disorders, not language disorders. They often result from the same type of brain damage as aphasia–which is why they often occur simultaneously. The muscular and respiratory mechanisms that control the production of speech in these two conditions are also related to swallowing (Hedge, 1994). Patients who are experiencing difficulties with swallowing after a stroke are said to be experiencing dysphagia. This is a serious medical condition and must be treated immediately in order to avoid aspiration pneumonia or other respiratory disorders or possible dehydration or serious weight loss (ASHA Supplement, 24, 77–92, 2004 & www.ancds.org/practice.html).

Speech Disorders

Articulatory function represents a system that relates meaning to sound. True meaning arises with an individual's language; however, when we want to convey the meaning of the rule-structured language, we must rely on phonology (rules of the sound system) to express the sounds of our language. Phonology is a learned system of sounds that is used systematically and in a rule-governed manner for the purpose of communicating with others. It is but one component of the language system. It is important to remember that children learn their sound system in a predictable developmental way. The sounds generally learned first are those that are produced more visibly or in the anterior portion of the mouth (i.e., /p/, /m/, /h/, /n/, /w/) and are typically produced well by about three years of age. On the other hand, sounds that are more complex or are produced less visibly (i.e., /r/, /l/, /s/) may be acquired as late as six years of age, and /z/, /v/, and "zh" may not be fully mastered until eight years of age (Sander, 1972).

Children and adults may experience disorders of articulation for a variety of reasons. Developmental problems are the primary reason for articulation problems in young children. However, both children and adults can suffer from disorders that are either structurally or neurologically caused (Love, 2000).

Structural variation may influence an individual's ability to produce sounds. Cleft lip and/or palate are the most common structural disorders contributing to articulatory disorders. These craniofacial anomalies, if left unrepaired, are likely to influence articulatory function as well. Children born with cleft lip or cleft palate will require early and effective medical, surgical, and behavioral intervention in order to prevent permanent communication disorders and facial deformities. This complex condition requires the work of an effective team. Team members typically include, at a minimum, a surgeon, speech-language pathologist, audiologist, orthodontist, nursing staff, pediatrician, and dentist (Scheuerle et al., 2000).

Two other conditions that affect speech should be mentioned briefly: disorders of voice and fluency. Vocal disorders are often associated with laryngeal problems or may indirectly be related to one's respiration, nasal and sinus health, or vocal usage. Voice disorders may be functional, implying there is no structural or physical basis for the problem and no discernable pathology found. Fluency is a disruption in the rhythm of speech often resulting in repetition of sounds, syllables, or words; secondary manifestations such as facial gestures and postural changes, or avoidance behaviors and struggle. In most instances, stuttering or fluency disorders are considered developmental in nature since they begin in early childhood and without appropriate intervention may persist throughout one's lifetime.

Hearing Disorders

About 28 million people in the United States have some degree of hearing loss, and of these, 80 percent have irreversible hearing loss (www.asha.org). Furthermore, over one million children in the United States have hearing loss and of these, 83 out of every 1000 children have a hearing loss that can interfere with their ability to learn in school (U.S. Public Health Service, 1990). Hearing loss that is acquired early will have a significant and negative impact on a young child's ability to learn to read, write, and produce language. Therefore, early diagnosis and treatment are very important to assure success.

There have been many advances in hearing aids in the past 20 years. Some of the most outstanding changes have been in the development of cochlear implants and digital hearing aids. Despite these changes and dramatic improvements in the quality and amplification of sound, only about 20 percent of all people who could profit from amplification actually get a hearing aid. Successful hearing aid users are those who are motivated to improve their communication by improving their listening and hearing capability. The audiologist will not only make recommendations about whether a hearing aid will benefit the individual with a hearing loss, but also determine which, if any, assistive devices might be helpful.

A cochlear implant is a device that provides direct stimulation to the auditory nerve. This device is sometimes useful when there is damage to the tiny hair cells in the cochlea because with this type of damage, sound may be received by the eardrum and the ossicles (tiny bones in the middle ear) but cannot be sent through the cochlea. In these instances, the cochlear implant may be successful in stimulating the cochlea and going directly to VIII cranial nerve (auditory nerve). The use of this device will not result in a restoration of hearing, but may allow for greater sensation of sound and improved perception. In all areas of hearing loss, it is not enough to fit someone with a hearing aid, assistive listening device, or cochlear implant; training is required to maximize the potential of the device. This process is usually referred to as aural rehabilitation and may be provided by an audiologist or speech-language pathologist. The overall goal of aural rehabilitation is to maximize communication success in everyday situations. Several goals of training may include learning how to listen; learning what to do when the message is not clear; learning how to advocate; learning how to best use the device; and learning skills in using speech reading, facial expression, gestures, and body language to enhance the total communication. Aural rehabilitation is certainly important for the success and continuation of the effective use of all assistive devices.

SUMMARY

The relatively new discipline of communication sciences and disorders is an exciting and challenging frontier. Professions within the discipline offer many opportunities for employment and lifetime careers, working in a variety of environments, and working with a wide range of individuals with communications disorders or differences across the life span. Graduates entering these professions are afforded the opportunity to make a difference in clients' quality of life. Communication is our most human characteristic. Communication is essential to learning, working, playing, and enjoying a full and rich quality of life. Careers in communication sciences and disorders are both challenging and rewarding, and provide flexibility in work environments. The development of this discipline has been so dramatic in the twentieth century that it has proven difficult to predict the amount or directions of growth and development that will occur in this century. There seems no doubt these professions will remain strong, grow, and will continue to need outstanding and dedicated professionals.

REFERENCES

Beebe, S. A., Beebe, S. J., & Redmond, M. V. (1996). *Interpersonal communication relating to others*. Boston: Allyn & Bacon.

Billeaud, F. P. (1998). *Communication disorders in infants and toddlers* (2nd ed.). Boston: Butterworth-Heinemann.

Chapey, R., & Hallowell, B. (2001). Introduction to language intervention strategies in adult aphasia. In R. Chaped (Ed.), *Intervention strategies in aphasia and related neurogenic communication disorders* (4th ed.). Baltimore: Lippincott, Williams, & Wilkins.

Denes, P., & Pinson, E. (1973). *The speech chain: The physics and biology of spoken language*. New York: Anchor Press.

Gillam, R. B., & Bedore, L. M. (2000). Communication across a lifespan. In R. B. Gillam, T. P. Marquart, & F. N. Martin, *Communication sciences and disorders: From science to clinical practice*. San Diego, CA: Singular.

Hedge, M. D. (1994). *A coursebook on aphasia and other neurogenic language disorders*. San Diego, CA: Singular.

Hinckley, J (2007) Problem Solving and Treatment Integrity In A.M. Guilford, S.V. Graham, & J. Scheuerle, *The speech-language pathologist from novice to expert*. Upper Saddle River, NJ: Pearson.

Love, R. J. (2000). *Childhood motor speech disability*. Boston: Allyn & Bacon.

Malone, R. L. (1979). Speech-language pathologist may be a mouthful but . . . *Asha, 20,* 788.

Moeller, D. (1976). *Speech pathology and audiology: Iowa origins of a discipline*. Iowa City, IA: University of Iowa Press.

National Institute on Deafness and other communication disorders. (1995). Research on human communication. Bethesda, MD: Author.

Newby, H. (1958). *Audiology: Principles and practice*. New York: Appleton-Century Crofts.

Owens, R., Metz, D., & Haas, A. (2001). *Introduction to communication disorders: A life span perspective*. Needham Heights, MA: Allyn & Bacon.

Powers, G. (2000). Communication sciences and disorders: The discipline. In R. Gillam, T. Marquardt, & F. Martin (Eds.), *Communication sciences and disorders from science to clinical practice*. San Diego, CA: Singular.

Rosa-Lugo, L., & Champion, T. (2007). The influence of knowledge and experience on responding to cultural diversity in speech-language pathology. In A.M. Guilford, S.V. Graham, & J. Scheuerle, *The speech-language pathologist from novice to expert*. Upper Saddle River, NJ: Pearson.

Sander, E. (1972). When are speech sounds learned? *Journal of Speech and Hearing Disorders, 37*(1), 55–63.

Scheuerle, J., Guilford, A., Habal, M., Abdoney, M., Boothby, R., Frans, N., Ford, C., & Constantine, J. (2000). Cleft palate: Modern technology and neuroscience merge. *The Journal of Craniofacial Surgery, 11*(1), 66–70.

U.S. Public Health Service. (1990). Healthy people 2000. Washington, DC: Government Printing Office.

WEBSITES

American Academy of Neurology–www.aan.com
National Aphasia Association–www.aphasia.org
American Speech-Language-Hearing association
  –www.asha.org

Chapter 4

CASE MANAGEMENT

Robynanne Cash-Howard

Case management is the ongoing process of planning, coordinating, evaluating, and monitoring clients' programs, services, and needs. Case managers utilize professional rehabilitation and mental health knowledge and skills, including networking, relationship building, and leveraging of community resources to ensure that the best interest of the client is met and their rights are respected. Client advocacy is a strong underlying theme of all case management activities. Case management is a practice that has been discussed throughout the human service literature for decades. A variety of definitions of case management have appeared in the literature over time.

The Third Institute on Rehabilitation Services (1965) defined case management as the use of techniques "to control the distribution, quality, quantity and cost of all aspects of case work activities in order to accomplish the program goals or the agency" (p. 12). Thompson, Kite, and Bruyere (1977) further defined case management as "the process of ensuring that clients move sequentially through the appropriate statuses without undue delay" (p. 3). The Commission for Rehabilitation Counselor Certification (2003) has defined case management as "a systematic process merging counseling and man-

agerial concepts and skills through the application of techniques derived from intuitive and researched methods, thereby advancing efficient and effective decision-making for functional control of self, client, setting, and other relevant factors anchoring a proactive practice. In case management, the professional's role is focused on interviewing, counseling, planning rehabilitation programs, coordinating services, interacting with significant others, placing clients and following up with them, monitoring progress, and solving problems" (p. 2). Lastly, The Commission for Case Management Certification (2005) defined case management as "a collaborative process that assesses, plans, implements, coordinates, monitors, and evaluates the options and services required to meet an individual's health needs, using communication and available resources to promote quality, cost-effective outcomes" (p. 2).

These definitions indicate that not only does case management involve the process of coordinating multiple services on behalf of the client, but they also indicate that case management has been practiced for several decades (Hershenson, Power, & Waldo, 1996).

BACKGROUND

The practice of case management is intricately woven within the history of public sector rehabilitation. Its origins can be traced back to the 1940s when it became apparent that the medical model of solely attending to, or "fixing," an injury or disabling condition was insufficient to meet the needs of persons with disability. During the early history of rehabilitation (consult Rubin & Roeseller [2008] and Wright [1980] for a detailed discussion of the history of rehabilitation), the standard practice of service delivery involved "fixing" the injury and sending the individual on his or her way. However, during the 1940s, people who acquired serious injuries or disabilities were more likely to survive due to the era's medical advances and the discovery of antibiotics. Consequently, simply fixing the disabling condition no longer proved to be adequate, and it became evident that a more comprehensive approach to meeting the needs of persons with disabilities was necessary. This notion of a comprehensive approach not only took into consideration the impact of the disability or injury but also began to recognize the psychosocial (social, vocational, leisure, family, etc.) implications as well. Moreover, because of attempts to meet the needs of the whole person, it became clear that a variety of services would need to be provided by multiple agencies. Attaining the necessary services from various agencies required knowledge and skills that the typical client did not possess. Consequently, there was a need for someone to assist persons with disabilities in identifying and accessing the services offered by these agencies. It was out of this need that the position of case manager and the practice of case management began. The Commission for Case Management Certification (2005) is a certifying body for case managers, as healthcare professionals responsible for coordinating the care delivered to an assigned group of patients based on diagnosis or need. This organization also certifies that a case manager is qualified to deal professionally with many aspects of patient/family education, advocacy, delay management, and outcomes monitoring and management as a part of the overall service provision to the client.

Today, case management has evolved into an extremely varied profession, one that incorporates aspects of rehabilitation, nursing, social work, psychology, and business. Its mission, although implemented differently depending upon the work setting, is to assist clients in achieving the highest level of independence possible. Case managers serve a variety of clients, depending on their work setting. Examples include (a) an injured worker who needs help in identifying retraining options due to physical restrictions resulting from an accident or injury; (b) a hospice patient needing coordination of end-of-life medical services; (c) a client with mental health issues who needs assistance with medication management and counseling follow-up; (d) a developmentally delayed couple expecting their first child and needing housing; or (e) a person recently paralyzed who needs appropriate home modifications.

Due to the comprehensive nature of rehabilitation services and the involvement of multiple agencies in meeting the needs of people with disabilities, planning, coordinating, monitoring, and evaluation of these services have become an essential component in the successful rehabilitation of clients. The case manager engages in the planning process via the development of the client's Individual Plan for Employment (IPE) or Treatment Plan. The IPE or Treatment Plan serves as a contract that outlines the goals, objectives, services, service providers, and projected timeframes that will be required in order for the client to achieve a successful outcome. The IPE or Treatment Plan also outlines who is responsible for each of the above activities and further indicates the criteria by which the Plan will be evaluated. Once the Plan has been developed, the case manager begins the process of coordinating, monitoring, and evaluating these services to ensure compliance with the established Plan. Coordination of services is a primary step in implementing the Plan. For example, a Plan may call for adjustment counseling, home modifications, transportation assistance, and weekly physical therapy in order to assist a client reach a successful outcome. The case manager would be required to coordinate or schedule all of these services to best fit the client's needs to ensure compliance with the established Plan. The case manager would then be required to monitor these activities to ensure: (1) appropriateness and compliance; (2) that intended outcomes are being achieved; and (3) whether or not services are being terminated, extended, or changed as needed. In the event that services are not being provided as identified in the Plan, the case manager, along with other relevant staff, would need to revise or amend the Plan. This latter step is known as evaluating and ensures quality and consistency with the Plan for desired outcomes. This process of planning, coordinating, evaluating, and monitoring of client services came to be known as case management.

According to Cassel, Mulkey, and Engen (1997), the goals of case management (as reported by the Case Management Society of America [1995] in *The Standards of Practice for Case Management*) are as follows:

- to ensure that services are generated in a timely and cost-effective manner through early assessment;
- to assist clients to achieve an optimal level of wellness and function by facilitating timely and appropriate health services;
- to assist clients to appropriately self-direct care, self-advocate, and make

decisions to the degree possible;
- to maintain cost effectiveness in the provision of health services;
- to appropriate expenditure of claims dollars and timely claim determinations; and
- to enhance employee productivity, satisfaction, and retention, when applicable.

Since case management has been recognized as an area of practice, the role of the case manager is to help those served. The manner in which this help is provided has changed over time and continues to evolve and vary. A prime example is *The Standards of Practice for Case Managers* as it has been updated in year 2002 and is currently under evaluation for update now (2008) in order to keep up with the ongoing changes with the occupation as practiced in many different settings. However, constants remain (e.g., the ethical principles of autonomy, beneficence, nonmaleficence, justice, veracity, and distributive justice).

Within the broader context of rehabilitation, the evolution of case management theory is somewhat recent, and like the profession of rehabilitation, it too has its roots in the medical model. This model, though not a theory of practice per se, is the foundation from which case management's structure began. Within the medical model, there is an assumption that the case manager knows best how to direct the care of a client and should therefore be the primary decision-maker. However, this assumption is in direct conflict with the need to educate and assist the client in making decisions for him or herself and fails to uphold the ethical principle of autonomy. This process of allowing and encouraging the client to make his or her own decisions also is at the core of client empowerment and self-advocacy. Resolution to this dichotomy is being accomplished through the tenets of higher education in the disciplines encompassed in case management delivery (rehabilitation counseling, nursing, psychology, etc.) and in the enforcement of each professional's code of ethics. The latter has become more important in the recent past as many certifying agents have become watchdogs for their individual disciplines and have taken a more responsible role in ensuring that professional standards are upheld.

ROLES, FUNCTIONS, AND COMPETENCIES

Based on a recent, ad hoc review of job descriptions for the position of case manager from various human service agencies (State of Florida, Department of Children and Families, Mental Health Care, Inc., Genex Services, Inc., Coventry Health Care) the following roles and functions have been identified:

- Review and maintain case files to ensure accurate case recordings/reporting/billing
- Coordinate client services
- Schedule appointment and ensure client compliance
- Arrange transportation
- Monitor medication compliance
- Monitor compliance with treatment plan
- Schedule and attend staffings/treatment team meetings
- Develop Individual Plan for Employment

In addition to the above, Leahy, Shapson, and Wright (1987) identified the following necessary skills of the case manager: (1) referral of clients to appropriate specialists and/or special services; (2) identification of and arranging for functional or skill remediation services for successful job placements; (3) collaboration with other providers so that

services are coordinated, appropriate, and timely; (4) informing clients and other service providers about the organizations; (5) interpreting organizations' policy, laws, and regulations to clients and others; (6) selecting appropriate adjustment alternatives such as counseling centers or educational programs; (7) coordinating activities of all agencies involved in a counseling plan; (8) using functional assessment information in determining counseling services needs; (9) clearly stating the nature of clients' problems for referral to service providers; (10) consulting with medical professionals regarding functional capacities, prognosis, and treatments plans for clients; (11) identifying and challenging stereotypic views toward persons with disabilities; (12) obtaining regular client feedback regarding satisfaction with services delivered and suggestions for improvement; (13) explaining the services and limitations of various community resources to clients; (14) educating clients regarding their rights under federal and state laws; (15) understanding the applications of current legislation affecting the employment of individuals with disabilities; (16) reading professional literature related to business, labor markets, medicine, and rehabilitation; and (17) applying principles of community mental health and career/employment legislation to daily practice.

In order to perform the skills outlined above, the case manager must possess competencies in the following areas: (a) knowledge of the rehabilitation process; (b) knowledge of counseling theories and approaches; (c) knowledge of community resources; (d) knowledge of where to find information about such resources; (e) effective networking skills; (f) knowledge of disability laws (Rehabilitation Act of 1973, ADA); (g) knowledge of various disabilities, prognosis, medication, side-effects; (h) knowledge of assessment and evaluation tools and methods; and (i) have an understanding of the impact of multicultural influences on the client's rehabilitation outcome.

It has also become a necessity for case managers to be able to utilize the latest in online or computer-based technologies. These resources offer a wide variety of information and time saving tools. The need for case managers to be computer savvy has arrived and will become more of a vital component in the case manager's skill toolbox. (A list of web-based resources can be found later in this chapter.)

information
- Ability to work well with other disciplines
- Ability to clearly summarize pertinent clinical information via written correspondence
- Medical records documentation
- Ability to address and prioritize multiple task demands within established timeframes
- Ability to utilize computer technology, available online resources and related software.

PREFERRED QUALIFICATIONS

A further review of recent job descriptions for the position of case managers revealed the following preferred qualifications at entry:

- Master's degree in a human service related discipline. (It is important to note that, although some employers of community-based rehabilitation and mental health agencies are willing to accept a candidate with a bachelor's degree in a human services-related discipline, a master's degree is preferred).
- Ability to assess and record observations.
- Ability to solve practical problems and deal with a variety of concrete variables in situations where only limited standardization exists
- Good organizational and time management skills
- Excellent oral and written communication skills
- Ability to work as a team player
- Exceptional interpersonal skills
- Skills in case management, crisis intervention, conflict management
- Skills in maintaining highly confidential

AREAS OF APPLICATION

Within the context of a case management, the client and the case manager are typically engaged in a one-to-one relationship. The client enters this relationship with a problem and is in need of assistance in order to determine and/or implement a successful solution. The case manager conveys empathy regarding the situation and in so doing enhances the client's feelings of acceptance and being understood. This practice of listening to the client and conveying empathy is consistent with Carl Rogers' client-centered counseling approach. Carl Rogers' notion of client-centered counseling has been employed by case managers because it allows for clients to move toward their innate desire to be realistic and forward moving. The client-centered counseling approach has been found to promote improved client decision-making and to increase client's perception of having more control over their lives. This approach can easily be applied in a variety of situations. The client-centered approach can be, and is, employed within a hospital environment, rehabilitation facility, mental health situation, within the client's home, and even at a job site, with successful outcomes. Assisting the client in making good, solid decisions regarding health care, employment, and/or personal life is the ultimate goal of case management services.

Reality Therapy (RT) is another approach used by case managers when dealing with a client who may be noncompliant with treatment or who fails to follow through on planned activities. The case manager's goal in utilizing an RT approach is to encourage the client to act in a realistic and responsible manner in order to promote positive outcomes. This theory enables the case manager to be verbally active and sometimes confrontational with the client in order to direct his or her attention toward specific behaviors and to increase awareness of how these behaviors may affect immediate outcome. This approach often is used to increase clients' personal responsibility. Oftentimes in the provision of case management services, the case manager recognizes client behaviors that are detrimental to successful outcomes and must employ a variety of communication methods to educate the client and to assist him or her in making more effective choices, thereby increasing the probability of positive outcomes. This theory can be wonderfully helpful in cases where the client needs a more forceful approach in order to understand the detriments of his or her behavior on his or her health, employment status, and/or financial situation.

EMPLOYMENT SETTINGS AND EARNINGS

The position of case manager is found in a plethora of settings. These include, but are not limited to, state and federal vocational rehabilitation agencies; community mental health centers; community rehabilitation facilities; addictions facilities; state, local, and psychiatric hospitals; group homes; correctional facilities; insurance companies, attorney offices; and in other private, for-profit entities.

Within the state and federal VR programs, newly hired vocational rehabilitation counselors are required to have a master's degree in rehabilitation counseling. They must be Certified Rehabilitation Counselors (CRC) or be eligible to sit for the CRC exam within six months of employment. The starting salary within the state VR agency ranges between $28,000 and $31,000. The starting salary within the federal vocational rehabilitation agency ranges between $38,000 and $52,000.

State/Federal Vocational Rehabilitation Agencies

Within the state and federal vocational rehabilitation agencies, case management activities are integrated into the responsibilities of the vocational rehabilitation counselor. In other words, there may not be a separate position for the duties of the case manager. Counselors perform the duties of the case manager under the title of vocational rehabilitation (VR) counselor. However, this has not always been the case. According to Lee Ann Brumble (personal communication, January 16, 2002), the state VR agency began contracting out case management services to private vendors in the mid- to late 1980s. During the same period, a similar process also was occurring within the federal VR system (Ruth Fanning, personal communication, January 16, 2002). The contracting out of case management services within both agencies continues to date, though the federal VR program stopped renewing such contracts in 1999–2000. It is still possible to find private vendors conducting case management services for state and federal agencies under longstanding contracts. The contracting-out for case management services seems to occur in cycles and may become standard practice again in the future.

Community-Based Rehabilitation Facilities

Within community-based mental-health agencies, addictions facilities, rehabilitation facilities (Goodwill Industries, Abilities Inc., etc.), assisted and supervised living facilities, and some correctional facilities, case management activities are conducted by an identified professional case manager. Within these settings, newly hired case managers are typically required to have a bachelor's degree in a human service-related field with several years of experience, or a master's degree in counseling, rehabilitation counseling, or psychology. The starting salary, depending on the size of the agency, ranges between $18,000 and $28,000 per year.

Hospitals, Assisted Living Facilities, and Insurance Companies

Case managers are employed in hospitals, assisted-living facilities, insurance companies, managed care organizations, attorney offices, private nonprofit companies that serve people with disabilities, hospice agencies, and national organizations that serve people with specific disabling conditions (United Cerebral Palsy Association, National Spinal Cord Injury Association, American Diabetes Association, etc.). Within these settings, case management services are conducted in much the same way as previously outlined but with a greater focus toward medical management. Salaries within these settings tend to be somewhat higher than those in community-based rehabilitation facilities, with starting salaries ranging between $38,000 and $50,000. Many of the case management services within these settings are conducted on a contractual basis and require a master's degree along with related certifications.

With regard to typical work setting, the majority of employers who hire case managers house them within an office building with set work hours. However, there are increasing numbers of employment settings where the case manager may be required to work in a field setting. In these instances, the case manager may travel locally or regionally to meet with clients. They set their own work hours dependent on case load needs and may work from home. This flexibility is often a selling point for an employer and has appeal for professionals who desire more autonomy in their employment settings.

Medical Case Management

As the medical community broadens its scope of service and areas of application, so to does the field of case management. Case management has been demonstrated to be an effective tool in ensuring successful transitions from injury and hospitalization to home, work, and/or school settings. Mullahy (1995) indicated that case management is viewed as a valued tool from a business perspective due to cost savings reported by insurance companies, employers, and governmental agencies. Medical case management services can increase the client's ability to: (1) return to work faster; (2) successfully complete educational and/or vocational endeavors in a timely manner; (3) recuperate medically via the identification and implementation of a solid treatment plan; and, (4) apply learned occupational and physical therapy skills at home to increase self-sufficiency (Mullahy, 1995).

Interventions employed through medical case management are aimed at assisting the client to reach a maximized state of independence; not only is the client assisted, but the payor (insurance company, employer, self-insured employee) and the community also benefit. Such benefits include savings recognized by the termination of payments/support no longer needed by the client and the individual's subsequent ability to contribute to the tax base rather than to take indefinitely from tax-sponsored programs.

Opportunities for advancement in the field of medical case management are increasing. Once hired into the industry, the Medical Case Manager will find opportunities for upward mobility into supervisory and managerial positions. According to the Department of Labor, Occupational Employment and Wages (04/03/08), the median salary for those employed in the field ranges from $19,610 to $53,580. The median wage (middle 50%) can expect a salary of $29,630. The bottom 10 percent would earn $19,610 and the top 10 percent would earn $53,580. These figures do not take into account self-employed case managers who typically command a substantially higher wage, which reflects their level of education and specialization within the medical field.

PREPARATION AND CREDENTIALS

Education and experience are paramount in becoming a skilled case manager. One can prepare for this occupation in different ways depending upon the desired work setting. Most case managers have academic training in the following areas: rehabilitation counseling, nursing, social work, counseling or educational psychology, gerontology, or criminal justice.

As previously stated, the work setting will determine the amount and type of academic training required. It is noteworthy to mention that a master's degree in rehabilitation counseling from an accredited CORE (Council on Rehabilitation Education) program or completion of a bachelor's degree in nursing seems to provide the most latitude and opportunities within the for-profit arenas of case management today. In addition to educational attainment, work experience

is crucial to success in the field. Experience can be gained through participating in internships during graduate school, volunteer work, continuing education courses, and on-the-job training, all of which enhance the likelihood of further success in the field. Knowledge acquired postdegree is most often just as important as that acquired during graduate school. Postgraduate training or continuing education affords the case manager the opportunity to keep abreast of new technology, treatments, licensure/certification requirements, computer and internet-based resources, and legislative changes, thereby ensuring continued success in the field.

In order to maximize one's marketability in the field of case management, one of the following certification and licenses is needed: Certified Rehabilitation Counselor, Certified Case Manager, State and/or National Nursing license, and Licensed Social Worker. Some additional credentials that might prove beneficial and can be acquired over time include Licensure as a Marriage and Family Therapist or Mental Health Counselor, certifications as a Vocational Evaluator, Rehabilitation Registered Nurse, Disability Management Specialist, Life Care Planner, Nurse Life Care Planner, and/or Certified Addictions Professional.

PROFESSIONAL ORGANIZATIONS

The following is a list of professional organizations that pertain to case management, depending on one's employment setting. For more information, access the websites for each of these organizations online. This list is not exhaustive but will provide the reader with a beginning for career exploration and for additional information on certification/licensure applicable to the field of case management:

- American Association of Occupational Health Nurses–www.aaohn.org
- American Counseling Association (ACA)–www.counseling.org
- American Nurses Association (ANA)–www.nursingworld.org
- American Rehabilitation Counseling Association (ARCA)–www.arcaweb.org
- Association of Rehabilitation Nurses (ARN)–www.rehabnurse.org
- Commission for Case Manager Certification (CCMC) – www.ccmcertification.org
- Commission on Certification of Work Adjustment and Vocational Evaluation Specialists (CCWAVES)–www.ccwaves.org
- Commission on Rehabilitation Counselor Certification (CRCC)–www.crccertification.org
- International Association of Rehabilitation Professionals (IARP)–www.rehabpro.org
- National Association of Social Workers–www.socialworkers.org
- National Council on Rehabilitation Education (NCRE)–www.rehabeducators.org
- National Rehabilitation Association (NRA)–www.nationalrehab.org
- National Rehabilitation Counseling Association (NRCA)–http://nrca-net.org
- United States Social Security Administration (SSA)–www.ssa.gov

OUTLOOK AND FUTURE TRENDS IN CASE MANAGEMENT

According to Rubin and Roessler (2008), the number of case management positions has increased significantly over the last four decades. Growth projections regarding the broad field of case management have increased exponentially as new service area needs (forensic, life care planning, guardianship, employment discrimination, etc.) and client populations (aging, severely disabled, pediatric, etc.) have been identified. Farr and Ludden (2000) identified the field of case management as one the top growing occupational areas in the nation, and it is growing above the national average rate. The percentage of growth is taken from the three main job titles held by case managers: counselor, social worker, and nurse. The United States Department of Labor, Bureau of Labor Statistics recently reported a 21 percent increase in case managers and related occupations through the year 2016. This is classified as a much faster than the average rate when compared to all occupations.

SUMMARY

The need for case managers and case management services continues to increase as new service needs, and populations are identified. Clients served, service needs and technology may change, but the principle goal of case management remains constant. Case managers will continue to promote the greatest level of independence possible with the client, being always mindful of the ethical considerations needed to ensure the best possible service provision for all involved and to remain vigilant in maintaining and updating skills and education.

REFERENCES

Bureau of Labor Statistics, U.S. Department of Labor. (12/18/07). *Occupational outlook handbook, 2008-09 edition.* Retrieved May 16, 2008 from www.bls.gov.

Case Management Society of America. (1995). Standards of practice for case management. *Journal of Case Management, 1*(3), 7, 9–12, 15–16.

Cassell, J. L., Mulkey, S. W., & Engen, C. (1997). Systematic practice: Case and caseload management (pp. 214–233). In D. R. Maki & T. F. Riggar (Eds.), *Rehabilitation counseling: Profession and practice*. New York: Springer.

Commission for Rehabilitation Counselor Certification (2003). Scope of Practice for Rehabilitation Counseling. Retrieved May 16, 2008 from www.crccertification.com.

Commission for Case Management Certification (2005), Glossary of Terms. Retrieved May 16, 2008 from www.ccmcertification.org.

Farr, J. M., & Ludden, L. L (2003). *Enhanced occupational outlook handbook* (4th ed.). Indianapolis, IN: Jist Works.

Hershenson, D. B., Power, P. W., & Waldo, M. (1996). *Community counseling: Contemporary theory and practice*. Needham Heights, MA: Allyn & Bacon.

Leahy, M. I., Shapson, P. R., & Wright, G. N. (1987). Professional rehabilitation competency research: Project methodology. *Rehabilitation Counseling Bulletin, 31*, 94–106.

Mullahy, C. M. (1995). *The case manager's handbook*. Gaithersburg, MD: Aspen.

Rubin, S. E., & Roessler, R. (2008). *Foundations of the vocational rehabilitation process* (6th ed.). Austin, TX: PRO-ED.

Third Institute on Rehabilitation Services. (1965). *Training guides in caseload management for vocational rehabilitation*. Washington, DC: Vocational Rehabilitation Administration, DHEW.

Thompson, J. K., Kite, J. C., & Bruyere, S. M. (1977). Caseload management: Content and training perspective. Paper presented at the American Personnel and Guidance Association Annual Convention, Dallas.

Wright, G. N. (1980). *Total rehabilitation*. Boston: Little, Brown.

Chapter 5

CLINICAL PSYCHOLOGY

VINCENT E. PARR

Clinical psychology as a profession has two important advantages as a choice for one's lifetime work. First, there are many options, variability, and flexibility in the work that one can choose. A clinical psychologists can function as a professor at a university or community college; a consultant to a hospital, mental health clinic, private industry, local, state, and federal law enforcement agencies; an expert witness in forensic cases for civil and criminal court; an employee of the federal government; or operate a private practice full or part time. In any of these settings, they can engage in research related to their personal areas of interest or those of their employer. They also can be involved in psychological assessment in a number of areas including intelligence, personality, psychopathology, neurological and fitness-for-duty testing. In addition, clinical psychologist can also specialize in biofeedback, neuropsychology, geriatric psychology, sports and/or health psychology. Finally, they can provide community service in a variety of ways, serving on committees or boards of universities, health care organizations, and community agencies.

Clinical psychology offers an advantage as a lifetime endeavor that few other professions can. Gandhi's challenge to the human race was "to turn the spotlight inward." In facing this challenge, clinical psychology is ahead of most in its inherent ability to do just that. One reason for the unhappiness and suffering on this planet is that we, in Western and European societies in particular, typically have the spotlight directed outward. If we can make a certain amount of money, get a particular mate, succeed in our jobs, have a near perfect family, etc.–then we can be happy! Good luck. Clinical psychology can open the door to a level of self-understanding that most people never discover.

HISTORY AND DEVELOPMENT

The word "psychology" was derived from ancient Greek and is composed of two words: *psyche*, which means the soul or mind and *logos* meaning study or knowledge. Literally it means the study or science of the mind. Philip Melanchthon (1497–1560), a collaborator of Martin Luther, coined the word. However, it did not come into general use for more than 100 years. Aristotle has often been called the originator of psychology because he presented the first complete systematic discussion of fundamental psychological issues.

There has been a long and close association between psychology and philosophy. The development of Western philosophy, with which psychology is most associated, began in ancient Greece in 700 B.C. The great syntheses in ancient thought were accomplished by Democritus (460-370 B.C.), Plato (427–347 B.C.), and Aristotle (384–322 B.C.). Later philosophers, from Descartes (1596-1650) through Kant in the eighteenth century, continued to debate the "mind" and "thought" and other psychological principles from a purely philosophical or metaphysical perspective.

Examples of the philosophical exploration of psychological thought had its early roots ancient Greek philosophy. The entire range of psychological inquiry in Greek philosophy included virtually all the fundamental problems addressed in modern psychology: learning, memory, perception, sensation, motivation, emotions, sleep, dreams, temperament, personality, and the mind as it relates to health and sickness. Aristotle, Plato's well-known student, is given credit as the originator of psychology. In his De anima ("On the Soul"), he presented the first complete system of fundamental psychological issues. He believed the human soul to be the highest kind of soul because it has the ability to think. Rene Descartes believed that the subject of psychology was not man but the spiritual mind of man and its contents. John Locke (1632-1704) stated that the human mind was like a "blank slate," and that all ideas come from the senses and through reflection. George Berkeley (1685-1753) believed that the material world is made or generated by the mind and something exists only if it is perceived. David Hume (1711-1776) said that we couldn't know anything at all about universal truths, the nature of things, causes or the self–we can only know what is in our consciousness

and that the only two sources of knowledge are impressions and ideas. All these philosophical ideas, among many others, contributed to the study of the mind and to the development of psychology.

In the nineteenth century, the study of physiology was the single most important factor contributing to the development of a science of psychology. With the establishment of laboratories and utilizing the scientific method to look at psychological issues, psychology separated from philosophy. The two founders of what was considered the new science of psychology were Wilhelm Wundt (1832–1920) in Germany and William James (1842–1910) in the United States. In 1879, Wilhelm Wundt established the first psychological laboratory in Leipzig, Germany. This has been universally accepted as the birth year of psychology, and Wundt became known as the first psychologist. Francis Galton (1822–1911) introduced the use of statistical methods to psychology. This grew mainly out of mathematics and the discovery of the normal curve. Adolphe Quetelet (1796–1874) demonstrated that the normal curve and statistical methods could be applied to biological and social data. Karl Pearson (1857–1936) developed the mathematical procedure for finding the correlation coefficient now called the "Pearson r." The British psychologists Charles E. Spearman (1863–1945), Cyril L. Burt (1883–1971), and Godfrey H. Thomson (1881–1955) developed factor analysis–the most widely used method in psychological research on abilities and personality. Another British statistician, R.A. Fisher (1890–1962), created a statistical procedure called the analysis of variance for use with small sample sizes. American psychology researchers enthusiastically adopted statistics. This began when James McK. Catell (1860–1944), a student of Galton, brought statistics to the United States in 1887 and is considered the foremost figure and originator of psychometrics–the theory and methods of psychological measurement. E.L. Thorndike (1874–1949) also applied these statistical methods to education and educational psychology. Through the use of his methods of measurement and tests further advanced statistics and psychometrics. In 1886, Lightner Witmer (1867–1956) opened the first psychological clinic in Philadelphia and offered clinical services to the city's school children. While the above is but a very brief account of the early history of psychology from which modern clinical psychology developed, persons interested in more of psychology's historical development are encouraged to consult Hothersall (2003) and Schultz and Schultz (2007).

Modern clinical psychology developed between World Wars I and II. During the first quarter of the twentieth century, clinical psychology largely dealt with psychometrics. This was followed closely by the development of clinical tests and measurements and the professional delivery of these services. For example, during World War I the first mass applications of clinical psychology occurred, especially in the use of psychological tests. The success of psychology testing in screening newly recruited soldiers produced a rapid expansion of the use of standardized tests, particularly intelligence test. Between 1920 and 1940, clinical psychology continued to advance and expand beyond its historic emphasis on children and juvenile problems, which was largely educational in nature but was then being utilized in clinics, hospitals, courts, and prisons. In 1931, the Clinical Section of the American Psychological Association (APA) named a special committee to set standards for the training of clinical psychologists. In 1936, the Psychology Department of Columbia University proposed a tentative curriculum for clinical psychology. In the decade between 1930 and 1940, the total number of psychological clinics almost doubled and totaled 150 by 1941 (Goodwin, 2005).

Just as World War I produced a breakthrough for clinical psychology, World War II created a turning point in its history. Some 1,500 clinical psychologists served in the armed forces during World War II. By war's end, Veterans Administration (VA) hospitals needed more services from clinical psychologists—more than 50 percent of the patients in VA hospitals were described as neuropsychiatric patients. During this era, clinical psychologists were being called upon to provide services which previously had been denied to them. In 1946, clinical psychology celebrated its fiftieth anniversary and by mid-century, clinical psychology was in the throes of a struggle for professional respect. The gap between the science of psychology and its clinical practice was considerable. Today, however, this gap has narrowed significantly and clinical psychology as a science and clinical practice is almost universally respected.

PHILOSOPHICAL ASSUMPTIONS

Paul Tillich stated, "No therapeutic theory can be developed without an implicit or explicit image of man" (Thomas, 2000). There are five basic questions that clinical psychologist and all counselors face:

1. *What is the nature of man?* It is important that the psychologist be optimistic in the belief that through education, man can become "himself" in a manner that will bring satisfaction and a sense of accomplishment. This could be the meaning of existence—that man continues to strive to become "himself."
2. *What is the nature of human development?* Is man basically good or bad? Is he a "Tabla Rosa" or blank slate that nature and experience writes on? Freud's

view of human nature was that man is basically "bad." Carl Rodgers believed man to be basically "good." Rousseau believed that man is born "good" (born with a clean slate) and that society corrupts him. Albert Ellis believed that man is born neither good nor bad, but fallible and capable of both good and bad behavior.

3. *What is the nature of the good life?* This has been a problem of the ages. What will determine the "best possible" or "good" form of human nature? One concept is arête, which means excellence in all aspects of human development. Bertrand Russell said, "The good life is one inspired by love and guided by reason" (Russell, 1967).

4. *Who determines what is good?* Parents, teachers, society, culture, and governments all have a say in this. Each may either foster or hinder the true student's search for the good life, or maybe the search itself is the good life.

5. *What is the nature of the universe and man's relationship to it?* Here it is up to each of us individually to formulate our own conception or personal cosmology including psychologist and his/her clients.

MISSION AND OBJECTIVES

The mission and objectives of clinical psychology are ultimately to relieve the suffering of the human condition. The clinical psychologist approaches this challenging task through the gathering of information from research, observation, education, assessment, testing, and treatment. This approach informs the practice of therapy and ultimately leads not only to better mental health for the individual, but also for the family, the community, the nation, and hopefully to a healthier world community.

MAJOR THEORIES

There are scores of texts written on the various theories in psychology and counseling such as Patterson and Wilkins' *Theories of Counseling and Psychotherapy* (1997). What follows is a very brief overview of the major theories. Four theories will be singled out for a brief synopsis: psychoanalysis, behaviorism, humanism, and cognitive behavior therapy.

Psychoanalytic Theory

Sigmund Freud has been one of the most influential theorists in the history of psychology (and in the history of thought). His theories fundamentally changed how people viewed the self, the mind, and the body. Freud's model of the mind was quite revolutionary and the most comprehensive of its time. His model divides the mind into three parts. The first is the conscious mind, the smallest but most accessible component of psyche. The second is the preconscious mind and consists of material that is not readily accessible but is available if the person is relaxed or focused. Objects such as childhood memories exist in the preconscious mind. The most critical for analytic theory is the unconscious mind. This aspect is the largest part of the mind but is not available to the conscious mind. It contains what Freud considered instinctual energy, which fuels the entire system of self. One can experience pieces of the unconscious mind through dreams, neurotic symptoms, and what Freud called parapraxis ("slips of the tongue," written errors or errors in remembering). Freud's notions of the unconscious changed how people viewed others and themselves (Schultz & Schultz, 1987).

Freud also posited what is known as a structural model of personality, positing three highly interactive systems called the id, ego, and superego. The id is the most primitive of the three, containing instinctual energy. It is completely unconscious, and uses primary process through the pleasure principle, a drive for immediate gratification of tension or need. The ego is often called the executive of the personality. It develops to mediate the gratification of the needs of the id, taking into account the environment. It utilizes secondary process, attempting to find a match between the id's image of the object needed to reduce tension and the actual object in the real world. Finally, the superego develops as the person is socialized and internalizes the values, norms, and beliefs of society. The superego is as irrational as the id, striving for perfection as seen by its socialization, operating on the morality principle. It consists of the conscience, from the internal representation of being punished, and of the ego ideal, from the internal representation of being punished. The id and the superego are often seen as being in conflict as their needs are not the same, leaving the ego to attempt to resolve their needs as experienced in the real world. The strength of the ego directly affects its ability to function effectively despite competing demands from the id and superego. If the ego cannot resolve these conflicts, anxiety results (Freud, 1964; Hall, 1954).

Defense mechanisms are created to deal with anxiety. Here we briefly describe some of the most common. Repression, perhaps the most basic defense, is the mechanism by which thoughts or feelings that create anxiety are kept in the unconscious. Denial is the process by which anxiety-creating events in the external environment are blocked from awareness. Projection occurs when a person attributes to others thoughts or feelings that provoke anxiety in the self. Reaction formation is expression of the opposite of anxiety-producing unconscious impulses (e.g., consciously professing fondness for someone whom you despise). Rationalization offers a logical explanation for something although it is really not the case. Displacement substi-

tutes a less anxiety-provoking behavior for an unacceptable unconscious impulse (e.g., kicking the cat rather than hitting your boss). Intellectualization occurs when one avoids anxiety-provoking material by focusing upon the intellectual at the expense of the threatening emotional aspects of the situation. Regression is returning to an earlier stage of development rather than facing conflicts as an adult. Freud considered sublimation the most evolved defense. This mechanism involves changing unacceptable impulses into socially acceptable and productive work, such as transforming sadistic impulses into a career as a successful surgeon (Hall, 1954).

Freud also postulated that all people develop through psychosexual stages. The oral stage, which occurs between birth and 18 months, is characterized by a focus on oral gratification. The anal stage, from 18 months to three years, brings a focus on anal gratification. Toilet training is a major developmental task in this stage. The phallic stage, from three to five years old, shifts focus to the genitals. In the phallic stage, the child experiences the Oedipal conflict, which is characterized in males by the wish to possess mother and get rid of father. However, as the father is too powerful, the child fears that his father may actually take away the child's penis. Freud's postulated an analogous situation for girls at this developmental stage: the Electra complex. However, this aspect of his theory has received little subsequent support and criticism, and has contributed to the impression that Freud believed women are not as fully developed as men. The latency stage begins at the close of the phallic stage and lasts until roughly 12 years. In this period, both sexes find peers of the same gender and renounce sexuality for a time. Finally, the genital stage begins at approximately age 13. Freud characterized this final psychosexual stage as the desire to find mates of the opposite sex and procreate (Freud, 1961; Schultz & Schultz, 1987).

Freud's theories have been widely influential but have also received considerable criticism over time. His basic tenets, however, have become part of our culture. Freud's view of women has proved especially problematic, and this part of his theory has been subject to perhaps the most criticism. Freudian thought has spawned a great number of intellectually descendent psychoanalytic theorists. Indeed, neo-analytic theorists continue to change and expand Freud's original conceptualizations. These approaches, as well as classical psychoanalytic therapy, remain widely influential in current psychotherapy. Psychoanalysis is often identified as the "first force" in psychology, a testament to the foundational influence of Freudian thought (Schultz & Schultz, 1987).

Behavioral Theories

Behaviorism emerged in the 1960s to challenge psychoanalysis as the leading theory in psychology and has been called the "second force" in psychology. Behaviorism rejected the notion of subjective experience, such as free association and the study of dreams as the proper study for psychology, because it did not provide supporting scientific data. The assumptions of psychoanalysis were criticized as they could not be not verified and observed by other investigators. Behaviorists believe the only method for the study psychology should be the observation of behavior, the stimuli preceding the behavior and the reinforcing conditions that control it. This serves as the basis for formulating scientific principles of human and animal behavior. The central theme of behaviorism is the role of learning in human behavior. Behaviorists' initial success came in large part from extensive research done in laboratories. Its usefulness for explaining and treating behavior disorders soon became evident.

The origins of behaviorism were in the work of Russian physiologist Ivan Pavlov

(1849–1936). Its elaboration and refinement are largely due to three American psychologists: E.L. Thorndike (1874–1949), J.B. Watson (1878–1958) and B.F. Skinner (1904–1990) (Hothersall, 2003).

A central theme of behaviorism is that most human behavior is learned. Behaviorists focus on how learning takes place and emphasize the effects of stimuli from the environment on response patterns, i.e., how they are acquired, modified, or eliminated in both adaptive and maladaptive behavior. Moreover, the terminology of behaviorism separates it from other theories (Skinner, 1969). Several key ones follow:

1. *Classical conditioning* is best represented by Pavlov's famous experiment of the dog salivating to food. The food is the unconditioned stimulus and the salivation is the unconditioned response. Through conditioning the same response can be elicited by a wide range of other stimuli, e.g., the ringing of a bell. This form of conditioning is called respondent or classical conditioning.
2. *Operant conditioning* explains how an organism "operates" on the environment, i.e., or what it has to do to obtain a goal that is rewarding or avoid something that is aversive. In operant conditioning the response precedes the stimulus as when a person pulls the lever on a slot machine and gets a reward.
3. *Reinforcement* is the strengthening of a new response by repeated association with some unconditioned stimulus. Such a stimulus is called a reinforcer and can be either positive or negative. In Pavlov's dog, the reinforcer was the bell in association with the presentation of food. In operant conditioning, the response is strengthened because it is repeatedly associated with a reward. In the beginning, a high rate of rein-

forcement may be necessary to elicit a response, but far fewer rates are needed to maintain it. When reinforcement is consistently withheld, the behavior is eventually extinguished or ceases to occur.

4. *Generalization* occurs when a response which has been conditioned to one stimulus becomes associated with another stimulus. For example, Pavlov's dog originally became conditioned to the sound of the footsteps of his trainer when he was to be fed. Later this sound generalized to the sound of a bell. Generalization allows us to learn from the past by sizing up new situations; however, there is also the possibility of making inappropriate generalizations as when a child of wealthy parents learns to disregard others as unworthy.

5. *Discrimination* is a complementary process to generalization and occurs when an organism learns to distinguish between similar stimuli and to respond differently to them. For example, an individual can learn (be conditioned) to respond to middle C being played on a piano and not the key next to it.

6. *Modeling* involves the imitation of a desired response patterns as exhibited by parents, teachers, peers, etc. The individual is rewarded for the new behavior and it can be learned rapidly. Parents are important models in a child's early development; however, children may also imitate destructive and disturbed behavior of others.

7. *Shaping* is the process of reinforcing successive approximations of a desired behavior. This is often necessary, for example, when a child does not have the behavior desired in their repertoire. In the process of shaping, the behavior not desired is not reinforced and therefore is extinguished and the desired behavior is reinforced in increments and ultimately achieved.

8. *Learned drives* are acquired by a pairing something with a limited number of primary biological drives such as hunger, thirst, the elimination of waste, etc. When primary drives are associated with something like parental approval, an infant learns that parental approval, a secondary drive, leads to the gratification of bodily needs and thus learns to seek their parents' approval.

9. *Cognitive Mediation* involves "self-statements" that occur between the stimulus and response. Behavioral researchers found that this internal dialogue would often determine the response. (This we will be discussed in more detail in the section on rational emotive behavior therapy.)

Humanistic Therapy

Carl Rogers (1902-1987) is the best-known figure in the "third force" of psychology. Humanistic approaches emerged in reaction to psychoanalytic theory and behaviorism, which had given personal growth little attention and downplayed the role of free will in human behavior. Humanism as a theoretical orientation affirms the innate potential for positive growth in human beings (Rogers, 1961). Rogers and most humanistic psychologists believe that human beings develop in positive, healthy ways in the absence of environmental opposition. The goal of self-actualization is the promotion and perpetuation of a healthy self, characterized by greater autonomy and self-sufficiency. This innate drive toward self-actualization promotes wholeness, congruence, and integration. Rogers assumed that self-actualization was a natural and normal tendency to create fully functioning people open to new experiences filled with meaning, challenge, and personal excitement (Rogers, 1961).

Unconditional positive regard by others who are important to us is a key component of self-actualization. Unconditional positive regard is acceptance of a person without placing contingencies on his or her behaviors. Conditional positive regard is more coercive, because behavioral conditions are placed on a person's worth. That is, the person receives positive regard only if certain preconditions, or contingencies, are met. These problematic contingencies might include expectations regarding intelligence, physical appearance, or "perfection." After years of experiencing conditional worth, a person may apply internalized conditions to one's self. Self-acceptance is then possible only if one satisfies all the conditions of behavior that others have communicated as necessary for worthiness. Attempts to comply with these conditions create unhappiness, self-doubt, and difficulties in living (Rogers, 1951).

Rogers viewed psychotherapy as an effort to assist others in self-actualization. Therapeutic interventions are grounded in the notion that no person is inherently bad or incapable and that free will is a positive force for growth. Humanistic approaches emphasize difficulties encountered in normal living and hold that resolution of these problems is rooted in each person's innate capacity for personal growth. Therefore, the therapist's task is to provide an environment of genuineness, empathy, and unconditional positive regard for the client. This therapeutic environment provides a context for the client to discover solutions to present difficulties and their potential for positive future growth (Rogers, 1961; Schultz & Schultz, 1987).

Cognitive-Behavioral Therapy

The cognitive behavioral movement is the "fourth force" in psychology. The grandfather of cognitive behavioral therapies was Albert Ellis (1913–2007). Originally called Rational Therapy (RT) and then Rational-Emotive Therapy (RET), later Ellis emphasized that the system he developed was always rational, emotive and behavioral. Fittingly, he changed the name to Rational Emotive Behavior Therapy (REBT). REBT's main function is to change a person's irrational thought processes through reason, logic, and active disputing so that he or she can lead a more productive and happy life.

Basic principles of REBT emphasize that (1) *we are all fallible human beings (FHB)*, and (2) *the ABCDE's of rational living*. In this latter context:

A is the action, the activating event, or the adversity;

B is the belief, the self-statements, or the thoughts that a person is telling themselves about the event. At this point an individual can have either a rational and/or irrational belief about events that happened to them;

C is the emotional consequences, of the belief e.g., frustration and/or anger;

D is disputing irrational beliefs occurring at (B) that a person tells themselves about the event (A). The desired result is that a person will be left with a rational (or healthy) belief. If a person learns to effectively dispute and does so vigorously, they eventually achieve rational beliefs; and,

E represents an effective, efficient, and eloquent philosophy of life. For example, a person has a have a flat tire (A), and immediately he or she may have two feelings: frustration and anger (C). Most people report that about 99 percent of the time the flat tire made them angry. Ellis argued that a tire can not "cause" a human emotion, and if it did then everyone would have to be angry when they had a flat tire. The flat tire and anger are correlated, meaning they happen close in time, but the tire does not cause the anger.

Ellis described three insights and skills necessary to achieve emotional peace and without them, peace of mind is practically impossible: (a) you create and maintain 100 percent of your thoughts, feelings, and behavior; (b) you understand how you create your feelings; and (c) you know how to get rid of these feelings rapidly.

The ultimate goal in REBT is to give up all ratings of personal worth and "only" rate the behavior. Based on the tenet that a person can change his or her behavior, in REBT, the client learns to dispute his or her basic irrational beliefs until he/she no longer believes them. What remain are the rational beliefs. For example, it is appropriate not to like having a flat tire and thus to feel frustrated (still caused by us), but then we have a magical belief, that it shouldn't happen to us! Why should you be spared having flats when the rest of us are not (disputing)? Ellis believed that a well-functioning individual was one who thought and behaved rationally and was in tune with the outside world. Most importantly, the REBT therapist strives to assist clients in replacing "rating" with "acceptance" and teaches "unconditional" self, other and World acceptance–as it is –not as we want it to be. While this above section focused on REBT (Ellis, 1996), persons interested in other forms of cognitive behavior therapy and an extensive list of resources and related links are encouraged to consult Marshall (1997) and: www.nacbt.org.

CLIENTS TYPICALLY SERVED

Clinical psychologists serve clients from many walks of life. Clients vary depending on the setting in which the psychologist practices. For example, they may see anyone from small children to elder adults. Moreover, they may work in elementary and secondary schools, colleges, and universities. When employed in hospitals, they typically see patients with more serious mental disorders, such as schizophrenia. As consultants their clients may be police officers, city managers, spouses, family members, workers, and owners of companies, etc. In clinics, they may work with persons who are alcohol and/or drug dependent, anorexic, or bulimic. Some psychologists in clinics administer biofeedback and neurofeedback testing with a variety of different patients. In private practice, they may see any and/or all of these types of clients who effectively work and live in the community.

WORK SETTINGS

Work settings for clinical psychologists vary widely, depending upon the interest and training of the professional. Some clinicians work in hospital or clinic settings where the focus is usually on assessment or psychotherapy. Neuropsychology is an area of specialization increasingly in demand, often linking clinical psychologist with neurology departments in medical schools or hospitals. As discussed earlier, VA hospitals have long-standing psychology departments that became common practice settings after World War II. Clinical psychologists are also frequently found in traditional college and university psychology departments. They serve as teaching faculty for undergraduate and graduate students, conduct research in their areas of expertise, and provide community service and work in counseling clinics that serve students in need. Many psychologists turn to administration, utilizing their skills in the management people and services. Finally, most clinical psychologists work independently in private practice settings. They function as autonomous practitioners of mental health services, providing psychological assessments and psychotherapy to children, adolescents, adults, couples, and families within the ethical guidelines of the profession.

HOW SERVICES ARE UTILIZED

Clients

Clients are primary mental health consumers. They are usually referred by other professionals or nonprofessionals or may come independently to seek services. Clients are typically seen for individual, couple, or family treatment.

Agencies and Businesses

Agencies hire clinical psychologists to act as service providers, doing assessments, psychotherapy, or organizational consultations. In addition, as previously noted, clinical psychologists may serve in administrative positions.

Colleges and Universities

Colleges and universities most often hire clinical psychologists as faculty members but also hire them as direct service providers to students. In educational settings, psychologists often occupy hybrid positions combining teaching, research, and clinical service.

Other

Health organizations such as hospitals and clinics frequently utilize clinical psychologists as service providers, supervisors of other mental health providers, and administrators. Forensic psychologists working in the legal system, provide evaluation and expert testimony in the courts.

PREPARATION AND DEVELOPMENT TO WORK IN FIELD

Clinical psychology initially adopted the scientist-practitioner model, first articulated at a conference in Boulder, Colorado (1949). The model holds that clinical psychologists will be trained first as scientists (in a university psychology department), where their work as clinicians is predicated on this scientific base. The degree (Ph.D.) and a clinical internship are required components of the training experience. Psychologists thus should be competent in research, diagnosis, and psychotherapy.

A 1973 conference in Vail, Colorado expanded this model, recognizing other modes of training in which greater focus is given to preparation of practitioners. This training philosophy, sometimes termed the practitioner-scholar model, requires that psychologists develop research knowledge relevant to clinical practice. However, this approach emphasizes preparation of practitioners who apply research, not scientists who do research. This approach has been termed the practitioner-scholar model. This training philosophy forms the basis for Doctor of Psychology (Psy.D.) programs. Both types of programs coexist at present, and the number of Psy.D. programs has increased dramatically in recent years.

To become a clinical psychologist, one must complete an undergraduate degree in psychology or an allied field. This is usually a B.S. or B.A. degree, depending on which department psychology is in at the individual's university. The average is four years of study at the university to be eligible for the degree. Then the individual will be required to apply to a university for the M.S. or M.A. degree (master of science or master of arts). This graduate degree can be obtained at the same university or a different one. The M.S. typically requires a master's thesis as a requirement for the degree. A student who stops after the master's degree can work in a clinical setting often doing testing under the supervision of a licensed clinical psychologist.

After the master's degree, which will take on average one to two years, one must apply for the doctorate degree. This is usually a Ph.D. (Doctor of Philosophy) or a Psy.D. (Doctor of Psychology) degree. The Ph.D. requires a wide knowledge of not only psychology in general, but also, philosophy, physiology, learning theories, history of psychology, experimental design, statistics, developmental psychology, social psychology, and clinical psychology. The Ph.D. also requires the successful completion of a comprehensive doctoral exam and the independent production of an original research contribution to the field (a dissertation). The Psy.D. is most often based in schools of professional psychology and requires classroom, research, and clinical experience. Some universities do not like a student to get three degrees from the same university and may require that one obtain the masters or doctorate from a different school. Many others, nonetheless, require a commitment from a prospective student with a bachelor's degree to begin with the masters degree and stay on until the completion of the doctoral degree.

Doctoral students are required to successfully complete a one-year clinical internship before they graduate. After receiving their doctoral degree, one or two years of supervised clinical experience is then required. Once completed, an individual can sit for the state licensure examination. After these requirements are successfully completed and if they pass the examination, the person then can call themselves a "clinical psychologist."

It is important for interested students to apply for doctoral programs and internships that have been approved by the American Psychological Association (APA). (A list of APA approved doctoral programs can be obtained at APA's website: www.apa.org.) Many state licensing boards require that both doctoral coursework and internships be from universities, hospitals, or other settings that have been accredited by the APA.

PROFESSIONAL ORGANIZATIONS

For clinical psychologist, the primary professional organization is the American Psychological Association (APA). Division 12 of the APA is dedicated specifically to clinical psychology. It is also important for the clinical psychologist to belong to the state psychological association in the state in which they practice. In addition, there are many postdoctorate degrees which may require special training for membership. Clinical psychologist may also be members of other professional organizations such as the American Association for the Advancement of Science (AAAS), the American Humanist Association (AHA), the Center for Inquiry (CFi), or the New York Academy of Science (NYAS). Membership in other organization will depend on the professional interest of the individual psychologist. It may also be important to join regional psychological organizations; this information can be located at the National Register of

Health Service Providers in Psychology or the American Board of Professional Psychology (ABPP) (www.abpp.org).

CAREER OPPORTUNITIES AND SALARY

The clinical psychologist has many career options from which to choose. The setting in which they work will be a factor in salary. Also, the beginning salary for clinical psychologist providing direct service to clients ranges considerably depending on geographic location. Beginning salaries range from $55,000 in hospitals and elementary and secondary schools to $80,000 for those employed by the federal government. The median beginning salary for clinical psychologist in 2007 was $70,000. Clinical psychologists in private practice can often make considerably more ranging from $100,000 to over $300,000 depending on areas of specialization and demographics. However, this may take some time to achieve because of competition in the marketplace and managed care. (For additional salary information, consult: http://www.payscale.com/research/US/Job=Clinical Psychologist? Salary.)

FUTURE OUTLOOK

The future of clinical psychology looks bright. It is universally respected as a profession and it offers a great deal of freedom and variability in work settings. Data from the 2008 U.S. Department of Labor, *Occupational Handbook* indicates that the employment of clinical psychologists is expected to grow as fast as the average for all occupations through 2010. Employment in healthcare will grow the fastest in outpatient mental health and substance abuse treatment clinics. Many job opportunities will be found in schools, public and private social services agencies, and in management consulting services. Business and industry will use psychologists' expertise in survey design, analysis and research to provide marketing evaluation, and statistical analysis. The increased utilization of employee assistance programs (EAPs), which offer employees help with personal problems, should also provide opportunities for employment. Employment for psychologists holding doctorates from leading universities in areas with an emphasis, such as counseling, health, and educational psychology, should also be good. Psychologists with extensive training in quantitative research methods and computer science may find they have a competitive edge over applicants without this background.

Graduates with a master's degree in psychology may qualify for positions in school and industrial-organizational psychology. Others may find jobs as psychological assistants or counselors providing mental health services under the direct supervision of a licensed psychologist. Still others may find jobs doing research, data collection, and analysis at universities, government agencies, or private companies.

Fewer opportunities directly related to psychology will exist for bachelor's level degree holders. Many find employment in such jobs as assistants in rehabilitation centers and halfway houses, etc., or in jobs involving data collection and analysis. Those who meet a state's certification requirements may become high school psychology teachers. A bachelor's degree in psychology, moreover, also provides an excellent foundation for graduate training in other human service fields, many of which are featured in this book.

SUMMARY

Clinical psychology is one of the most rewarding professions persons can choose for their lifetime's work. There are so many varied and exciting opportunities that are available to a professional psychologist. There are few professions that are as rewarding financially and personally as can be found in clinical psychology. Through the observation, research, and study of human behavior, the clinical psychologist learns about him or herself and the ones they love. Further, few professions can offer the peace of mind knowing that one is involved in an effort to relieve the suffering of others. In the end, we all turn the spotlight inward and we have the fortunate opportunity to experience inner peace.

REFERENCES

American Psychological Association (1992). Ethical principles of psychologists and code of conduct. *American Psychologist, 47*, 1597–1611.

Ellis, A. (1996). *Better, deeper, and more enduring brief psychotherapy: The rational emotive behavior therapy approach.* New York: Brunner/Mazel, Inc.

Freud, S. (1961). *The ego and the id and other works.* (Standard Edition, vol. A9). London: Hogarth.

Freud, S. (1964). *New introductory lectures on psycho analysis* (standard edition, vol. 22). London: Hogarth.

Goodwin, C. J. (2005). *A history of modern psychology* (2nd ed.). Hoboken, NJ: John Wiley & Sons.

Hall, C. S. (1954). *A primer of Freudian psychology.* New York: Mentor.

Hothersall, D. (2003). *History of psychology* (4th ed.). New York: McGraw-Hill

Marshall, S. (1997). *Cognitive behavior therapy: An introduction to theory and practice.* Philadelphia: W.B Saunders.

Patterson, C.H., & Watkins, C.E. (1997). *Theories of counseling and psychotherapy* (5th ed.). New York: Harper & Row.

Rogers, C. R. (1951). *Client centered therapy.* Boston: Houghton Mifflin.

Rogers, C. (1961). *On becoming a person: A therapist's view of psychotherapy.* Boston: Houghton Mifflin.

Russell, B. (1967). *Autobiography* (vol. 1). New York: George Allen and Unwin.

Schultz, D.P., & Schultz, S.E. (1987). *A history of modern psychology.* New York: Harcourt Brace Jovanovich.

Skinner, B.F. (1969). *Contingencies of reinforcement: A theoretical analysis.* New York: Appleton-Century-Crofts.

Thomas, J.H. (2000). *Tillich.* New York: Continuum International Publishing Group.

WEBSITES

American Board of Professional Psychology www.abpp.org

American Psychological Association www.apa.org

National Association of Cognitive-Behavioral Therapy (CBT) www.nacbt.org

Salary Survey Report for the United States http://www.payscale.com/research/US/Country=United_States/Salary

Chapter 6

COLLEGE STUDENT DEVELOPMENT AS A PROFESSIONAL CAREER

Mary Finn Maples & Peggy A. Dupey

Since its inception, college student development (CSD) has evolved to meet the needs of students in increasingly diverse higher educational environments. The profession's growing utility and visibility on campuses throughout the United States can be attributed to the CSD profession's expansion to include all aspects of counseling, addressing the vocational, personal, and developmental needs of students. This broader role requires professionals who possess an understanding and commitment to the more complex environments in which students learn and live (Stone & Archer, 1990). Those who choose a career in CSD can be assured of working with individuals who have intentionally and willingly placed themselves in a college or university environment, almost guaranteed to promote developmental change (Astin, 1993).

Student development work in higher education has been defined as "the application of knowledge and principles derived from the social and behavioral sciences, particularly from psychology (educational and counseling) and sociology as well as business administration" (Maples, 1996, p. 6). Student development professionals can be found in virtually all postsecondary educational environments and in almost every office utilized by students, ranging from admissions and orientation to financial aid, from residence life to counseling and testing. Student development professionals have a dizzying range of titles, from Vice Presidents for Student Development or Student Services to Advisers in Residential Life, Judicial Affairs, and Academic Planning. Regardless of their area of expertise, CSD professionals share a common goal of assisting students as the students seek meaning, establish and achieve goals, and clarify values.

The CSD profession is multifaceted, recognizing and appreciating the rich diversity of students, as well their intrinsic ability to attain goals, despite hardships and obstacles. In addition, the profession of CSD supports, complements, and supplements the pursuit of knowledge by students in higher education. It is a comprehensive, integrated, and interdependent network of programs and services designed to facilitate the progress of students in their pursuit of higher education (Maples, 1996).

HISTORY AND DEVELOPMENT

The first recorded college student development specialist was the *Dean of Student Relations* appointed by Harvard University in 1870 (Rudolph, 1965). Prior to this formal title and function, however, a patriarchal or "in loco parentis" (i.e., serving in place of the parent) was the prevalent model of student development (Fitzpatrick, 1968). Fitzpatrick (1968) stated, "If the early college was alma mater to her students, clearly the president was "pater familiaris" (p. 5). Faculty served the dual roles of professor and parent, which in the twenty-first century may prompt ethical questions of dual relationships and conflicts of interest.

Beginning in the early to mid-twentieth century, American higher education was challenged by considerable change, including the introduction of elective subjects beyond the prescribed curriculum, pluralism in higher education, coeducation, increase in knowledge and application of individual differences, and increasing cultural diversity and socioeconomic backgrounds among students. The changing educational landscape necessitated the formalization of student development beyond the classroom.

Perhaps the most prominent pioneer in the field of CSD was Esther Lloyd-Jones. Dr. Lloyd-Jones earned the first doctorate in Student Personnel Administration in Higher Education from Columbia University in 1929 and wrote the seminal work on the profession, *A Student Personnel Program for Higher Education* in 1938. While many noted authors and practitioners have contributed significantly to the profession since 1938, "none have provided definition and leadership to the field as much as Lloyd-Jones" (Meadows, 2001).

The University of Minnesota, Indiana University, and Columbia University were among the most prominent institutions in the development of the CSD movement. Not coincidentally, the profession has been closely aligned and has somewhat paralleled the profession of counseling and counselor education. These institutions most noted for CSD also produced many leaders in counselor education and counseling psychology. Prominent leaders in all three professions include C. Gilbert Wrenn (who was contributing continuously and notably to higher education until his recent death, at the age of 99, in December, 2001); E. G. Williamson, Ralph Berdie, Charles Warnath, Donald Super, and Arthur Chickering (Dean & Meadows, 1995). Most recently, the technological expansion of the late twentieth and early twenty-first centuries has created expanded communication tools and increased career opportunities, extending the role of college student development and its component services exponentially.

MISSION AND OBJECTIVES OF COLLEGE STUDENT DEVELOPMENT

While there are abundant models and theories of student development, the mission of the profession is largely consensual: "Student Development reflects theories of human growth and environmental influences as applied to in-class and out-of-class personal learning opportunities" (Center for Advising and Student Advancement [CASA], 2008).

If college student development is indeed a "network of programs and services designed to facilitate the progress of students in their pursuit of higher education" (Maples, 1998), practitioners who find their work positive and gratifying provide the best possible support for students. Many aspiring student development professionals gain awareness of the profession from student development role models while they are students. Encouragement by people already in the field often results in young people choosing the college student development profession. According to Hunter (1992), students "look to those already engaged in student affairs work and watch for signs, both subtle and overt, that tell them whether to join the ranks" (p.185). Additionally, many discover the profession through experiences they described as "accident, odd fate, magical, fallen into, thunderbolt, stumbled upon and destined" (Hunter, 1992, p. 183).

PREDOMINATE PROFILES OF CLIENTS SERVED BY COLLEGE COUNSELORS

College students today are as diverse as the backgrounds from which they come to our campuses. In 1971, 90.9 percent of first-time, full-time freshmen were white, while the percentage of white freshmen decreased to 76.5 percent in 2006. Since 1971, students of color have become an essential population on American campuses (Higher Education Research Institute [HERI], 2007). Despite becoming culturally and ethnically more diverse, the majority of today's college students come from middle to upper income families, a trend that is cause for concern among advocates for equal access to postsecondary educational opportunities regardless of socioeconomic status. Females now outnumber males on college campuses throughout the U.S., making up 57 percent of new freshmen in 2006 (HERI, 2007).

According to the National Center for Education Statistics (2008), college enrollment is expected to continue setting new records through 2016. Enrollment is projected to increase by 14 percent between 2007 and 2016. Full-time students outnumber part-time students; between 1995 and 2005 the number of full-time students increased

by 33 percent compared to a 9 percent increase in part-time students (HERI, 2007).

Other trends among college students include increased interest in community service, the desire to earn high incomes, a more polarized political orientation than their predecessors, and a decreased likelihood to identify with a particular religious orientation.

PHILOSOPHICAL ASSUMPTIONS AND PRE-EMINENT THEORIES

Models adopted and created within the CSD profession are integrative, requiring equality, collaboration, and understanding among all components and participants in students' experiences. CSD professionals, along with faculty, staff and administrators, are all essential in supporting students as they seek meaning through their personal, academic, and professional experiences.

The concurrent development of the field of psychology, led by such theorists as Carl Rogers and B.F. Skinner, influenced the student development profession (CASA, 2008). Based on the social sciences and counseling, the psychological paradigm has become a foundational element of the profession.

Because CSD remains a relatively young profession, theoretical bases are still being developed, tested, and implemented. However, as with most theories and models, each new one tends to build on the strengths of its preceding theories. For example, the Maples' Holistic Adult Development Model (1996) is an expansion of Chickering's Vectors of Adult Development (Chickering, 1969; Chickering & Reisser, 1993). Arthur Chickering researched and formulated a series of directional states by studying traditional-aged college students at a nontraditional college in the late 1960s. A quarter century later, Chickering and Reisser revisited the Vectors, having expanded the research population to include some culturally diverse students, as well as some students beyond the traditional college ages of 18–25 (Chickering & Reisser, 1993).

The essence of Chickering's theory is based on Seven Vectors: (1) Developing Competence; (2) Managing Emotions; (3) Moving through Autonomy Toward Interdependence; (4) Developing Mature Interpersonal Relationships; (5) Establishing Identity; (6) Developing Purpose; and (7) Developing Integrity. Although not proposed to be in rigid sequence, the vectors tend to build upon earlier experiences. Advocates of Chickering's theory maintain its sound rationale and applicability to students of all ages and can be a solid tool in helping them understand themselves by describing the vector(s) relevant to their experiences.

Chickering's vectors can serve as a framework through which adults view their development. While Chickering himself adheres to the theory as "Vectors of Adult Development," some consider his theory as one of "identity development" (Von Steen, 2001, p. 123).

The global, developmental nature of Chickering's theory allows its application to more than one generation of adults. While some models are limited to specific stage-orientation (Perry, 1981) or problem-orientation (Chandler & Gallagher, 1996), Chickering's model is applicable to all adults, not simply those in higher education.

Maples' Holistic Adult Development Model (1996), in Figure 6–1, builds upon Chickering's theory, by including more specific aspects of adult development.

The Holistic Adult Development Model (1996) assumes the spirit (personhood) as the focus of adult development and includes the developmental aspects of religious/aesthetic, career, intellectual, physical, emotional, and social. Maples has applied the Holistic Adult Development Model since its earliest unpublished years to judicial education participants in numerous workshops sponsored by the National College of Juvenile and Family Law, as well as the her coursework in College Student Development and in Law and Ethics.

Expanding beyond Chickering's global theory are several more specialized developmental approaches including *ethnic identity* (Cross, 1995; Helms, 1993; Phinney, 1989),

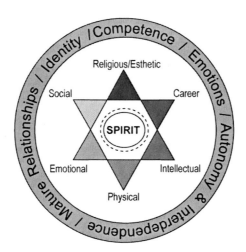

Figure 6-1. Holistic Adult Development by Mary Maples, Ph.D.

homosexual identity (Cass, 1979, 1984; D'Augelli, 1994), and *women's development* (Belenky, Clinchy, Goldberger & Tarule, 1986). While the benefits of specified models may be helpful in working with students, it is essential for both practitioners and students to examine theories and models to determine the validity of the research supporting them. Questions asked should include: (1) what were the numbers of human subjects involved in the studies? and (2) what were the demographic elements? By seeking and conducting valid and efficacious research, college student development professionals and students can contribute to the growing literature in this dynamic profession.

APPLICATION IN THE REAL WORLD

In 2008, Maples and Han examined the emerging technological advances of student development and college counseling. In their article, published in the "flagship journal" of the American Counseling Association, *The Journal of Counseling & Development*, they suggest that South Korea appears to be more advanced than the United States in providing counseling via the Internet (McGowan, 2008). The second author of this chapter has been conducting *cyber-counseling* since 1996 in Korea, and to Korean college students via the Internet from the United States, since 2002.

Another sign of the growing popularity of distance counseling is Ready Minds, Inc. (2006), an organization recognized by the National Board of Certified Counselors that has been training professionals to become Distance Certified Counselors (DCCs) since 2002. For college students who are off-campus during breaks, the longest during the summer months, this is an invaluable service. Students are in instant communication with their mentors, advisors, counselors, and other helpers.

Further driving an appreciation of real world applications of College Student Development is the dramatic increase in culturally diverse college students in the United States. The most prominent representation appears to be Latino(a) students from Puerto Rico, Cuba, Caribbean nations and Central and South America, as well as Mexico, with Latina women now being seen as the "Latino Majority in College" (Torres, 2004). Because advanced graduate preparation in College Student Development is still in a stage of relative infancy (Meadows, 2001), many educational programs are expanding to meet the need for training.

Prior to the end of World War II, there were few scientific studies of applications of student development to the real world. Even today, many College Student Development training programs include the works of pioneers like Esther Lloyd-Jones, who calls *her* predecessor "pioneers"—Frank Parsons(e.g., in 1907) and Clifford Beers "certain great personalities" (Meadows, 2000, p.17). While certainly meritorious in their time, too many College Student Development training programs continue to rely on the contributions of these early pioneers in an attempt to meet the needs of current Student Development graduate students, and, ultimately, new generations of college students, without attending to the well-researched contributions of later, more current authors.

Consider, for example, the fact that television, email, fax machines, iPods, voice mail (in some cases, even telephones), computers, chat rooms, You Tube, and dozens more technological communication devices did not exist in those earlier days. Yet, educators continue to rely on them to help graduate students to understand and work with *contemporary* students, often referred to in the majority as Millennials (Howe & Strauss, (2003). Traditional College Student Development professors are relying on the outdated and outmoded theories of the past to attend to the increasing technological needs of the Millennials. As graduate students are acknowledging, because they attend the workshops and conferences sponsored by contemporary training organizations (Ready Minds, Inc., for example), professors need to "get with the program." It is anticipated that the new generation of professors in the field will have training and access to both the technological advances ("smart classrooms") that will help to advance their graduate students into meeting the needs of those whom they serve as well as training to understand the developmental characteristics of this new generation of both graduate students and the diversity of college students whom they serve.

SALARY INDICES

Compensation and specific salary ranges are not feasible due to the considerable number of specialties within the profession. The College Student Personnel Workers Fact Sheet (2008) includes such titles as "vice presidents of student life, deans of students, directors of student life, counselors, residential life, intramurals, admissions, international student services, health and counseling services, career services, financial aid, academic advisors, recruitment and retention advisors" (p. 1).

In 2007, the Economic Research Institute Survey of Salaries estimated the following salary ranges for the "typical College Student Development Specialist," which includes, but is not limited to all of the above positions to be with a master's degree nationally:

Starting Salary	$38,500– 42,500
Average	$65,000–72,000
Salary with Experience	$95,000- 120,000

The national average for all College Student Personnel workers was $73,000 in these categories.

The U.S. Bureau of Labor Statistics (2007) estimated that the average salary of College Student Personnel Workers was $66,500. The USBLS also indicated that "benefits are usually very good for college student personnel workers, who may get 4–5 weeks of vacation per year with very generous health and pension programs" (p. 3).

Perhaps the most comprehensive study regarding compensation for College Student Development/Counseling personnel was conducted by the National Association of Student Personnel Administrators (NASPA) in 2006. As stated earlier, there are a multitude of student development positions and the NASPA study highlights only the senior (vice presidents, deans, associates, and directors of various services). Of the 50+ positions compared between 2002 and 2005, 10 were compensated at a figure in excess of $100,000 in 2005 compared with only one in 2002. The lowest average salary in 2005 was for Director of Student Employment ($43,892)–the same position being compensated in 2002 at $46,703, a loss of 6 percent in three years. Only six of the positions compared over the three-year period noted a loss. All others had significant gains, with the highest percentage of gain for the assistant to the SSAO (Senior Student Affairs Officer) with a 52 percent gain. There was no description or explanation as to the cause of the gain. It should be noted, nonetheless, that 2005 was the last year these data were available (consult: http://www.naspa.org/).

PROFESSIONAL PREPARATION AND DEVELOPMENT

In the early history of colleges and universities in the United States, there were no specialists assisting students in their non-classroom or cocurricular lives and activities. However, as with all other advances in higher education, College Students Development generalists and specialists have become better educated, more regulated, and more visible.

Before examining how graduate students are prepared to work in the varied environments within higher education, it is crucial for the potential applicant to possess one important personality characteristic: a *passion* for college students from diverse backgrounds. The potential graduate student must be able to interact with non-traditional, culturally and ethnically diverse, differently abled students from a variety of backgrounds. Personal interviews with each applicant to graduate programs conducted by faculty are essential to select people best suited for the profession. Applicants should seek graduate programs which are nationally accredited (Maples, 2001).

According to the Standards Manual of the Council for the Accreditation of Counseling and Related Educational Programs (CACREP, 2001), "Accreditation is a process and a condition. The process entails the assessment of educational quality and the continued enhancement of educational operations through the development and validation of standards. The condition provides a credential to the public-at-large which attests that an institution's programs have accepted and are fulfilling their commitment to educational quality" (Maples, 2001, p. 58). Robert O. Stripling, often referred to as the father of accreditation, stated in 1975 that "accreditation may not guarantee qualification, but qualification is unlikely without some form of accreditation" (Maples, 1979).

Change in 2009 Standards

As noted above, the nationally recognized accrediting body for graduate programs in College Student Development (CSD), called "Student Affairs Practice in Higher Education" and "College Counseling" (CLC), is the Council for the Accreditation of Counseling and Related Educational Programs (CACREP). In the 2001 Standards Manual, these programs are considered to be separate areas of study. However, although these standards only require 48 semester credits of study for a master's degree, many noteworthy graduate programs have increased their requirements, some to as many as 66 semester credits (for example, the University of Nevada, Reno), allowing for CSD and CLC accreditation standards to be met simultaneously. In the 2009 CACREP standards, these separate, but not necessarily distinct, programs are being combined into one area of emphasis, now entitled College Counseling and Student Development (Third draft–2009 CACREP Standards). Though the credit hour requirement has not yet been determined at this writing, the requirement seems likely to increase when the two program emphases are combined.

Is Accreditation Really Necessary?

In this time of budget cutbacks, staff reductions, decreasing services to students, and increasing cost of living, almost all institutions are seeking ways to reduce educational costs. Despite the temptation to reduce graduate credit requirements, graduate program directors are wise to keep in mind the long-term value of their degrees and the depth of knowledge imparted to their graduates. Graduates of CACREP accredited master's degree programs benefit from the following courses, not generally a part of nonaccredited programs with fewer credit hours:

Counseling Theories and practicum–6
Addictions Counseling–3

Legal & Ethical Issues in Counseling–3
Appraisal & Assessment–3 (emphasis in higher education)
Group Counseling–3
Multicultural Counseling–3
College Student Development–3
Issues & Trends in College Student Development–3
Counseling in Higher Education–3
Media & Presentation Technology–3
Service Internship in Higher Education–3 to 6 (600-900 clock hours)
Administration in Higher Education–3
Curriculum in Higher Education–3
Internship in College Counseling–3 to 6 (600-900 clock hours)
Electives in Area of CSD Specialty–3 to 6 (Maples, 2001, pp.64-65)

In addition to the required coursework, there are several essential competencies which should be guaranteed by graduate programs. Blimling and Alschuler (1996) referred to CSD professionals as Student Development Educators:

> Student development educators are those people in student affairs (development) engaged in promoting the growth, development and learning of students. . . . The primary role of student development educators is to teach through experiences and activities inside and outside the classroom–skills that empower students with self-knowledge, self-awareness and enhance the quality of lives now and later. (p. 207)

WORK SETTINGS

Perhaps one of the most important influences upon the work settings of CSD professionals is the massive contribution of technology in the last part of the first decade of the third millennium. As early as 2000, Engels, Jacobs, and Kern identified signifi-

cant competencies that would be needed by College Student Development and Counseling personnel in current and future work venues. They include, but are not necessarily limited to:

- *Resources*–identifying, organizing, planning, and allowing time, money, material and human resources;
- *Interpersonal*–working with others as a team member, a teacher, a service provider, a leader, a negotiator who works effectively with men and women from diverse backgrounds and cultures;
- *Information*–using computers and other means for acquiring, evaluating, maintaining, interpreting, and using information;
- *Systems*–understanding, monitoring, correcting, designing, and improving social organizational, technological, and other complex interrelationships;
- *Technology*–selecting applying, and maintaining technological tools and equipment (p. 190).

The physical setting of the preponderance of CSD professionals is higher education. According to the Chronicle of Higher Education (1999), there are six types of academic, post-secondary institutions in the United States (see Table 6–1). There are currently more than 5,000 institutions, many developed in the twenty-first century, to accommodate working adults. The University of Phoenix, with an emphasis on programs for working adults, has 190 locations throughout the United States. Additionally, there are online, degree-granting institutions such as Capella University. Currently, CSD professionals tend to work in the settings described in Table 6–1.

Today's college students are likely to encounter CSD professionals in almost every student services division on campus, including but not limited to Enrollment

Table 6-1
Types and Numbers of Institutions of Higher Education in the United States

Public, 4 year	615
Public, 2 year	1,092
Private, 4 year (nonprofit)	1,536
Private, 4 year (for profit)	200
Private, 2 year (nonprofit)	184
Private, 2 year (for profit)	700

Services (Recruitment, Admissions, Orientation), Financial Aid , Academic Advising Residential Life, Student Activities, Student Union, Career Development, Counseling. Multicultural Programs, and Inter- national Student Service.

In addition to the variety of CSD positions mentioned above, there is a plethora of opportunities available to the graduate of a "Counseling and College Student Development" program (wording in CACREP 2009 Standards Manual). Specialized opportunities exist in *Peer Programs; Disabled Services* (or Differently-Abled, Univeristy of Oregon terminology); *Student Government & Leadership Training.*

All of the services and programs listed above require preparation beyond the classroom. Intensive internships and graduate assistantships are common, usually a minimum of 300 hours, half of which requires that the graduate learn *about* the service or program, and half of which the student provides assistance and help to the professional personnel who run the program or service.

The most outstanding value of this type of career for the master's or doctoral graduate is the tremendous number of careers within a career. There are more than 35 different positions for graduate student alumni to work in a community college or university setting upon which to build a lifetime career.

PROFESSIONAL ORGANIZATIONS

When the profession of Counseling and Student Development was originated in the early twentieth century, there really were no special interest organizations. As with any profession, organizations and affiliations provide numerous benefits to their members. Among them are: (a) regulating the profession; (b) development of professional relationships and networks; (c) providing learning and continued training opportunities for members; (d) maintaining and upgrading ethical and behavioral standards as the customs and mores of the country changes; (e) reasonable charges for membership to maintain programs and services; and (f) mandating professional qualifications of members (Maples, 2001).

With these characteristics in mind, it is important to note that each of the various specific "careers within a career" listed above has its professional identity in small associations. The following are more "global" and unifying in essence:

- *American Counseling Association* (ACA). This is the umbrella organization encompassing 16 smaller divisions, ranging from the first, established in 1914 as the National Vocational Guidance Association (NVGA), to the newest, the Association for Gay, Lesbian, Bisexual and Transgender Counseling (AGLB TC), established in 2000.

The organizations most closely associated with the College Student Development profession are:

- *The American College Counseling Association* (ACCA), established in 1991 as an "outgrowth" of the *American College Personnel Association* (ACPA), once an originating division of the American Counseling Association. ACPA was a founding division of the American Personnel and Guidance Association (now ACA) when it was founded in 1952.
- *The National Association of Student Personnel Administrators* (NASPA), comprised primarily of mid- and senior-level administrators in institutions of higher education.

FUTURE OUTLOOK

Perhaps the greatest influence upon the direction of College Counseling and Student Development, as the third millennium leaves its infancy and becomes a teenager, is *technology*. Also, as the competition for traditional-aged students (18–23) becomes more challenging, *effective enrollment management*, including recruitment, admissions, financial aid, orientation, academic advising, and other services, takes on greater meaning. Accountability through action and outcome research will effectively utilize scarce resources.

Finally, there are many indications that the future of higher education will depend upon cooperation and collaboration among Student Development professionals, academic faculty, and administrators. The future of effective Counseling and Student Development will continue to call for talented professionals who possess a *passion* for college students of all ages, and who are willing to work 24/7 for those college students for whom the passion exists. Counseling and Student Development are intrinsically and extrinsically rewarding careers for the right person. As the first author of this chapter is fond of telling her students on the first day of class, College Student Development can be compared to an erupting volcano: You never know what will happen next!

REFERENCES

Astin, A.W. (1993). *What matters in college? Four critical years revisited.* San Francisco: Jossey-Bass.

Belenky, M., Clinchy, B., Goldberger, N., & Tarule, J. (1986). *Women's way of knowing: The development of self voice and mind.* New York: Basic Books.

Blimling, G., & Alschuler, A. (1996). Creating a home for the spirit of learning: Contributions of student development educators. *Journal of College Student Development, 37*(2), 203–216.

CACREP. (2001) *Standards manual.* Alexandria, VA: ACA Press

Center for Advising and Student Advancement (CASA). (2008). Colorado State University. http://www.casa.colostate.edu/advising/Faculty_Advising_Manual/Chapter1/theories.cfm.

Chandler, L., & Gallagher, R. (1996). Developing a taxonomy for problems seen at a university counseling center. *Measurement and Evaluation in Counseling and Development, 29*(1), 4–12.

Cass, V. (1979). Homosexual identity formation: A theoretical model. *Journal of Homosexuality, 14*, 219–235.

Cass, V. (1984). Theories about college students, environments and organizations. In S.R. Komives & D.B. Woodward, Jr. (Eds.), Student services: *A handbook for the profession.* San Francisco: Jossey-Bass.

Chickering, A. (1969). *Education and identity.* San Francisco: Jossey-Bass.

Chickering A., & Reisser, L. (1993). *Education and identity* (2nd ed.). San Francisco: Jossey-Bass.

College Student Personnel Workers Fact Sheet. Retrieved April 23, 2008 from http://www. spe.edu/pages/1795.asp.

Cross, W.E. (1995). The psychology of nigrescence: Revising the Cross model. In J. Ponteretto, J. Casas, L. Suzuki, & C. Alexander (Eds.), *Handbook of multicultural counseling*. Thousand Oaks, CA: Sage.

D'Augelli, A. (1994). Identity development and sexual orientation. Toward a model of gay, lesbian and bisexual development. In E. Trickett, R. Watts, & D. Berman (Eds.), *Human diversity: Perspectives of people in context* (pp. 312–333). San Francisco: Jossey-Bass.

Davis, D.C., & Humphrey, K.M. (2000). *College counseling: Issues and strategies for a new millennium*. Alexandria, VA: ACA Publications.

Dean, L., & Meadows, M. (1995). College counseling: Union and intersection. *Journal of Counseling and Development, 74*(2), 139–142.

Economic Research Institute. (2007). *Survey of salaries*. Washington, DC.

Engels, D.W., Jacobs, B.C., & Kern, C.W. (2000). Life-career development counseling. In D.C. Davis & K.M. Humphrey (Eds.), *College counseling: Issues and strategies for a new millennium*. Alexandria, VA: American Counseling Association.

Fitzpatrick, R. (1968). The history of college counseling. In M. Siegel (Ed.), *The counseling of college students* (pp. 1–14). New York: Free Press.

Gross, L. (2004). Creating meaning from intersections of career and cultural identity. In A. Ortiz (Ed.), *Addressing the unique needs of Latino American students: New directions for student services, 105,* 63–78.

Helms, J. (Ed.). (1993). *Black and white racial identity: Theory, research and practice*. Westport, CT: Praeger.

Higher Education Research Institute (HERI). (2007). *The American freshman–Forty year trends*. http://www.gseis.ucla.edu/heri/40yrtrends. php.

Howe, N., & Strauss, W. (2003). *Millenials go to college*. Great Falls, VA: American Association of Registrars and Admissions Officers and Life Course Associates.

Hunter, D. E. (1992). How student affairs professionals choose their careers. *NASPA Journal, 29,* 181–188.

Lloyd-Jones, E. (1938). *A student personnel program for higher education*. New York: McGraw-Hill.

Maples, M. (1979). *Reflections on the father of accreditation*. Speech delivered at the Robert O. Stripling retirement celebration, University of Florida, Gainesville, April.

Maples, M. (1996) Cornerstones of a civilized society: Law, ethics, morality, faith, spirituality. *Juvenile and Family Court Journal, 3, 26,* 127–150.

Maples, M., (2000). Professional preparation for college counseling: Quality assurance. In D. Davis & K. Humphries (Eds.), *College counseling: Issues and strategies for the new millennium*. Alexandria, VA: ACA Publications.

Maples, M. (2001). Professional preparation for college counseling: Quality assurance. In D. Davis and K. Humphrey (Eds.), *College counseling: Issues and strategies for a new millennium*. Alexandria, VA: ACA Publications.

Maples, M. (2002). College Student Development Services Course Handbook. Unpublished manuscript, University of Nevada, Reno.

Maples, M., & Han, S., (2008). Cybercounseling in the United States and South Korea: Implications for counseling college students of the Millennial generation and the networked generation. *The Journal of Counseling & Development, 86*(2), 178–183.

McGowan, A.S. (2008). Farewell. *The Journal of Counseling & Development, 86*(2), 2.

Meadows, M. (2001). The evaluation of college counseling. In D. Davis and K. Humphrey (Eds.), *College counseling: Issues and strategies for a new millennium*. Alexandria, VA: ACA Publications.

National Center for Education Statistics. (2008). *Digest of Education Statistics 2007*. http://nces. ed.gov/programs/digest/d07/.

Perry, W. (1981). Cognitive and ethical growth: The making of meaning. In A. Chickering & Associates (Eds.), *The modern American college: Responding to the new realities of diverse students and a changing society*. San Francisco: Jossey-Bass.

Phinney, J. (1989). Stages of ethnic identity development in minority group adolescents. *Journal of Early Adolescence, 9*(1–2), 34–39.

Ready Minds, Inc. (2006). *Training manual-Distance counseling credential*. Greensboro, NC: Center for Counseling Credentials.

Rudolph, F. (1965). *The American college and university: A history.* New York: Knopf.

Stone, G.L., & Archer, J.A., Jr. (1990). College and university counseling centers in the 1990s: Challenges and limits. *The Counseling Psychologist, 18*(4), 539–607.

Torres, V. (2004. The diversity among us: Puerto Ricans, Cuban Americans, Caribbean Americans and Central and South Americans. In A. Ortiz (Ed.), *Addressing the unique needs of Latino American students: New directions for student services, 105*, 5–16.

U.S. Bureau of Labor Statistics. (2007). *Current professional salaries.* Washington, DC: U.S. Government Printing Office.

Von Steen, P. (2001). Traditional-age college students. In D. Davis & K. Humphrey (Eds.), *College counseling: Issues and strategies for a new millennium.* Alexandria, VA: ACA Publications.

Chapter 7

COUNSELING PSYCHOLOGY

DESTIN N. STEWART & BRENT MALLINCKRODT

The field of Counseling Psychology is an applied specialty accredited by the American Psychological Association (APA). Graduates of accredited programs who receive a doctoral degree, complete an approved internship, and meet the requirements for postgraduate training specified in a given jurisdiction are eligible to be licensed as psychologists in all 50 states. Counseling psychology is distinguished from other helping professions by five themes evident in its history and contemporary practice (Gelso & Fretz, 2001). Although none of these themes is unique to counseling psychology, no other helping profession emphasizes this combination of elements. Thus, it is the unique mixture of these five fundamental characteristics that sets counseling psychology apart from other people-oriented professions.

First, counseling psychologists tend to work with higher functioning clientele than many other specialties. Although some counseling psychologists do work with profoundly impaired persons (for example, in inpatient hospital settings), generally, because many counseling psychologists are employed in university and college counseling centers, their clientele tend to present with acute rather than chronic problems.

The second key theme is a focus on each client's assets and strengths. Counseling psychologists tend to focus on coping and resilience regardless of the degree of impairment and tend to think less in terms of using their skills to repair damage or remediate deficits–although they can work effectively with clients in severe crisis. Their ultimate goal is to help clients mobilize their own coping resources and gain skills within a positive psychology framework. Their work emphasizes well-being and the more healthy aspects of personality. This perspective requires counseling psychologists to think of healthy functioning as more than the absence of all symptoms of illness but rather also as the affirmative presence of competencies, skills, and life satisfaction.

The third theme of counseling psychology implies that psychotherapy or counseling interventions are usually brief. Practitioners are skilled in a variety of effective time-limited approaches.

The fourth theme identified by Gelso and Fretz is an emphasis on person-environment interactions, as opposed to an exclusive focus on either the person or the environment. Counseling psychologists are skilled in assessing both client characteristics and aspects of the environment, and provide interventions at both the individual and the group or systems level.

The fifth theme is a developmental focus which, in turn, leads to an emphasis on educational interventions and on career counseling. Counseling psychologists are skilled at working with issues–be they academic, vocational and/or occupational that occur in their clients' lives. Although some counseling psychologists focus exclusively on career development, most do not specialize in this area but rather integrate these skills into everyday practice. Their training in career development allows counseling psychologists to help clients who might present initially with social or emotional problems to also find a sense of meaning and purpose in life through vocational exploration.

An understanding and appreciation of these five themes helps differentiate counseling psychology from other specialties (Gelso & Fretz, 2001). For example, historically, clinical psychology has been more concerned with the study of abnormal behavior and underlying pathology than counseling psychology. Attention to educational and vocational issues and interventions has not been a primary focus for clinical psychologists. In the past, clinical psychologists typically worked in inpatient or psychiatric hospitals, whereas counseling psychologists would more likely be found at universities and college campuses. Counseling psychologists and school psychologists both work with children in educational settings. However, the interventions of counseling psychologists are less likely to be exclusively targeted at improving the child's academic performance.

Although the unique mixture of these five themes does differentiate counseling psychology from other specialties to some degree, it is important to note that in recent years, these distinctions have become more blurred than in the past. For example, the typical work day of a counseling psychologist in private practice compared to a clinical psychologist in private practice typically have much more in common than the work days of two psychologists in the same field, but one teaches in a university psychology department and the other is in private practice. In other words, today there are generally many more differences between two psychologists in the same field but in different work settings than there are differences between two psychologists from different fields working in the same setting.

HISTORY AND DEVELOPMENT

The earliest roots of counseling psychology can be traced to the first decade of the 1900s to efforts by the pioneering social reformer Frank Parsons to develop career counseling services in Boston (Gelso & Fretz, 2001). However, the birth of the profession is generally attributed to the years immediately following World War II. In the late 1940s, U.S. colleges and universities experienced a huge influx of former soldiers pursing the educational opportunities made possible by Veterans Administration (VA) benefits. In response, postsecondary educational institutions hired a new type of professional counselor to assist these veterans with services provided through expanded counseling centers. Eventually this new specialization would be called *Counseling Psychology*. The foundations of several of the five themes previously described can be seen in these early developments, including a focus on career development, serving relatively high functioning clients with "intact personalities" (Gelso & Fretz, 2001, p. 31), and brief interventions delivered in educational settings.

In 1946, the 17th Division of the American Psychological Association was organized to serve this new specialty, although it was not until 1953 that its name became the "Division of Counseling Psychology." A series of conferences and meetings among early leaders of Division 17 resulted in a formal definition of the specialty, including the first guidelines for training (Gelso & Fretz, 2001). In 1952, the first three counseling psychology training programs were accredited by APA (Teachers College–Columbia University, Ohio State University, and the University of Minnesota), followed in the next five years by seven others. Another sign of the maturing field coming into its own was the publication in 1954 of the first issue of the *Journal of Counseling Psychology*, which signaled that the field was now producing a significant body of its own specialized scientific research.

Growth in the discipline leveled off in the 1960s and early 1970s, a period marked by some anxieties over the proper role and function of counseling psychologists. However, when these issues of professional identity were largely resolved, a new period of rapid growth began in the mid-1970s as increasing numbers of graduates began working in a broader range of settings. Counseling psychologists branched out in large numbers from their traditional careers in university teaching and counseling or in service at VA hospitals. This trend has continued into the present, with an increasing proportion of Counseling Psychology graduates embarking on careers in private practice, health care settings and as consultants in business and industry. As we will describe below, one hallmark of the specialty is the tremendous diversity of settings and services that employ counseling psychologists.

By 2008, there were 68 APA accredited counseling psychology programs admitting students. These programs graduate approximately 350 students per year. Of the total number of doctoral students applying for accredited internships in 2007, 13 percent

(about 1 out of 6) were trained in counseling psychology programs. Of the remainder, 79 percent were from clinical psychology programs, 5 percent from school psychology programs, and 3 percent from combined or "other" programs (http://www.appic.org/match/5_2_2_4_9a_match_about_statistics_surveys_2007a.htm retrieved June 13, 2008). Another indicator of the vitality of the field is its premiere scientific journal. Of the 28 primary journals published by APA, the *Journal of Counseling Psychology* (JCP) has the second highest number of individual subscribers (APA, 2007), and it is ranked first among 54 journals in applied psychology with regard to "impact factor"–that is, the number of times its articles are cited in other publications.

MISSIONS AND OBJECTIVES

One of the earliest statements that set forth objectives for the profession is still a fairly accurate description more than 50 years later:

> The professional goal of the counseling psychologist is to foster the psychological development of the individual. This includes all people on the adjustment continuum from those who function at tolerable levels of adequacy to those suffering more severe psychological disturbances. (APA, 1952, p. 176; cited in Gelso & Fretz, 2001. p. 34)

The five core themes we have described are also key influences on the methods and approaches that counseling psychologists use to achieve these goals.

Another core objective, which could be regarded as a sixth theme that influences every aspect of contemporary counseling psychology, is an emphasis on cultural diversity and on developing specialized skills to serve oppressed populations who lack access to services (Heppner, Witty & Dixon, 2004). Developing multicultural competencies is a core component of graduate training. Counseling psychologists are trained to work with clients whose cultural worldview and life experiences differ from their own. This specialized training includes, but is not limited to, working with racial/ethnic minorities, women, gay men, lesbian women, bisexual persons and other sexual minorities, persons with disabilities, clients of all ages, and persons whose religious beliefs are very different from the psychologist's. Upon beginning graduate training, many programs require students to make a commitment to a formal statement of training values that emphasizes goals of self-exploration and willingness to work on understanding one's own biases, as well as developing multicultural competency to serve a diverse clientele (see http://www.ccptp.org/trainingdirectorpage6.html, retrieved 6/10/08).

Finally, counseling psychology as a helping profession has long been committed to fostering social justice. However, a relatively new development is the explicit inclusion in a few graduate programs of training components designed to build students' skills as advocates for social change or to help these students learn ways to empower clients to work for change in their own social contexts (Toporek, Gerstein, Fouad, Roysircar & Israel, 2006). Students who seek a combination of traditional skills for helping individual clients but also skills to change the social conditions of oppression and inequality that contribute to many clients' presenting problems might find these counseling psychology programs to be an especially good match for their interests.

CLIENTS TYPICALLY SERVED

Many students are drawn to the field by the tremendous variety of clients served by counseling psychologists. Students have a wider range of possibilities when they begin their training than in almost any other specialty. Like school psychologists, counseling psychologists work with children in educational settings; like industrial/organizational psychologists, counseling psychologists work in business settings–either as consultants or as "in-house" psychologists in human resources; like clinical psychologists, some counseling psychologists work with severely disturbed clients in hospitals or outpatient clinics. In terms of the greatest numbers of clients served in the "modal" setting, perhaps the college or university student seeking counseling for a relatively short-term adjustment problem comes closest to fitting the definition, but strictly speaking, there is no "typical" counseling psychology client. Counseling psychologists work with clients of all ages and demographic characteristics. They work with individuals, couples, families, groups, and entire organizations.

Although it is impossible to distinguish counseling psychologists from other specialties on the basis of the clients they serve, their approach to working with clients often does set counseling psychologists apart. Thus, whether working with children, adults, or frail elderly clients, counseling psychologists tend to take a developmental approach and use interventions that emphasize learning new coping skills. Whether working with extremely high functioning clients or those severely debilitated by mental illness, the interventions of counseling psychologists tend to emphasize building strengths rather than repairing deficits. The commitment of the profession to social justice and to multiculturalism, together with the emphasis on person-environment interaction, prompts counseling psychologists to consider the social context and cultural values of all clients they serve. This focus means that counseling psychologists are especially likely to work with clients who lack access to traditional mental health services and who have experienced societal oppression, including racial and ethnic minority persons; gay, lesbian, or other sexual minority persons; immigrants; women; and persons with disabilities–to name a few types of clients.

PHILOSOPHICAL ASSUMPTIONS AND PREEMINENT THEORIES

Given the diversity of counseling psychologists' professional roles, no single theory or small set of theories dominates the field. However, given the five themes identified by Gelso and Fretz (2001) and the emphasis on multicultural diversity and social justice, it is possible to identify a collection of theories and key concepts that have had a very strong influence on counseling psychology as it is practiced today. The description that follows is not meant to imply an order of priority, nor should it be considered a complete list. Our intention is to briefly convey some idea of the many theories that have influenced the field.

In terms of approaches to counseling, client-centered (Rogers, 1951), interpersonal (Teyber, 2005), cognitive-behavioral (Beck, 1976), short-term dynamic therapy (Strupp & Binder, 1984), emotion-focused process experiential therapy (Elliott, Watson, Goldman & Greenberg, 2004), and feminist approaches (Brown, In Press) have been influential models. In the realm of career development, John Holland's (1973) theory of person-environment match has been tremendously influential. Albert Bandura's (1986) theory of social learning, particularly the concept of self-efficacy, also has had a great influence

on understanding the process of career choice (Betz & Hackett, 1981; Lent, Brown & Hackett, 2000).

Some theories have had a broad influence over many aspects of counseling psychology practice and research. Among these are the model of interpersonal communication and social influence developed by Stanley Strong (Strong & Claiborn, 1982), which led to a stage model of counseling change (Tracey, 1993). Other broadly influential theories are the models of problem-solving skills and coping (Heppner, Witty & Dixon, 2004) and models of the counseling relationship conceived as a "working alliance" (Bordin, 1979; Horvath & Greenberg, 1994). Wampold's (2001) research on the importance of therapist effects and on development of a contextual model for understanding how clients change has recently had a profound impact on the field. Helms' stage model of racial identity development (Helms & Cook, 1999) and Berry's (2001, 2007) two-dimensional model of acculturation and immigration experience have provided valuable frameworks for multicultural research and practice. Graduate training has been influenced by models of multicultural competencies (Sue, Arredondo & McDavis, 1992; Worthington, Soth-McNett & Moreno, 2007) and theories of how therapists develop their skills, which inform theory and research on clinical supervision (Bernard & Goodyear, 2003).

Given that the field is constantly evolving, counseling psychologists continually apply new models–or they apply longstanding models in new ways–to gain a better understanding of clients and counseling processes. Among the concepts that have become highly influential in recent research and practice are: the theory of minority stress applied to gay, lesbian, and other sexual minority persons (Meyer, 2003; Herek & Garnets, 2007); the concept of racial/ethnic microaggressions (Constantine & Sue, 2007); and the application of attachment theory to understand the psychotherapy relationship (Mallinckrodt, Porter & Kivlighan, 2005) and healthy personality (Lopez & Brennan, 2000).

PROFESSIONAL PREPARATION AND DEVELOPMENT

Graduates of counseling psychology programs must complete a doctoral degree, either the Ph.D., the Psy.D., or the Ed.D. (The Ed.D. has been phased out in most contemporary programs.) Roughly half of all students enter counseling psychology programs with a bachelor's degree, whereas the remainder has earned a master's degree in psychology or a related discipline. Some of the 68 programs admitting students prefer one type of applicant over another, but many admit a mixture of students with and without master's degrees. Some of the students with master's degrees have been working in a "people profession" for several years before deciding to return for doctoral training. Other students are admitted directly after finishing their undergraduate work. At many counseling psychology programs, 10 to 20 percent of those admitted are international students. Although many applicants did not major in psychology as undergraduates, successful applicants must have a strong background in psychology. Broad survey courses in abnormal psychology, human development, personality, statistics, and research methods are especially valuable.

All APA accredited counseling psychology programs have endorsed some variation of the "scientist-practitioner" training model, whose basic assumption is that research skills and counseling practice skills strengthen one another. Research is most applicable when the studies are designed by researchers who are skilled practitioners themselves. Similarly, counselors deliver the most effective services when they apply the rigorously disciplined thinking of a scientist in their field. Thus, all graduates of counseling psychology programs receive training in both research skills and skills necessary to be an effective practitioner. However, the balance between research and practice training varies across programs (Gelso & Fretz, 2001). Programs that describe themselves as following a "practitioner-scholar" model tend to emphasize practice skills, whereas those who follow the "scientist-practitioner" model tend to be more balanced. The "clinical scientist" model emphasizes research skills. Programs offering the Psy.D. degree generally have less emphasis on research training than those offering the Ph.D. Of those programs offering the Ph.D., about 20 percent are housed in departments of psychology, with the remainder in colleges of education. Perhaps the most consistent difference between these two academic settings is that counseling psychology students in departments of psychology will generally have more opportunities to serve as teaching assistants and instructors. Regardless of the setting and training model, it is vitally important for applicants to acquire both research experience and volunteer counseling opportunities before they apply. Although there is no requirement that applicants profess interest in a research career after graduation, applicants must possess a genuine scientific curiosity that is demonstrated through active involvement in research prior to applying to a counseling psychology program—particularly those that offer the Ph.D. Many undergraduate students acquire this experience by completing an honors thesis or through volunteering to join a research team of faculty and students.

Students who enter a counseling psychology program without previous graduate course work typically require five to six years to complete their training. Those who enter with relevant master's-level training, generally require four to five years. In either case, the first two to three years emphasize coursework in basic counseling skills, supervised practica, professional ethics, research methods, and foundations of psychology. Near the end of this period many students transition from campus-based beginning level practica to more challenging advanced practica and field placements. Virtually all programs also require courses in supervision so that advanced students acquire the skills they will need to teach practica if they choose a faculty career or to supervise trainees if they choose a career in a community agency or campus counseling center.

Trainees receive research experience throughout this period, but the extent will vary by program. Most programs require a master's-level or "predissertation" research project. The third or fourth year of training features intensive work on a research dissertation, completion of comprehensive examinations, and applications for predoctoral internship. This internship usually occurs at the end of the trainee's program and involves an additional application procedure. The applicant is matched to an internship site through a rigorous process of submitting applications and attending interviews. Not unlike medical training, the intern will then become a paid full-time member of the agency or facility staff and complete an entire calendar year of training before graduation.

WORK SETTINGS AND SALARY PROJECTIONS

Counseling psychologists work in a variety of settings and can obtain employment in the same fields as most any other type of psychologist, which is one of the most appealing aspects of counseling psychology for many students. A report of survey data collected in 2000 by the APA reported that counseling psychologists employed full time worked in the following settings: 38.7 percent independent practice; 34.9 percent higher education; 19.8 percent clinic or other human service agency; 6.2 percent hospital; 3.5 percent government; 2.2 percent schools or other educational setting; and 0.9 percent business and industry. Among the 34.9 percent who work in a university or college setting, 12.2 percent of the total sample reported working in a counseling center (Munley, Pate & Duncan, 2008). Thus, in simple terms, for every ten counseling psychologists working full time in 2000, four were in private practice, three worked in a college or university (one of these at a counseling center and two elsewhere on campus or as a faculty member), two worked at a community agency, and one of the ten worked in a hospital, school, or government service position.

These data can be somewhat misleading, because the flexibility of their training allows counseling psychologists to pursue many activities simultaneously. For example, many faculty members and college counseling center staff maintain a part-time private practice. Those in independent practice may teach occasionally as adjunct faculty members at a local university. Counseling psychologists in any of these roles may also serve as consultants. This variety of roles and opportunities can lead to greater employment satisfaction. The majority (55%) of counseling psychologists, in a recent survey, reported relatively high career satisfaction and mentioned that if they had to choose careers again, they would choose counseling psychology (Goodyear et al., 2008).

In terms of salary expectations, 2007 data collected by the APA suggest that the median salary for counseling psychologists who are licensed psychologists at university/college counseling centers with five to nine years of experience was $53,000; with 10 to

14 years experience, $62,000; and with 20 to 24 years of experience, $67,000. For faculty positions in colleges of education, the comparable median salaries were for six to seven years experience, $58,252; 11 to 13 years experience, $62,375; and 20 to 24 years experience, $78,068. Income in a private practice career is more variable and often involves considerable out-of-pocket costs (e.g., malpractice insurance). APA data report a median for five to nine years in private practice of $77,500; 10 to 14 years, $60,000; and 20 to 24 years of experience, $82,000 (http://research.apa.org/facsal06/t09.pdf and http://research.apa.org/t6 salaries07.pdf retrieved June 13, 2008). For updates in this information, consult periodic reports released by the American Psychological Association, Center for Workforce Studies (http://research.apa.org/).

PROFESSIONAL ORGANIZATIONS

By far, the most important professional organization for the field is the Society of Counseling Psychology (SCP), Division 17 of the American Psychological Association (see www.div17.org). In 2007, more than 9300 APA members (9.6% of the total) identified themselves as counseling psychologists (research.apa.org/profile2007t3.pdf retrieved June 13, 2008). However, less than half of all APA members belong to any of its divisions. Of the 39,000 members who do belong to one or more APA divisions, about 6 percent (2320 to be exact) were members of SCP Division 17 in 2006 (see http://research.apa.org/profile2006t5.pdf, retrieved June 13, 2008). Thus, in terms of membership Division 17 was the ninth largest of APA's 53 divisions in 2007. Graduate and undergraduate students are enthusiastically welcomed to join as affiliates of SCP (http://

www.div17.org/about_membership.html). All SCP members receive the organization's newsletter, published three times per year, and *The Counseling Psychologist*–the scholarly journal published by SCP.

Because counseling psychology is such a diverse field, members of SCP–its one official professional organization–often actively participate in a wide range of other organizations including: APA Division 29 (Psychotherapy), Division 35 (Psychology of Women), Division 42 (Independent Practice), Division 44 (Psychological Study of Lesbian, Gay, and Bisexual Issues), Division 45 (Psychological Study of Ethnic Minority Issues), and Division 51 (Psychological Study of Men and Masculinity). Many counseling psychologists have held leadership roles in these organizations.

OUTLOOK

An excellent resource for expected job prospects and salary data is the U.S. Department of Labor, Bureau of Labor Statistics "Occupational Outlook Handbook" (see www.bls.gov/oco/). The 2008–09 edition had this to say about the job outlook for psychologists:

Faster-than-average employment growth is expected for psychologists. Job prospects should be the best for people who have a doctoral degree from a leading university in an applied specialty, such as counseling or health, and those with a specialist or doctoral degree in school psychology. Master's degree holders in fields other than industrial-organizational psychology will face keen competition. Opportunities will be limited for bachelor's degree holders . . . Employment of psychologists is expected to grow 15 percent from 2006 to 2016, faster than the average for all occupations. Employment will grow because of increased demand for psychological services in schools, hospitals, social service agencies, mental health centers, substance abuse treatment clinics, consulting firms, and private companies. (Retrieved June 16, 2008).

Considering the specific job settings of counseling psychologists, we turn first to independent practice. Since the early 1990s, the movement toward managed care, which Gelso and Fretz (2001) term the "industrialization of health care" (p. 90) has had a profound influence on the way mental health services are delivered. In a nationwide survey of more than 15,000 psychologists in full-time and part-time private practice, four out of every five respondents reported that managed care had a negative impact on their practice (Phelps, Eisman & Kohout, 1998). Because counseling psychologists tend to work with higher functioning clients whose presenting problems may not be covered by third-party payments, the managed care movement has probably influenced this opinion of respondents to greater extent than for those who work with the more severely mentally ill. On the other hand, the ability of counseling psychologists to work in a time-limited framework has helped them adapt to these changes. Although these economic forces show no signs of abating, more than one in three counseling psychologists report working in private practice. Therefore, it seems safe to conclude that many graduates are able to survive and even flourish in a managed care environment. It is undeniably more difficult now than in the past to begin earning an income entirely from private practice shortly after graduation. Consequently, many recent graduates work first at a counseling center, community agency, or hospital to further develop a practice specialization that is in demand in their area. After a few years of honing their skills, these counseling psychologists may then make the jump to full-time private practice

or take a transitional step to part-time private practice while continuing to work for a few more years in their "day job."

The outlook for private practice careers as well as for positions in community agencies with mental health service delivery contracts will be greatly affected depending on whether Congress passes the "Mental Health Parity" act, which would require insurance companies to offer mental health treatment commensurate with benefits for physical illness. In March of 2008, the House of Representatives passed a version of this bill. The Senate passed its own version earlier in the year, but there were major differences between the versions that remain to be resolved as this chapter was written in June, 2008. President Bush announced his opposition to the House version which is generally regarded as offering more generous benefits to the 35 million Americans with disabling mental disorders (*New York Times*, "House Approves Bill on Mental Health Parity" March 6, 2008). Passage of this legislation, depending on the particular version that is adopted, could lead to a significant expansion in mental health services.

In regard to faculty positions, the good news for new graduates is a general concern about the "graying" of the faculty, with a wave of retirements expected over the next decade. The massive hiring of the 1960s followed by slower growth thereafter has contributed to a gradual increase in the mean age of faculty in all disciplines. One survey reported that in 1999, 32 percent of all full-time faculty were 55 years or older (cited in Fleck, 2001). Consequently, the coming years may be an especially good time for graduates seeking a faculty career in counseling psychology. However, current economic conditions have resulted in flat budgets or deep cuts in higher education in many states. Under these circumstances new faculty hiring may well be curtailed. Counseling psychology programs themselves also may be vulnerable in times of budget auster-ity. Five programs that were APA accredited 10 years ago are no longer admitting stu-dents in 2008. Students seeking a faculty career will be most successful if they remain flexible and think broadly about teaching opportunities at a range of institutions not limited only to the 68 counseling psychology programs presently accredited and admitting students.

College and university counseling centers experience many of the same problems with flat or reduced budgets as do academic pro-grams in times of economic recession. How-ever, there is a growing realization among many administrators about the crucial role that counseling centers play in retention of ethnic minority students and in helping all students realize their full academic potential. Counseling psychologists with strong multi-cultural skills and an emphasis on career development and coping strengths are ideal-ly suited to be at the forefront of such efforts. On campuses led by these enlightened administrators and on campuses in states where support for higher education remains strong, job prospects for counseling psychol-ogists will remain quite promising. A huge "wild card" for these prospects involves the 1.5 million U.S. troops who have served thus far in Iraq or Afghanistan. If even a small proportion of these veterans make use of "GI Bill" educational benefits–and especial-ly if current calls to expand these benefits to World War II era levels are enacted into law, college campuses could see a huge influx of military veteran students. It is possible that the field of counseling psychology is poised for a period of expansion reminiscent of the late 1940s. Of course, this will depend on whether the federal government increases veterans' educational benefits to 1946 levels and whether campus counseling services receive a commensurate increase in funding.

Careers in VA hospitals for counseling psychologists will be similarly affected by federal policy. Of the 1.5 million military personnel deployed to Afghanistan or Iraq, 100,000 have sought help for emotional problems, more than 30,000 have been diag-nosed with PTSD, and 750,000 have already left the military and are eligible for VA health care (*USA Today*, 10/22/07, Veteran stress cases up sharply). Counseling psychol-ogists with specialized skills in trauma and rehabilitation will be well prepared to serve as staff in the expanded "Wounded Warrior Rehabilitation" centers. Apart from serving veterans, predictions forecast in the federal *Occupational Outlook Handbook* cited above suggest that careers in health care settings may be the fasting growing segment of employment for counseling psychologists in the coming decade.

Thus, the outlook for counseling psychol-ogists in what has traditionally been three of the largest employment sectors–indepen-dent practice, higher education faculty, and counseling center positions–all could be pro-foundly influenced by policy decisions which remain unresolved as of this writing. The growing economic recession will defi-nitely pose challenges as it leads to budget tightening in government at all levels and on college campuses. On the other hand, either passage of Mental Health Parity legislation or an expansion of veterans' educational benefits could lead to an explosion in demand for the services that counseling psy-chologists are well equipped to provide–and an increased demand for faculty to train them. Apart from these three traditional work settings, there will certainly be an in-creased demand for counseling psycholo-gists to serve military veterans and to work as a vital component of interdisciplinary health care delivery teams serving a broad range of patients (DeAngelis, 2008). In the increasingly global economy, counseling psychologists with strong multicultural com-petencies are well equipped for careers to meet the expanding demand for diversity and cultural sensitivity training through human resources to meet the demands of doing international business. As has been true in the past, counseling psychology graduates who are flexible and resourceful in their career preparation strategy will no doubt continue to find highly satisfying positions. Counseling psychologists will continue to be in demand in the coming decade because the are highly regarded for their in-depth knowledge of human behavior, coping, and processes of change; they bring a combination of effective practitioner skills, the disciplined critical thinking of a research scientist, and a high level of multicultural competencies; they are skilled at both prevention and remediation and bring both research skills and teaching expertise to develop these interventions; their unique perspective on human development, career satisfaction, strengths, resilience, and coping are rare among other professions–in short, their multifaceted skills lead counseling psychologists to be regarded as the "Swiss Army Knife" of the people professions.

REFERENCES

American Psychological Association. (2007). Summary report of journal operations. *American Psychologist, 62*, 543–544.

Bandura, A. (1986). *Social foundations of thought and action: A social cognitive theory.* Englewood Cliffs, NJ: Prentice-Hall.

Beck, A. T. (1976). *Cognitive therapy and the emotional disorders.* New York: New American Library.

Bernard, J. M., & Goodyear, R. K. (2003). *Fundamentals of clinical supervision* (3rd ed.). Boston: Allyn & Bacon.

Berry, J. W. (2001). A psychology of immigration. *Journal of Social Issues, 57*, 615–631.

Berry, J. W. (2007). Acculturation. In J. E. Grusec & P. D. Hastings (Eds.), *Handbook of socialization: Theory and research* (pp. 543–558). New York: Guilford.

Betz, N. E., & Hackett, G. (1981). The relationship of career-related self-efficacy expectations to perceived career options in college women and men. *Journal of Counseling Psychology, 28*, 399–410.

Bordin, E. S. (1979). The generalizability of the psychoanalytic concept of the working alliance. *Psychotherapy: Theory, Research & Practice, 16*, 252–260.

Brown, L. S. (in press). *Feminist therapy: Not for women only.* Washington, DC: American Psychological Association.

Constantine, M. G., & Sue, D. W. (2007). Perceptions of racial microaggressions among black supervisees in cross-racial dyads. *Journal of Counseling Psychology, 54*, 142–153.

DeAngelis, T. (2008). Psychology's growth careers. *Monitor on Psychology, 39*, 64–71.

Elliott, R., Watson, J. C., Goldman, R. N., & Greenberg, L. S. (2004). *Learning emotion-focused therapy: The process-experiential approach to change.* Washington, DC: American Psychological Association.

Fleck, C. (2001). Faculty retirement: The issue, the predictions, and the effects on campuses. Briefing papers, Association of American Colleges and Universities. (http://www.greater expectations.org/briefing_papers/FacultyRetir ement.html, retrieved June 17, 2008

Gelso, C. J., & Fretz, B. R. (2001). *Counseling psychology* (2nd ed.) Fort Worth, TX: Harcourt College.

Goodyear, R. K., Murdock, N., Lichtenberg, J. W., McPherson, R., Koetting, K., & Petren, S. (2008). Stability and change in counseling psychologists' identities, roles, functions, and career satisfaction across 15 years. *The Counseling Psychologist, 36*, 220–249.

Helms, J. E., & Cook, D. A. (1999). *Using race and culture in counseling and psychotherapy: Theory and process.* Upper Saddle River, NJ: Prentice-Hall.

Heppner, P. P., Witty, T. E., & Dixon, W. A. (2004). Problem-solving appraisal: Helping normal people lead better lives. *The Counseling Psychologist, 32*, 466–472.

Herek, G. M., & Garnets, L. D. (2007). Sexual orientation and mental health. *Annual Review of Clinical Psychology*, 353–375.

Horvath, A. O., & Greenberg, L. S. (Eds.) (1994). *The working alliance: Theory, research and practice.* New York: Wiley.

Lent, R. W., Brown, S. D., & Hackett, G. (2000). Contextual supports and barriers to career choice: A Social cognitive analysis. *Journal of Counseling Psychology, 47,* 36–49.

Lopez, F. G., & Brennan, K. A. (2000). Dynamic processes underlying adult attachment organization: Toward an attachment theoretical perspective on the healthy and effective self. *Journal of Counseling Psychology, 47,* 283–300.

Mallinckrodt, B., Porter, M. J., & Kivlighan, D. M. Jr. (2005). Client attachment to therapist, depth of in-session exploration, and object relations in brief psychotherapy. *Psychotherapy: Theory, Research, Practice, and Training, 42,* 85–100.

Meyer, I. H. (2003). Prejudice, social stress, and mental health in lesbian, gay and bisexual populations: Conceptual issues and research evidence. *Psychological Bulletin, 129,* 674–697.

Munley, P. H., Pate, W. E., & Duncan, L. E. (2008). Demographic, educational, employment, and professional characteristics of counseling psychologists. *The Counseling Psychologist, 36,* 250–280.

Phelps, R., Eisman, E. J., & Kohout, J. (1998). Psychological practice and managed care: Results of the CAPP practitioner survey. *Professional Psychology: Research and Practice, 29,* 31–36.

Rogers, C. R. (1951). *Client-centered therapy.* Boston: Houghton-Mifflin.

Strong, S. R., & Claiborne, C. D. (1982). *Change through interaction: Social psychological processes of counseling and psychotherapy.* New York: Wiley.

Strupp, H. H., & Binder, J. L. (1984). *Psychotherapy in a new key: A guide to time-limited dynamic psychotherapy.* New York: Basic Books.

Sue, D. W., Arredondo, P., & McDavis, R. J. (1992). Multicultural counseling competencies and standards: A call to the profession. *Journal of Multicultural Counseling and Development, 20,* 64–88.

Teyber, E. (2005). *Interpersonal process in therapy: An integrative model* (5th ed.). Belmont, CA: Brooks/Cole.

Toporek, R. L., Gerstein, R. H., Fouad, N. A., Boysircar, G., & Israel, T. (Eds.). (2006). *Handbook for social justice counseling psychology: Leadership, vision and action.* Thousand Oaks, CA: Sage.

Tracey, T. J. (1993). An interpersonal stage model of the therapeutic process. *Journal of Counseling Psychology, 40,* 396–409.

Wampold, B. E. (2001). *The great psychotherapy debate: Models, methods, and findings.* Mahwah, NJ: Erlbaum.

Worthington, R. L., Soth-McNett, A. M., & Moreno, M. V. (2007). Multicultural counseling competencies research: A 20-year content analysis. *Journal of Counseling Psychology, 54,* 351–361.

Chapter 8

CRIMINAL JUSTICE

DONNA M. MASSEY-ANDERSON & COURTNEY A. WAID

On a daily basis, laws change, ground-breaking scientific discoveries are revealed and utilized, and new police practices are implemented. When we speak of *criminal justice*, we are referring to the three major components that comprise the criminal justice system: Law Enforcement, the Court System, and Corrections. Each of these subfields is dynamic in nature and is constantly changing, has its own areas of responsibilities, and is inter-related—what occurs in one field often affects what happens in the other two. Perhaps this is most evident in the area of law enforcement—often we see the blending of science and human service in order to improve and enhance public safety, such as in the use of DNA profiling in criminal trials which enhances the courts ability to conclusively convict or exonerate accused persons. Then there are technologies such as Kevlar, closed-circuit monitoring, and stun guns (tazers) which help protect our public safety officials as they conduct their jobs on a daily basis.

A large increase in the number of arrests instigated by law enforcement officers impacts the caseloads in the criminal court system. A large number of convictions by the courts impacts the number of people sent to prison. The general public however, does not typically differentiate between the three subfields. If we were to ask John Q. Public his opinion of crime rates in the United States and what should be done with law violators, we could expect to hear that the criminal should be locked up and the key thrown away. In this fashion, the public expects law enforcement officers to protect the public by arresting wrongdoers, the courts to convict criminals and send them to prison, and prisons to keep criminals locked away from law-abiding society. The public doesn't often question how police officers do their jobs, yet they are disturbed when criminals are released early from prison or not convicted due to technicalities and become quite upset if any criminal doesn't serve his or her full prison term or escapes from custody.

There is no doubt that several of the aforementioned issues have crossed your mind at some point, perhaps while watching the news or reading your local newspaper. The purpose of this chapter is to inform the reader of the broad array of subjects and issues dealt with by criminologists and criminal justice practitioners. Once familiar with the many aspects discussed, the reader will be able to make a more informed decision regarding a career in criminal justice.

HISTORY AND DEVELOPMENT

Law Enforcement

Many of today's criminal justice policies developed from earlier established English law. For instance, modern law enforcement is rooted in the development of the first paid police force in England in 1829. Named after their creator, Sir Robert Peel, these first police officers were referred to as *bobbies*. County sheriffs derived their names from the term *shire reeve*, law enforcement agents of early English society. The first police departments in America were established in Boston in 1838, New York in 1844, and Philadelphia in 1854 (Senna & Siegel, 2002).

Early police agencies were reactive in nature and did little to prevent crimes within the community. This reactive approach, coupled with foot patrols that impeded communication, hindered investigative methods necessary to control disorder, crime and social upheavals such as riots. Thus, early American police agencies focused on issues such as tax collections; social control within the community was often left in the hands of local citizens (Walker, 1999).

During the nineteenth century, due to immigration from Europe and the Civil War-torn South, cities began to grow larger and more diverse. Commensurately, formal police forces were established in large metropolitan centers, and by 1870, most cities had a formal, organized police force. These early departments placed an emphasis on disorder and crime prevention, as well as a quasi-military organizational structure. During the late nineteenth century, citizens elected police officers. Thus, it comes as no surprise that local politics was at the forefront of most departments, with corruption a probable and common repercussion (Walker, 1999).

The nineteenth century police were commonly seen as incompetent, primarily due to inadequate and inconsistent training. Supervision from administrative positions was also weak, which, in turn, led to poor communication of information. This lack of communication was evident in community relations as well. Coupled with the fact that officer response was reactive, their response to calls for service was very slow. This, as well as undue use of force, excessive corruption, and the bribing of administrators for promotions contributed to public dissatisfaction with police agencies. In a nutshell, the police were seen as social problems themselves and not very effective agents of problem prevention (Walker, 1999).

Throughout the early twentieth century, police organizations evolved through commissions on investigation and initiatives of reform. In the 1920s, for example, August Vollmer developed and implemented administrative missions that are still in use today. Other examples included the development of rigorous statistical data collection and maintenance (i.e., Uniform Crime Reports), implementation of strict officer policies and procedures, the pursuit of academic rigor in the field, and the development and use of technology (i.e., lie detector equipment) (Walker, 1999).

During the Depression, *professionalization* took hold of American law enforcement agencies. Emphasis was placed on enforcement of the law (versus social reform and service), bureaucracy, and the use of science and technology. Prohibition and social unrest, due to troubled economic times, contributed to the shift in work philosophy. After the Depression, professionalization was on the rise, as evidenced by the increased bureaucratization of police agencies, where officers followed a strict chain of command. As the 1950s approached, rapid development of American police forces was aided by the use of cars for patrol and the telephone for citizen summoning service, and the technology of fingerprinting (Walker, 1999).

In the 1960s, however, the public became critical of police forces and their bureaucratic structure. Police officers were seen as distant, and an "us vs. them" mentality developed between the police and the public. Furthermore, new issues arose in conjunction with the Civil Rights Movement and the Vietnam War, including protests and riots. In turn, increasing public dissatisfaction and the lack of officer effectiveness led to many U.S. Supreme Court decisions and federal commissions that changed the operation of modern police departments, such as the practice of reading an arrestee his or her rights and various commissions that focused on the increasing problems of drugs and violent crime. Many of these court decisions and legislative policies continue to guide the operation of police forces.

Nevertheless, several recent developments have taken the field of policing back to its Colonial American roots. Currently, many police departments have developed and implemented community policing endeavors. Reasons for such a shift include public and governmental dissatisfaction with the police, increased education of officers (and hence, the ability of officers to perform multiple, higher-level assignments), and the changing needs of communities (e.g., diversity) (Walker, 1999).

Corrections

As mentioned previously, prior to the development of prisons and jails, colonial America relied on the citizens in each community to identify and punish wrongdoers. Punishments such as banishment, stocks and pillories, and death were used to control individuals deemed as threats to public safety. Colonial American jails were used for the detention of the accused and as facilities to

house sentenced offenders; typically, the facility was the jailer's own home, with inmates paying a fee for services. Inmates shared rooms with inadequate ventilation and little heat, and many facilities very quickly became overcrowded. Nonetheless, in the 1770s, the Walnut Street Jail was opened in Philadelphia–documented as the first jail built on American soil (Blomberg & Lucken, 2000).

The first prisons in the United States were constructed in Pennsylvania and New York during the early 1820s. The Pennsylvania System was based on the Quaker religion; each inmate in the prison was segregated from other inmates in order for them to serve penitence for their misdeeds and to be removed from the contaminating presence of other criminals (hence the term *penitentiary*). The method developed in New York, known as the Auburn System, focused on the profit that could be made from prison labor. Inmates incarcerated in this type of facility were segregated at night, but were placed in each other's company during the day to work manufacturing jobs. They were not permitted to speak to each other, however, and structured living was required; they also wore prison-striped clothing and were marched throughout the institution in what has been termed "lock step" (Clear, Cole & Reisig, 2009; Welch, 2004). As society continued to develop, however, the brutal conditions of the first prisons were recognized. Thus, a new reform took place in America in the late 1800s, referred to as *the reformatory movement*. Based on an ideal of rehabilitation, the reformatories offered educational and vocational training to youthful offenders (Clear, Cole & Reisig, 2009; Welch, 2004).

The ideology driving the reformatory movement led to the development of other progressive penal reforms during the mid-nineteenth century. These reforms included indeterminate sentencing (whereby offenders would serve a range of years, rather than a specified amount of time); parole; probation; and the development of the juvenile court (a system designed to address the best interests of the child). Parole and probation were introduced in Boston in the 1840s. John Augustus, a shoemaker by trade, volunteered to supervise offenders sentenced to conditional, probationary terms in the community rather than having them serve prison or jail sentences. The use of parole was linked to the concept of the indeterminate sentence, as offenders continued to serve their sentence in the community upon release from prison (Clear & Dammer, 2003).

Practices such as the reformatory, the juvenile court, indeterminate sentencing, parole, and probation expanded in the early twentieth century. Importantly, each method placed a heavy emphasis on individualized treatment for the offender. Yet, many of the ideals and goals of the reformatory, parole, and probation never were realized in practice due to administrative resistance, overcrowding, and a lack of sufficient funding. Thus, many observers began to question the effectiveness of the rehabilitative penal system that was championed during the latter half of the nineteenth century and the first half of the twentieth century.

In the 1960s, community programs proliferated; however, the support for these programs was short-lived, as the conservative political ideology of the 1980s resulted in a correctional system that relied on prisons to warehouse offenders. Rehabilitation programs were eliminated, and offender populations began to increase dramatically. Furthermore, drug legislation and "three-strike laws" exacerbated overcrowding. And, unfortunately, these policies have led to more punitive sanctions and overcrowded correctional institutions in the past 30 years (Blomberg & Lucken, 2000).

MISSION AND OBJECTIVES

Law Enforcement

The general missions of law enforcement are to (1) provide public safety to the members of its communities; (2) reduce the fear of crime; and (3) maintain public order. Agencies may word their mission statements differently, but the objectives remain relatively consistent throughout the United States. For instance, the Los Angeles Police Department (http://www.lapdonline.org/search_results/content_basic_view/844) states on its website that "it is the mission of the Los Angeles Police Department to safeguard the lives and property of the people we serve, to reduce the incidence and fear of crime, and to enhance public safety while working with the diverse communities to improve their quality of life. Our mandate is to do so with honor and integrity, while at all times conducting ourselves with the highest ethical standards to maintain public confidence."

Corrections

The mission of the correctional field can be summed up as follows: the care, custody, and control of inmates; providing community safety; and respecting the rights of crime victims, as well as those under correctional supervision (probation, incarceration, and parole) (Welch, 2004). Although the mission statements of different state departments of corrections may vary somewhat, a central component of their existence is in the housing of people who have committed and been convicted of a criminal act. For instance, a visit to the Florida Department of Corrections (http://www.dc.state.fl.us/) website lists its mission as "to protect the public safety, to ensure the safety of Department personnel, and to provide proper care and supervision of all offenders under our jurisdiction while assisting, as appropriate, their reentry into society."

PREDOMINATE PROFILES OF CLIENTS SERVED

In all three areas of criminal justice, the typical consumer would be the general public, although each area is responsible for different aspects of the justice system. For example, law enforcement officials generally work with both victims of crime and the perpetrators of crime. Law enforcement agents are charged with identifying, investigating, and apprehending individuals accused of committing a crime. Nonetheless, they also may be asked to assist members of society in activities that have nothing to do with crime, such as providing assistance to stranded motorists and educating school children, as well as other types of service that aids the community.

Representatives of the court also work with both crime victims and offenders, but in a different way. The concern for court personnel is in determining whether or not the accused should be processed in a criminal court trial. The true victim may even take a back seat, so to speak, to the goals of the court. Recognizing that the victim is often "left out of the court process," many jurisdictions have implemented victim assistance programs within police departments and/or the state prosecutor's office. The objectives of such programs are to provide information and assistance to victims of crime–ensuring that not only the offender but also the victim is provided with certain rights in a criminal trial. For additional information on victims' rights, visit Tennessee's website: http://www.attorneygeneral.org/vicrigh.html.

Community corrections programs, prisons, and jails are charged with carrying out criminal sentences. Once an accused person has been convicted of committing an offense in question, jails and prisons house them–providing public safety through incarceration. Others, however, after conviction, remain in the community to serve their sentence; this includes probation, partaking in community service and other types of *intermediate sanctions*, which are typically more restrictive than probation but less severe than incarceration in prison (Clear & Dammer, 2003).

The typical clients in the criminal justice system often are thought of as *the crime victim* and *the criminal offender*. Recent suggestions have been made that in order to improve the quality of life for all community residents, efforts should be directed toward addressing the actions of the offender, the needs of the victim, and the needs of the community. This philosophy recognizes that criminal actions impact more than just those immediately involved (Clear, Cole & Reisig, 2009). When one expands the scope of the criminal act in this fashion, it is much easier to see that family members of both the victim and the offender are often impacted by the law violation and that the community at large may feel violated and less safe than they did prior to the act taking place. Therefore, more emphasis has been placed on the interactions and relationships of law enforcement officers with members of the community, often locating police substations in crime-prone areas to aid the residents and to develop a local understanding of diverse neighborhoods (Clear, Cole & Reisig, 2009).

PHILOSOPHICAL ASSUMPTIONS

Why are some people arrested, while others are released to return home with no further consequences? Why are some offenders sentenced to prison while others are not? What is the rationale of the American system of justice? Are prisons supposed to punish, deter, or rehabilitate? Are law enforcement officials supposed to protect the public? And if so–How should this be done?

For those who pay attention to the crime situation in the United States, one may think that our system advocates a "get tough" approach to dealing with crime and criminals. However, several philosophies and ideologies are operative in our current system of justice. At any one time, some modes of thinking are more popular with justice officials than others. Nevertheless, a basic review of each ideology will help in an overall assessment of the American system of criminal justice.

Criminal justice in the United States can be organized into three broad ideological models, each with a unique combination of philosophies relating to justice administration: (1) conservative, (2) liberal, and (3) critical. Conservative and liberal perspectives represent the traditional thought within the field, whereas the critical perspective can be described as a radical approach with alternative views and challenges to the traditional models.

The conservative model can be traced back to the first written codes of law and punishment. This model stresses *retribution, incapacitation,* and *deterrence. Retribution* is a justification for punishment based largely on the assumption that a punishment proportionate to the crime committed is just or deserved. Historically, retribution was based on revenge (and the age old idea of *lex talionis,* or "an eye for an eye"), whereas today the philosophy is rooted in the idea of equivalency (i.e., punishment is to be equivalent to the crime committed/harm done). *Incapacitation* states that punishment should decrease crime through incarceration, thereby making it impossible for offenders to commit more crimes. *Deterrence* is the tenet that crime can be discouraged with punishments that are certain, swift and just severe enough (but not too severe).

The conservative model advocates the ideals of accountability, justice, and fairness. Criminal acts, not criminal offenders, are the focus of this approach. However, individual offenders and their personal and social situations are a concern of the liberal perspective. Liberal scholars and practitioners advocate *rehabilitation*–which includes such things as providing education, vocational training, counseling, and other forms of self-improvement while offenders are incarcerated, thus improving their opportunities for leading crime-free lives once released. Rehabilitative measures, interestingly, are based on the assumption that crime will decrease if offenders are prepared to return to society and live in a law-abiding manner upon completion of criminal sentences.

The most recent ideological development in the field of criminal justice is the *critical perspective.* This branch of ideology is more concerned with disparate conditions in society than on crime, criminals, or institutions of the criminal justice system. Critical scholars claim that attempts to incapacitate or rehabilitate offenders are futile if unemployment, homelessness, poverty, inadequate health care, and punitiveness towards certain groups by the criminal justice system are not addressed.

Currently, the conservative model predominates due to disillusionment with the rehabilitative efforts of the mid-twentieth century. Retribution is evident in truth-in-sentencing, mandatory minimum sentences and three-strikes policies. Consequently, offenders are required to spend a specified amount of time behind bars prior to their release back into the community (often 85% of their sentences), justice officials are required to provide a minimum sentence prior to release, and serious/habitual offenders receive stiffer and longer prison sentences after a third felony conviction (Clear, Cole & Reisig, 2009; Welch, 2004). With an element of fairness highlighted, liberal thinkers are appeased, and hence, supportive of some current policies.

MAJOR THEORETICAL FRAMEWORKS

As a student of crime and justice issues, it is important to understand theories of crime and criminal behavior because they provide answers to questions about criminals and crime. Based on systematic research, theories inform us not only about behavior to be expected from those apprehended of crime, but also how to plan, implement, and carry out strategies for reforming offenders.

Within criminology and criminal justice, there are many theoretical perspectives. In fact, theories of crime are so vast in number and specificity that criminologists and criminal justice practitioners utilize frameworks, often referred to as paradigms or schools of thought, to organize specific theoretical perspectives within the field. Each framework represents shifts in the major propositions of previous crime theories, hypotheses of human nature and the structure of society, specific methods for conducting research, and public policy directives. Theories of crime come under one of three schools of thought: classical, positive, and critical.

Classical School

Prior to the American Revolution, crime was thought to be the product of the devil and/or demons. As society began to move away from the influence of religion, the principles of the exercise of "free choice in behavior and equality under the law" began to shape criminal justice philosophy and procedures. Theories that follow classical school principles highlight rational, calculating choices by individuals. Thus, within this school of thought, potential offenders weigh the costs and benefits of a crime prior to engaging in a specific criminal act (Akers & Sellers, 2009). In addition, justice models based on classical school theories place an emphasis on utilitarianism; thus, laws and punishments are developed to serve the greatest happiness for the greatest number. The goal of many policies based on the classical school is to prevent crime, and many punishments are based on aspects related to the crime itself, not the criminal (Welch, 2004).

Positive School

The middle of the nineteenth century brought discontent with rising crime rates. In addition, the advent of rigorous record keeping allowed criminologists and criminal justice practitioners to discern yet another problem: recidivism–offenders returning to crime. Understandably, professionals in the field began to question preventative polices developed and advocated by the classical theorists. The increasing crime problem, coupled with the rapid growth of large industrial centers and immigration, led scholars and policy advocates to reconsider the causes of crime (Blomberg & Lucken, 2000). From this shift in thinking, the positive school was born.

Many of the principles advocated by positive theorists are in direct opposition to the tenets of the classical theorists. For example, society and outside influences beyond one's control act upon the individual; thus, crime is not a product of the offender's free will and choice, but may occur as a result of psychological problems or blocked opportunities for conventional living in his or her environmental circumstances. Policy directives based on positive theories often are rehabilitative in nature, and punishment is based on the offender's characteristics and needs (Welch, 2004).

Critical School

Theories of crime following the positive school tradition predominated within criminology and criminal justice until the 1960s. However, with the advent of the Vietnam War and the Civil Rights Movement, people began to question forces in society–in particular, forces which sought, either consciously or unconsciously, to keep disadvantaged groups in society subjugated. Power structures, through their domination and repression, were seen as the cause of crime. Scholars who aligned themselves with this school of thought became critical of social situations and the criminal justice system (Akers & Sellers, 2009). Hence, this departure from positivistic theories was termed "the critical school." Critical theorists, for instance, question the lack of attention paid to white collar and corporate crime as well as reasons for a disparate number of minorities under correctional control (Welch, 2004).

APPRECIATION OF REAL WORLD APPLICATION

When law enforcement officers encounter someone in need of assistance, especially if that person has been the victim of a crime, one of their primary purposes is to determine if and when a crime has occurred, the extent of injuries to the victim and calling for assistance from medical personnel if needed, and to investigate and apprehend the offender.

Once an offender has been apprehended, the court system is called into action. Then the offender will be formally charged with a crime, and if serious enough, held in jail until trial. County and municipal jails have legally mandated processing requirements that they must follow in order to properly hold the accused for trial. In fact, the majority of people housed in jails today are *pretrial detainees* who have not yet been convicted of any criminal offense (Clear, Cole & Reisig, 2009).

After conviction in the criminal courts, the offender may receive a sentence of probation, any number of intermediate sanctions or be sentenced to jail (for a misdemeanor offense) or prison (for a felony offense). For those given a sentence of incarceration, however, many issues may arise. Those who were employed will lose their jobs, and those who were married or had a family will often lose those close ties and contacts. Being housed in an atmosphere where custody and control are the two main requirements of a hardware secure (locked) facility, will often force the newly convicted individual to associate with other offenders. Moreover, inmates also may have many issues to deal with in addition to the loss of family ties, loss of employment, and forced association. For example, they may have substance abuse problems (drug or alcohol addiction), mental illness (depression, schizophrenia, or a host of others), a low educational status, and/or other health issues, some of which may be treated quickly and easily, while others may be chronic or long-term, such as tuberculosis or HIV/AIDS (Clear, Cole & Reisig, 2009; Welch, 2004). What results from the needs of typical clients is that police officers, court and correctional personnel must be prepared and equipped to work with a wide assortment of people, each of whom has unique problems, issues, and needs.

PROFESSIONAL PREPARATION AND DEVELOPMENT

The field of criminal justice is unique as employees in this arena are charged with maintaining public safety in many different forms. As stated earlier, law enforcement is most responsible for meeting the safety needs of the public at large, investigating criminal activity, and apprehending law violators. However, they also are the most visible members of the criminal justice system—we see police officers at work while we continue with the routine of living our daily lives. Court personnel are responsible for ensuring that our system of justice continues to flow by processing offenders further into or out of the criminal justice system. Overall, the field of corrections is often the most invisible component of our system of justice as the sanction for committing a crime is often conducted behind fences and away from public view.

Students interested in a career in criminal justice have many options. Associates (AA) degrees are offered at many community colleges across the nation. Historically, the study of crime fell within the domain of sociology, but today the field of criminal justice is recognized as an area of study of its own. Because of funding by the U.S. government through such things as LEAA funds, colleges and universities offer criminal justice courses to assist in the development, preparation, and improved professionalization of this field through a four-year program that culminates in a bachelor's (B.A. or B.S.) degree. However, educational and work opportunities do not end at the associate's and bachelor's degree levels. Many universities offer master's degrees and doctorates in criminal justice and criminology.

While the majority of students who have earned associates and bachelor's degrees enter the field after graduation, additional educational opportunities exist. Many law enforcement, court, and correctional administrators have pursued and completed master's degrees. Master's degree programs typically require two additional years of education beyond the bachelor's degree. Doctoral students attend and participate in numerous specialized courses, and usually develop a specialization in one of the three subfields of criminal justice (i.e., law enforcement,

courts, or corrections). A major emphasis of the educational goals of the criminal justice doctoral program focuses on the theoretical and research aspects of crime. Students pursuing the Ph.D. degree can expect to spend a couple of years participating in advanced courses and must develop an original research project that culminates in the writing of a dissertation. Ultimately, Ph.D. students can spend between three and seven years completing all of the requirements for this degree. While those with associate's, bachelor's, and master's degrees may continue working in the field, those with Ph.D.'s typically teach and conduct research in colleges and universities or work for major research organizations.

WORK SETTINGS

Law Enforcement

As the field of criminal justice becomes more specialized, a greater number of law enforcement agencies are requiring applicants to have completed a minimum of two years of education beyond the high school level. Regardless of whether criminal justice students began their educational careers at the community college or university level, every student in this field must have developed a solid framework upon which to build his or her education. Because laws vary from state to state, those employed by law enforcement agencies are often enrolled in police academies—where new recruits are required to pass the courses and simultaneously successfully complete a physical training component and other things such as the successful negotiation of driving/obstacle courses and firearm training. Many agencies now assess new recruits in many areas, not just physical agility. For instance, new recruits may be required to complete a psychological assessment and criminal background check as conditions of employment.

Once training at a certified law enforcement academy is completed, new officers typically begin employment in one of a number of work settings, each varied in mission and structure. Generally, a new officer will be employed by either a local or state agency, such as a city police department or a county sheriff's office. Other specialized forms of law enforcement include the United States Capitol Police, police agencies serving state capitols, and college/university police departments. State level departments include highway patrol agencies and state-level investigative agencies.

Occasionally, a law enforcement officer's first job will be with the federal government; however, a majority of federal agencies require that new employees obtain several years of law enforcement experience prior to submitting an application. A common example of a federal agency is the Federal Bureau of Investigation. Other federal agencies include the U.S. Customs and Border Protection, United States Marshals Service, and the Drug Enforcement Administration. While many federal agencies maintain central offices in Washington, D.C., employees who work within federal law enforcement must be mobile, as employment opportunities and advancement are available throughout the United States.

As law enforcement officers conduct their jobs on a daily basis, they can be confronted with a number of different issues and situations. For instance, in any one day a police officer may be called upon to provide public assistance as he or she diverts traffic away from a motor vehicle accident, respond to a domestic violence call, provide directions to a lost motorist, and investigate the theft of one's personal property. One of the most interesting aspects of a career in law enforcement is the uncertainty of the daily routine, as situations occur in which the officer is provided with many opportunities to utilize a wide variety of problem-solving techniques.

Corrections

The field of corrections encompasses a multitude of work settings. For instance, prisons provide employment opportunities for correctional officers, teachers, counselors and mental health personnel, medical personnel, and administrators. Jails are typically operated by the county sheriff's department and are generally operated by county sheriff's deputies. Community corrections includes such employment opportunities as probation officers, or case managers, parole officers, intensive supervision probation officers, and treatment facility personnel. When the field of juvenile justice is included as a component of corrections, many jobs listed above are also offered; however, the clients in this case are under the legal age of 18 (typically considered the age one becomes an adult in most states). There are jobs available for youth/child service officers (the term used in the juvenile system to identify a correctional officer), juvenile probation officers or juvenile case managers, and aftercare officers (the term used in the juvenile system to refer to a parole officer). Many of the positions in the correctional field require a minimum of a bachelor's degree, in criminal justice or a related discipline (teacher, counselor, and mental health professionals, to name a few). Other positions, such as correctional officer, require a high school diploma or a G.E.D. The correctional officer position often has the most interaction with the inmate population and is responsible for security-related issues. All positions within a correctional setting, however, are responsible for maintaining institutional security.

Those entering the field of corrections are often enrolled in a state training academy in order to receive specialized instruction on the various aspects that their specific jobs entail. For instance, correctional officers will be instructed in the proper use of physical force and restraints; correctional law; state policy and procedure guidelines; and often courses on communication, social skills, and anger management techniques in order to assist inmates in improving their daily living skills and interactions (B. Fowler, personal communication, May 6, 2008). Probation officers and case managers may be provided training on counseling techniques, communication and interaction skills, policy and procedure regulations, and components unique to their job requirements. These may include supervisory techniques, utilizing community resources, and learning to complete state-mandated paperwork (B. Fowler, personal communication, May 6, 2008).

Individuals working in the correctional arena are also provided with a number of different situations. If one is working as a probation or parole officer, for example, the main work responsibilities include supervising offenders in the community. This entails keeping an eye on the offenders, as well as addressing situations that may occur as a result of employment, family, or education needs. To illustrate, a parolee may need assistance in locating employment and housing, assistance in obtaining health insurance, and possibly financial assistance such as food stamps, as well as participating in various counseling sessions—all of which are required to assist the parolee in successfully reintegrating back into society.

FUTURE OUTLOOK

The outlook for the field of criminal justice continues to be promising for students majoring in this discipline. The opportunities for employment as a police officer are projected to increase more than 10 percent by 2016, according to the Bureau of Labor Statistics (http://stats.bls.gov/), while the projected increase for correctional officers and jailers is 17 percent during the same time period. Future employment as probation officers and correctional treatment is expected to grow by 11 percent by 2016 (http://stats.bls.gov/).

Those individuals employed in the criminal justice system, regardless of area of specialization, have found that the majority of their work involves working with other people, such as the general public, victims of crime, fellow police or correctional officers, prosecuting and defense attorneys, court officials, and community corrections representatives. Thus, one should keep in mind that communication skills are very important in these subfields. If you are interested in helping other people in exciting and challenging ways, we invite you to explore this area in more depth and in greater detail.

PROFESSIONAL ORGANIZATIONS

Academic

Academy of Criminal Justice Sciences (ACJS) www.acjs.org
American Society of Criminology (ASC) www.asc41.com
Alpha Phi Sigma (APS) (Nat'l CJ Honor Society) www.alphaphisigma.com
Lambda Alpha Epsilon (LAE) (Nat'l CJ fraternity for students) www.acjalae.org/

General

Office of Juvenile Justice and Delinquency Prevention http://ojjdp.ncjrs.org/
Bureau of Justice Statistics (BJS) http://www.ojp.usdoj.gov/bjs/

Bureau of Labor Statistics
http://www.bls.gov/
National Criminal Justice Reference Service http://www.ncjrs.gov/
National Institute of Justice (NIJ)
http://www.ojp.usdoj.gov/nij/
Sourcebook of Criminal Justice Statistics
http://www.albany.edu/sourcebook/

Law Enforcement

Fraternal Order of Police (FOP)
http://www.grandlodgefop.org/
Federal Bureau of Investigation (FBI)
http://www.fbi.gov/
Drug Enforcement Administration (DEA)
http://www.usdoj.gov/dea/index.htm
U.S. Customs and Border Protection
http://www.cbp.gov/
U.S. Department of the Treasury
http://www.ustreas.gov/
United States Marshals Service
http://www.usmarshals.gov/
International Brotherhood of Police Officers http://www.ibpo.org/
Department of Homeland Security
http://www.dhs.gov/index.shtm

Corrections

American Correctional Association
(ACA) http://www.aca.org/
American Jail Association (AJA)
http://www.aja.org/
Federal Bureau of Prisons (BOP)
http://www.bop.gov/
National Institute of Corrections (NIC)
http://www.nicic.org/

REFERENCES

Akers, R.L., & Sellers, C.S. (2009). *Criminological theories: Introduction, evaluation, and application* (5th ed.). Los Angeles, CA: Roxbury Publishing Company.

Blomberg, T.G., & Lucken, K. (2000). *American penology: A history of control.* New York: Aldine de Gruyter.

Clear, T.R., Cole, G.F., & Reisig, M.D. (2009). *American corrections* (8th ed.). Belmont, CA: Wadsworth/Thomson Learning.

Clear, T. R., & Dammer, H. (2003). *The offender in the community* (2nd ed.). Belmont, CA: Wadsworth/Thomson Learning.

Senna, J. J., & Siegel, L. J. (2002). *Introduction to Criminal Justice* (11th ed.). Belmont, CA: Wadsworth/Thomson Learning.

Walker, S. (1999). *Police in America: An introduction.* New York, NY: McGraw-Hill.

Welch, M. (2004). *Corrections: A critical approach* (2nd ed.). New York,: McGraw-Hill.

WEBSITE SOURCES

Bureau of Labor Statistics (http://stats.bls.gov/). Retrieved May 6, 2008.

Federal Bureau of Prisons (http://www.bop.gov). Retrieved May 4, 2008.

Florida Department of Corrections (http://www.dc.state.fl.us/). Retrieved May 4, 2008.

Los Angeles Police Department (http://www.lapdonline.org/search_results/content_basic_view/844). Retrieved May 4, 2008.

Tennessee Attorney General (http://www.attorneygeneral.org/vicrigh.html). Retrieved May 4, 2008.

Chapter 9

GERONTOLOGY

WILLIAM E. HALEY, KATHRYN HYER & MARY F. MUSHEL

The world is in the midst of an amazing transformation–a longevity revolution (Butler, 2008) that has already changed ideas of aging, growth, and development. A baby born in the United States in 1900 expected to live until 49, but by 2004 a newborn could expect to live until 78 (Federal Interagency Forum on Aging Related Statistics (FIF ARS), 2008). The nearly 30 years of life expectancy gained in the United States in the twenty-first century is unprecedented in history, although increased life expectancy is a worldwide phenomenon dramatically changing all societies. The profound implications of longer life are beginning to be recognized, studied, and debated. Longer life changes family structure, economics, work, health care, business and political institutions. Starting in 2011, the baby boom generation–those born between 1946 and 1964–will begin to turn 65 years old. This cohort has 78-million members. America will require new services and the boomers will provide new models of aging and the changes to our culture; how we study and conceptualize aging should be profound. Indeed, it is an exciting time to enter gerontology.

The study of aging and its implication is called gerontology. Its focus is the scientific study of the process of human aging in all its many aspects: biological, psychological, and sociological. Along with the closely related field of geriatrics (which focuses on clinical aging), it is also concerned with ameliorating problems associated with physical, psychological, social, economic, and other changes with aging. Geriatrics is increasingly recognized as a specialty in medicine, nursing, psychology, and other professions providing healthcare, diagnosis, and/or treatment of older adults.

While views of older people are evolving and more positive images of older people are seen in magazines, newspapers, and on TV, many people have pervasive and persistent negative stereotypes. Students and professionals who work in gerontology recognize the range and diversity of elders and, contrary to stereotype, usually find their experiences very positive. Working with older adults provides helpers not only a sense of satisfaction from helping others, but many individuals also enjoy the stories and experiences that older adults can offer. Older adults and their families tend to be grateful for the help they receive, and a deep bond often develops between professionals and the older adults with whom they work.

BACKGROUND

Despite the growing numbers of elders throughout the world, there are people who fear the changes and there are various myths about older people. A negative stereotypical view of people–just because they are older–is "ageism," a term coined by Robert N. Butler in 1969 that is parallel to racism and sexism. Ageism can be a serious problem for older persons (Robb, Chen & Haley, 2002).

A common myth in our society is to regard older persons as a homogeneous–all alike and uninteresting individuals. However, people actually become more differentiated as they age which results in a more diverse population (Atchley, 1997)–the opposite of the myth. When examining social, physical, and psychological characteristics across age groups, the most common finding is that older persons show great variability. Health and well-being in later life varies from independence and activity to frailty and dependence in a nursing home, and economic situations vary from wealth to extreme poverty. Diversity, however, results in a more difficult task for planners, government and private agencies, as well as for health care and service agencies for older adults. Those who study aging, however, are able to explain why planners need to be more careful in differentiating young old (65–74), old-old (75–84), and the oldest-old (85 and above) who differ greatly in their needs. Furthermore, gerontology students learn the impact of experiences on aging and learn about cohorts. For example, a 60-year-old who grew up during the Depression may have very different savings habits than a 60-year-old who grew up during the boom years of the 1950s.

Other myths include the belief that older people cannot change or learn, are socially isolated and likely to be depressed, are severely disabled and live in nursing homes, and their problems are hopeless. However,

we will address each of these myths and refute them in the pages ahead.

Another factor deterring some students from working with older adults is the typical complexity of older persons' problems. It is important to recognize that almost 80 percent of older adults require care for chronic conditions such as hypertension, arthritis, and heart disease (Institute of Medicine [IOM], 2008). Importantly, 20 percent of Medicare beneficiaries have five or more chronic conditions (IOM, 2008). These diseases require ongoing care and daily decision-making by the patient, and the older adult and their families need to learn how to help their health care providers monitor and manage the condition. The patient also must understand the disease and play an active role in taking medications as prescribed and reporting conditions as they change if the patient is to be an effective member of the heath care team (Hyer, 2007).

Cognitive impairments and other mental health issues also complicate medical care. For example, depression in older adults is usually closely linked to coexisting medical and social problems that also require attention (Dyer et al., 2003; Hasche & Morrow-Howell, 2007).

Professionals arranging social services for older adults often encounter a complex, fragmented network. Without great skill and experience in aging, it is difficult to find information, much less to be able to refer clients, resulting in persistent problems, barriers, frustration, and, frequently, unmet needs (Wacker, Roberto & Piper, 1998). However, some professionals enjoy the complexity and challenge of working with older adults and working in teams to provide collaborative care, and recognize the value and importance of a specialization in aging services.

Old age is the last of the human developmental stages to be studied. This is in part due to the fact that, until more recent times, some persons lived to an advanced age but the great majority did not. As mentioned earlier, the life expectancy increase has meant that the world has seen a rapid increase in the number of older persons. In 1900, only 4 percent of the population of the United States was over 65; by 2005, this percentage had more than tripled to 12.4 percent and is projected to be 20 percent by 2030 (FIFARS, 2008). This can be attributed to such factors as a general improvement in conditions of life, declining mortality rates, and the baby boomers of 1946–1964, whose trailing and leading edge members will be 65 to 84 years of age in 2030.

The growth of the older adult population means that most health and human services professionals will work with older adults as a matter of course. Older adults account for a disproportionate share of health care services because age increases the risk for health conditions, especially chronic illness. The 12 percent of older Americans today account for 26 percent of all physician office visits, 35 percent of all hospital stays, 34 percent of all prescriptions, and 90 percent of nursing home use. Despite the prevalence of older adults in the system, the health-care workforce typically receives little geriatric training. According to a recent report, the United States is "not prepared to deliver the best care to older adults" (IOM 2008, p. 1). Older adults have multiple conditions and concerns, and professionals should have specialized training in aging in order to practice more effectively and ethically.

An old gerontology joke involves 95-year-old Morris who complains to the physician that his knee hurts. The physician sighs and says, "Morris, you are 95, what do you expect?" Morris retorts, "This knee is also 95 and it doesn't hurt." The physician does not seem to recognize that pain is not normal nor does the physician want to work with Morris to encourage Morris' continued mobility and desire to remain active.

Unfortunately, the most common pattern in many healthcare and human services professional education has been to provide little or no exposure to the special problems of older adults in their curricula. Thus, it is common that clinicians who work with older adults have very little knowledge about the elderly. Clinicians also receive little training in working together as a geriatric team even though multiple clinicians interact with patients across settings (Hyer, 1998). The Geriatric Interdisciplinary Team Training Program funded by the John A. Hartford Foundation demonstrated changes in attitudes, knowledge and team skills for the medical residents, nursing and social work students who completed the program (Fulmer, Hyer & Flaherty, 2005).

The IOM report indicates the dearth of geriatric training in virtually every health care profession. Less than 1 percent of physician assistants, pharmacists, or registered nurses specialize in geriatrics. In 1987, the National Institute on Aging predicted a need for 60,000–70,000 geriatric social workers by 2020, yet today only about one-third of the number needed specialize in geriatrics. Of the 633,000 physicians in the United States, 7,128 have a certificate in geriatric medicine and only 1,596 have a certificate in geriatric psychiatry (IOM, 2008).

Haley and Gatz (1995) distinguished between three levels of training in aging: exposure, experience, and/or expertise. All healthcare and human services professionals should receive some minimal *exposure* to geriatrics and gerontology content in their curricula. Improvements have been made in medicine; almost 98 percent of all medical schools have some exposure to geriatrics (Eleazer, Doshi, Wieland, Boland & Hirth, 2005). However, the exposure is frequently late and certainly is inadequate. Additional practicum *experience*, providing supervised training in working with older adults and working as a team member with other clinicians is also highly desirable if not crucial. A further level of training that may include exposure and experience might include completion of a Certificate in Gerontology. There is a tremendous need for professionals with *expertise*, or specialization, in geriatrics or gerontology. In some areas, such as Geriatric Medicine, practitioners can earn a specialized Board Certification; in others, such as Clinical Psychology, postdoctoral fellowships are available to provide specialty training in geriatrics and/or gerontology. A directory of geropsychology training programs, internships, and postdoctoral fellowship programs can be found online at http://gero psych.org/students.t.html. In other areas, specialization is generally accomplished in a more informal manner but should include in-depth study and supervision.

The previously noted demographic changes will make every aspect of life different. All jobs and services will be impacted by the aging of America and the world-wide growth in the numbers of older people. Gerontology knowledge may well-become a core component in most fields. Gerontology continues to include undergraduate or graduate degrees in the field (Peterson, 1987). Gerontology graduates should expect to play direct roles in managing or caring for older adults thorough diverse administrative roles, including nursing home administration and administrative positions in aging services, including adult day care, assisted living facilities, and public agencies (Giordano & Rich, 2001). Geriatric care management is another important role for gerontologists (Cress, 2001), as is the development and evaluation of programs, and entrepreneurship (Peterson, 1987).

Training and education in gerontology are also relevant and beneficial to diverse fields such as business, health care, medicine, law, research, social work, political science, public health, sociology, and education. For example, specialists in elder law and in financial planning issues for older adults, have many career opportunities. Because of the large number of older adults, gerontology

education can complement any other of the human services as well as being a distinct area of expertise in its own right. Just as the elder population itself is very diverse, those who study, practice, serve, or research this group are a multidisciplinary group.

HISTORY

Since life expectancy has increased so much in recent times, there has been a corresponding proliferation of interest in gerontological education, research, and human services. Gerontology courses began appearing in universities such as Duke and the University of Michigan in the 1950s, but the first universities to develop degree programs in gerontology were the University of South Florida and North Texas State University (now the University of North Texas) in 1967. Although many schools had "centers" or "institutes" devoted to some aspect of aging, they did not offer degrees. Students in these programs received certificates of study. Now, many universities have at least some coursework in gerontology, if not degree or certificate programs.

There is increasing attention to diversity, e.g., gender and race/ethnicity, and its effects on aging. The overall life expectancy in 2004 was 75.2 years for men but 80.4 years for women (FIFARS, 2008). Life expectancy for nearly all ethnic minorities in this country is less than for Caucasians. In 2004, the nation's minority population totaled 98 million, or 33 percent, of the country's total of 296.4 million. The US Census Bureau's national population projections suggest that 47 percent of the U.S. population will be from minority groups by 2050. The ethnic minority elderly population has been described as being in "double jeopardy" due to their minority and aging status, and the fact that older ethnic minorities have greater risk of poverty and poor health. On the other hand, minority older adults often have strong coping resources as "survivors" of disadvantage and discrimination, and may rely on faith and family support to cope effectively with the stresses of late life (Haley, Han & Henderson, 1998). Psychological interventions can be tailored to be culturally appropriate for diverse older adults and their families (Gallagher-Thompson et al., 2003).

The increasingly diverse population requires increased knowledge of different cultures, beliefs systems, and family interactions for the health worker to be effective. The study of ethnogeriatrics can be very important for those interested in preparing for the diversity of the aging population. It is important that workers gain knowledge of how health risk varies by ethnicity, how culture impacts health beliefs and behaviors, how family tradition may influence care giving and attitudes toward palliative care as well as develop skills that demonstrate culturally appropriate respect and appropriative assessments methods.

MISSION AND PHILOSOPHY

Human service workers need to understand older persons as well as show them respect, genuine concern, and appreciation. The Code of Ethics of the American Psychological Association (APA) describes six fundamental principles which include: competence, integrity, professional and scientific responsibility, respect for people's rights and dignity (assuring privacy and autonomy), and concern for others' welfare and social responsibility (Haley & Mangum, 1999). Because older adults may be vulnerable and subject to conflicting interests of family and/or society, providers must be especially alert to ethical dilemmas and those who

have such characteristics as warmth, sensitivity to others, loyalty, and commitment to others will be more likely to make caring, ethical decisions (Haley & Mangum, 1999).

As a rule the study of gerontology calls for multidisciplinary programs and services. What makes older patients unique is not their age; it is the high likelihood that they have multiple chronic conditions (comorbidity), functional disability, and coexisting problems that may include a number of pharmaceutical, psychological, and social problems. On the other hand, with optimal exercise, diet, and mental attitude, older adults can age successfully (Rowe & Kahn, 1998). One important concept is the goal of development of reserve capacity, e.g., working throughout our lives to enhance our strength, lung capacity, intellectual capacity, etc., beyond what is required to carry out our daily activities. If people can build up reserve capacity in these areas, then even with losses of strength, lung capacity, or neurons with aging, people can remain active and independent much longer than if they were sedentary and not building their abilities to their full capacity (Andel, Hughes & Crow, 2005; Saxon & Etten, 2002).

Clients or patients may be 65 (or younger) up to 100 (or older), and may be taking many prescribed medications as well as over-the-counter medications, or none at all. It is also common that older adults in good health are volunteering at the nearest nursing home or hospital, helping to take care of elder patients in poor health. Most older adults are independent and function effectively, with only 5 percent of Americans over age 65 living in nursing homes or other institutional settings at any one time. It is important to avoid stereotyping the needs of older persons since these can vary from needing total care to needing help with their golf swing! Typical needs of older clients in human services settings include the need for either formal or informal information, services such as those meeting social needs, psychological needs, health care, and advocacy, or to the most basic needs of food, shelter, and companionship.

Gerontology is based inherently on the belief that all life has value and that each person deserves being treated with respect and appreciation of their dignity and wisdom. Out of respect of their personal self and history, it is appropriate to ask their opinions, where possible, even in minor decision-making and to include holistic modalities which may take into account their younger years while being treated for their present biopsychosocial needs.

MAJOR THEORIES

Aging is often studied from biological, psychological, sociological, economic, and other perspectives, and these disciplines bring their own theoretical frameworks to bear on issues of aging. However several important perspectives that are relevant to human services workers who work with older adults will be mentioned.

Life Span Development

Earlier theories suggested that development was complete with adolescence, but, soon life stages were identified and life span development was recognized as intuitively significant. Adults realize that they can make decisions regarding the modification of behavior, life style, values, and activities. (Kart, 1994) This theory explores all stages of life; people are enriched and broadened by understanding all of life's stages in the complex relationship of age, social and economic status, and health in all of their life (Moody, 2000).

Family Systems Theory

Older adults usually function in a system of family relationships. Most older adults are not isolated, but live near a family member or are in frequent contact with family. When older adults experience disability, families provide over 80 percent of the care, and often do much to prevent institutional placement. Work with older adults involves not only helping the elderly, but also supporting their families (Knight, Kaskie, Shurgot & Dave, 2006). In many cases, families may have adaptive strengths, but aging families may have problems such as unfinished business, hierarchies, and the family's unique homeostasis including situational or developmental crises (Neukrug, 2000).

Stress, Coping, and Adaptation

This framework emphasizes the importance of focusing on environmental stresses and strains, and on individual differences in coping, as ways of understanding well-being and health in older adults. Coping with stressors and adapting to them results in the opportunity for individuals to make appropriate changes in elder years as well as in younger years (Kart, 1994). The theory indicates that stresses accompany role changes in life such retirement, widowhood, and health problems and disability, but that either positive or negative outcome can occur with stress depending on the individual's mental attitude and coping resources (Haley & Jang, 2002).

A particular level of stress is necessary to encourage reaction and function; too much or too little may hinder emotional and physical well-being. Significant events occur throughout life, both positive and negative. Contrary to stereotype, older adults experience fewer negative life events than younger persons, but face specific kinds of stresses including health problems, disability, and bereavement (Jang & Haley, 2002). The manner in which we respond to life events, role changes, and stress in life depends on personal and environmental factors both positive and negative. Personality further influences how people respond to stress (Hooyman & Kiyak, 1996).

Research indicates that high levels of stress lead to increased vulnerability of physical and psychological problems for the elderly. High levels of stressors, with few resources, will put these persons at high risk, while those with substantial psychological or social resources may be less vulnerable. Positive psychological resources such as optimism, self-esteem, internal locus of control, and mastery of skills affect appraisal and choice of coping responses. Spiritual beliefs and religious participation also promote successful coping (Haley & Jang, 2002).

One major theme of stress and coping research is that older adults can be helped to cope with stress through a variety of mechanisms. These may include direct stress reduction, teaching adaptive cognitive appraisals and coping techniques, and eliciting social support.

AREAS OF APPLICATION

Gerontology grew as a result of interest in improving the lives of older adults and their families. As its professional foundations were established in application, this is where it continues to excel. Currently there is a large range of opportunities for gerontologists to work with individuals ranging from the well elderly to the disabled. Although most older adults live in the community, some elders need full-time assistance, sometimes in institutions such as nursing homes and assisted living facilities, and hospice care may be useful at the end of life.

Caregiving has become a major issue for family members, usually spouses and daughters, which is fraught with stress related to economics, depression, and health problems. For example, caring for patients with Alzheimer's disease is extremely difficult for a family member. Appropriate interventions, such as support groups, psychotherapy, and respite care, are often helpful and satisfying for caregivers (Sörensen, Pinquart & Duberstein, 2002). Even when a family decision is made that a nursing home is required, the stress of the decision itself is often difficult for the caregiver.

In the area of mental health, there is a volume of impressive literature documenting that pharmacological and psychosocial interventions both are effective with a variety of late-life mental disorders (Bartels, Haley & Dumas, 2002). Of special interest is the fact that certain psychological therapies, including interpersonal therapy and cognitive-behavioral therapies, have been found to be equivalent in their effectiveness in treating late-life depression (as are treatments with antidepressant medications).

There is considerable evidence that even some of the most difficult problems encountered by older adults—Alzheimer's disease and related dementias—can be helped. There are medications that have been shown to improve cognitive functioning in Alzheimer's patients. Furthermore, both behavior management and pharmacotherapy can be used to manage behavioral problems in these patients (Bartels et al., 2002). Appropriate intervention with family caregivers can be effective not only in reducing caregiver depression, but even in delaying nursing home placement (Mittelman, Haley, Clay & Roth, 2006).

PREPARATION TO WORK IN THE FIELD

Preparation to work in the field of gerontology ranges from high school, to on-the-job training to a doctoral degree. The field is broad, as are requirements for positions in the field. Educational programs exist on a range from vocation, community college, to postdoctoral situations. For example, the M.A. program in Gerontology at the University of South Florida (USF) requires 36 graduate credit hours, and the Ph.D. in Aging Studies at USF requires 90 hours. Information on admissions requirements and other details can be found at http://www.cas.usf.edu/agingstudies/. There are noncredit programs, such as certificate programs, and continuing education programs that are especially valuable for practicing professionals.

The Association for Gerontology in Higher Education ([AGHE], 2004) has identified seven categories of professional roles:

1. **Direct Service Provision.** This can include institutional settings such as independent living in apartments, assisted living, nursing homes, even hospitals with extended care services in a dedicated area. Geriatric care managers coordinate care for older persons, to help them live independently as long as possible by arranging in home, supportive services (Cress, 2001). Other services could be daycare, transportation, meals on wheels, and almost any service imaginable. Some professionals work in private practice settings; psychologists can be reimbursed through Medicare for mental health services. There has also been a significant increase in private geriatric care management, usually paid for directly by older adults or their families, although businesses are increasingly providing elder care assistance comparable to child care support in the workplace, hoping to support women with caregiving responsibilities.

2. **Program Planning and Evaluation.** The major influence on programs for older adults has been the Older Americans Act (OAA) initially passed by Congress in 1965. A unique element of the act has been that all authorized programs and services are offered free of charge to all clients (Gelfand, 1999). There usually are short-term and long-term goals (plans), which need to be well defined to meet clients' needs. The evaluation process may apply to the agency as well as the individual worker.

3. **Management and Administration.** There are a myriad of administrative roles available for gerontologists (Giordano & Rich, 2001). Administrators need special expertise not only in administrative issues, but also specialized gerontological content so programs can meet the needs of older persons and their families. Careers as administrators of long-term care facilities require licensure but are well compensated with the mean national salary of $82,000 (McKnight's Career Guide, 2008).

4. **Product Development and Marketing.** Older persons are increasingly recognized as a large and important market force. Even industries such as those in the automotive and recreation fields, are increasingly devoting at least some of their efforts toward attracting older adult consumers. Hospitals and other organizations that serve older adults increasingly hire gerontologists to develop special aging services and promote these to the public.

5. **Advocacy.** Human service professionals often need to be an advocate, who acts on behalf of the client by negotiating appropriate services and making sure that rules and regulations benefit clients. Unfamiliar bureaucracy frequently intimidates elders; they, nevertheless, deserve fair treatment with dignity and respect. Many states have professional nursing home ombudsmen who protect the rights of institutionalized older adults.

6. **Education and Training.** There is a great need for trained faculty to provide education in gerontology including degree programs at colleges and universities, which can include associate degrees, bachelor's degrees, graduate and undergraduate certificates, and master's degrees. There are also currently a number of doctoral programs in gerontology or aging studies that typically focus on policy research, or research on health and aging (Haley & Zelinski, 2007). There is a particular shortage of specialists in gerontology within major professions such as social work, nursing, medicine, dentistry, psychology, and allied health fields (IOM, 2008). There are also many opportunities to provide continuing education programs. While not widely done at present, it is imperative that the educational process regarding older adults starts early in life. There is increasing interest in intergenerational programs that bring older people and children together for mutual benefit, whether these involve foster grandparenting, collaborative arts projects, collocation of daycare centers with adult daycare, and even creation of intergenerational community charter schools (Whitehouse, Benezu, Fallcreek & Whitehouse, 2000).

7. **Research.** Traditionally, gerontological researchers have completed doctoral degrees in an established academic discipline such as psychology or sociology, and then developed a specialization in gerontological research. A recent trend is the development of doctoral programs in gerontology, or aging studies. There are currently nine such programs in the United States (Haley & Zelinski, 2007). They may supply some of the greatest potential for research in aging with a new outlook on research as well as on education. Universities remain the most obvious centers for concentrated research, although skilled researchers can also find positions at foundations, state and federal government, and even within industries.

INTERVENTIONS

The usual range of interventions for older adults includes modifications of the assessment and treatment approaches used with younger adults. Comprehensive geriatric assessment is the cornerstone of effective intervention for older adults. Several guides to comprehensive assessment in geriatrics and clinical gerontology review assessment of medical, psychological, and social issues in older adults (Gallo, Fulmer, Paveza & Reichel, 2000; Lichtenberg, 1999). One important but relatively neglected area in gerontology is prevention of depression and disability, and promotion of successful aging (Rowe & Kahn, 1998). Results to date are promising that such interventions as exercise, proper nutrition, social support, and development of positive and adaptive attitudes promote health, effective functioning, and quality of life in older adults (Rowe & Kahn, 1998). "Use it or lose it" is a maxim common in gerontology applying to physical, psychological, and social aging. The skills and abilities we continue to use, we will maintain into older age (barring accident or disease) while those we do not continue to use we lose. As individuals, we can make significant choices to increase probability of healthy, positive aging (Saxon & Etten, 2004). Environmental changes in the home, such as use of improved lighting, handrails, and removal of throw rugs, can also be an important part of allowing older adults to remain functional and independent.

Special psychotherapies adapted to older clients, such as Life Review, may be effective. Although medication is frequently offered, older adults may often benefit from counseling, which is seldom offered. A recent review found that there is considerable evidence for the effectiveness of both psychosocial interventions and medications, either separately or in combination, for treating depression and dementia in older adults (Bartels, Haley & Dumas, 2002). Adequate self-help solutions may be used as well as peer therapy; mutual assistance may benefit those in an area where older persons frequently receive little counseling. A number of excellent self-help books are available to help families caring for older parents (Morris, 1996), specific conditions such as Alzheimer's disease (Mace & Rabins, 2006) and terminal illness (Lynn & Harrold, 1999).

In instances of crisis intervention, stabilization is the primary goal (Mehr, 2001). An overriding goal is to insure the self-image of the client by continuing to treat with respect and dignity to help achieve as much autonomy possible and in a careful manner. Services for elders will frequently take place in the home or place of residence although home health care is not as available or affordable as is nursing home care (which may be paid by insurance including Medicare and Medicaid). Services also take place in agencies, at a place of business, community colleges, daycare, or wherever elders congregate.

Blackburn and Dulmus (2007) provide a thorough review of clinical gerontology interventions. Of particular note is the importance of engaging interdisciplinary teams (Hyer, 2007; Zeiss & Steffen, 1996) to bring together the expertise of diverse professionals in resolving the multiple problems faced by elderly clients.

PROFESSIONAL ORGANIZATIONS

Most professions have organizations, which provide support to their members, continuing education, job possibility, credentials, and, not the least, camaraderie, recreation and friendship support. Many of these organizations also offer student membership at a greatly reduced rate so it behooves students to consider membership; the benefit for students is often immeasurable. Some of the organizations in the field of gerontology will be briefly noted.

1. The American Association of Homes and Services for the Aging is an organization of nonprofit long-term care facilities.
2. The American Geriatrics Society is an association of medical specialists who research, diagnose, and treat older adults.
3. The American Health Care Association is a similar organization within the for-profit sector. The Association for Gerontology in Higher Education works to advance gerontological education both in universities and through continuing education programs.
4. The American Psychological Association includes a large Division of Adult Development and Aging (Division 20), and the Section on Clinical Geropsychology (Division 12, Section II) is a home for clinical psychologists who work with older adults.

5. The American Society on Aging focuses on the needs of direct service providers and program administrators and provides extensive continuing education programs.

6. The Gerontological Society of America is a prestigious scientific organization that includes sections for biological sciences, clinical medicine, behavioral and social sciences, and social research, policy, and planning.

7. The National Association of Professional Geriatric Care Managers provides certification for gerontologists and other professionals who provide care management services.

A myriad of other organizations too numerous to mention allow professionals focused on areas such as administration to share knowledge and advance their specialties. Web addresses for the organizations described above are provided after the References of this chapter.

CAREER ADVANCEMENT, OPPORTUNITIES AND SALARIES

The level of a person's education tends to define career advancement as well as salary. The four levels of formal education (associate's, bachelor's, master's, doctoral) most closely reflect the starting salary for gerontologists, followed by experience. A detailed salary survey is provided by the Association for Gerontology in Higher Education (2004). In general, most students who study Gerontology are successful in finding positions and are highly satisfied with these positions (AGHE, 2004). Beginning salaries also are dependent of where one lives. Traditionally, salaries for service personnel are higher in the northern tier of states as

well as in the far West. Salaries are basically dependent on supply and demand. Gerontology is still an unfamiliar field; there is need for more recognition of the need for special training in gerontology to prepare professionals to work with older adults. Because of the general lack of awareness by employers about the importance and relevance of gerontology to diverse fields, it is essential that each student or practitioner in the field practice good public relations in this area.

Students who are innovative and entrepreneurial have the opportunity to invent new career paths and chart their own course in this area. Some of our recent graduates are working in diverse areas, such as grant writing for a local hospital's geriatrics program; providing massage therapy for older adults; developing specialized adaptive wheelchair seating for disabled older adults; and serving as administrators for nursing homes, hospices, and community agencies.

FUTURE OUTLOOK

The outlook for students specializing in geriatrics and gerontology is superb. The need for national education regarding gerontology is great, since again, the field is so new that many are not aware of its existence, much less the need. There is a national need –for more publicity, not only on the availability of educated persons in all areas of society but also on the need for gerontologically-educated persons in all areas of society (not only the "typically" age-related services, but also in all other areas where persons live, work, and recreate such as businesses, industries, and entertainment). Perhaps, with the advent of the baby boomers into status as older adults, this will happen.

There is great need for respect and acceptance of the older generation who experience the last of all "isms"–ageism; this may be alleviated, nonetheless, with the arrival of the "boomers" into a new and sometimes better time for the older retirees. Old age can be a time not only of loss, but also a time of growth and wisdom (Haley, Robb, Jang & Han, 2003), and opportunities are limited only by the imagination of gerontologists.

SUMMARY

Gerontology, the study of aging, is the last chapter in almost everyone's life; it is also the last life stage to be studied by scientists, researchers and scholars. Because this generation is benefiting from the research of the past, most elders are happy, healthy and independent. The beginning of the millennium is an appropriate time to renew interest, to excite young persons, and to inform the public about the potential field of aging. Professionals in the field of human services should make it a priority to develop expertise in gerontology as an important aspect of their professional practice.

REFERENCES

Andel, R., Hughes, T. F., & Crowe, M. (2005). Strategies to reduce risk of cognitive decline and dementia: A review. *Aging Health, 1,* 107–116.

Association for Gerontology in Higher Education (2004). *Careers in aging: Opportunities and options.* Washington, DC: Author.

Atchley, R. C (1997). *Social forces and aging: An introduction to social gerontology* (8th Ed.). Belmont, CA: Wadsworth.

Bartels, S. J., Haley, W. E., & Dumas, A. R. (2002). Implementing evidence-based practices in geriatric mental health. *Generations, 26,* 90–98.

Blackburn, J. E., & Dulmus, C. N. (Eds.) (2007). *Handbook of gerontology: Evidence-based approaches to theory, practice, and policy* (pp. 269–308). Hoboken, NJ: John Wiley & Sons.

Butler, R. N. (2008). *The longevity revolution: The benefits and challenges of living a long life.* New York: Perseus.

Cress, C. (2001). *Handbook of geriatric care management.* Gaithersburg, Maryland: Aspen.

Dyer, C. B., Hyer, K., Feldt, K. S., Lindemann, D. A., Busby-Whitehead, J., Greenberg, S., Kennedy, R., Flaherty, E., & Fulmer, T. (2003). Frail older patient care by interdisciplinary teams: A primer for generalists. *Gerontology and Geriatrics Education, 24,* 51–62.

Eleazer, G. P., Doshi, R., Wieland, D., Boland, R., & Hirth, V. A. (2005) Geriatric content in medical school curricula: Results of a national survey. *Journal of the American Geriatrics Society, 53,* 136–140.

Federal Interagency Forum on Aging Related Statistics (2008). *Older Americans 2008: Key indicators of well-being.* Washington, DC: Author.

Fulmer, T., Hyer, K., & Flaherty, E. (2005). Geriatric interdisciplinary team training: program results. *Journal of Aging and Health, 17,* 443–470.

Gallagher-Thompson, D., Haley, W.E., Guy, D., Rubert, M., Arguellas, T., Tennstedt, S., & Ory, M. (2003). Tailoring psychological interventions for ethnically diverse dementia caregivers. *Clinical Psychology: Science and Practice, 10,* 423–438.

Gallo, J. J., Fulmer, T., Paveza, G. J., & Reichel, W. (2000). *Handbook of geriatric assessment* (3rd ed.). Gaithersburg, MD: Aspen.

Gelfand, D. E. (1999). *The aging network: Programs and services.* (5th ed.). New York: Springer.

Giordano, J. A., & Rich, T. A. (2001). *The gerontologist as an administrator.* Westport, CT: Auburn House.

Haley, W.E., & Gatz, M. (1995). Doctoral training and methods for attracting students to work in clinical geropsychology. In B.G. Knight, L. Teri, J. Santos, & P. Wohlford (Eds.), *Applying geropsychology to services for older adults: Implications for training and practice* (pp. 113–118). Washington, DC: American Psychological Association.

Haley, W. E., Han, B., & Henderson, J. N. (1998). Aging and ethnicity: Issues for clinical practice. *Journal of Clinical Psychology in Medical Settings, 5,* 393–409.

Haley, W. E., & Jang, Y. (2002). Stress and coping. In D. J. Ekerdt, R. A. Applebaum, K. C. Holden, S. G. Post, K. Rockwood, R. Schulz, R. L. Sprott, & P. Uhlenberg, (Eds.), *Encyclopedia of aging* (pp. 1353–1360). New York: Macmillan Reference USA.

Haley, W. E., & Mangum, W. P. (1999). Ethical issues in geriatric assessment. In P. Lichtenberg (Ed.), *Handbook of assessment in clinical gerontology* (pp. 606–626). New York: John Wiley & Sons.

Haley, W. E., Robb, C., Jang, Y., & Han, B. (2003). The wisdom of years: Understanding the journey of life. In J.D. Robinson & L.C. James (Eds.), *Diversity in human interactions: The tapestry of America* (pp. 123–143). New York: Oxford University Press.

Haley, W. E., & Zelinski, E. I. (2007). Progress and challenges in graduate education in gerontology: The U.S. experience. *Gerontology and Geriatrics Education, 27,* 11–26.

Hasche, L., & Morrow-Howell, N. (2007). Depression. In J. E. Blackburn & C. N. Dulmus (Eds.), *Handbook of gerontology: Evidence-based approaches to theory, practice, and policy* (pp. 269–308). Hoboken, NJ: John Wiley & Sons.

Hooyman, N., & Kiyak, H. (1996). *Social gerontology: A multidisciplinary perspective.* Boston: Allyn and Bacon.

Hyer, K. (1998). The John A. Hartford interdisciplinary team training program. In E. Siegler, K. Hyer, T. Fulmer, & M. Mezey (Eds.), *Geriatric interdisciplinary team training* (pp. 3–12). New York: Springer.

Hyer, K. (2007). Geriatric team care. In K.S. Markides (Ed.), *Encyclopedia of health and aging* (pp. 242–244). London: Sage.

Institute of Medicine. (2008). *Retooling for an aging America: Building the health care workforce.* Washington, DC: National Academies Press.

Jang, Y., & Haley, W. E. (2002). Life events and stress. In D. J. Ekerdt, R. A. Applebaum, K. C. Holden, S. G. Post, K. Rockwood, R. Schulz, R. L. Sprott, & P. Uhlenberg (Eds.), *Encyclopedia of aging* (pp. 784-789). New York: Macmillan Reference USA.

Kart, C. S. (1994). *The realities of aging: An introduction to gerontology* (4th ed.). Needham Heights, MA: Allyn and Bacon.

Kastenbaum, R. (1995). Gerontology. In G. L. Maddox (Ed.), *The encyclopedia of aging* (2nd ed.) (pp. 416–17). New York: Springer.

Knight, B.G., Kaskie, B., Shurgot, G.R., & Dave, J. (2006). Improving the mental health of older adults. In J.E. Birren & W. Schaie (Eds.), *Handbook of psychology and aging.* Academic Press: New York, NY.

Lichtenberg, P. (Ed.). (1999). *Handbook of assessment in clinical gerontology.* New York: John Wiley & Sons.

Lynn, J., & Harrold, J. (1999). *Handbook for mortals: Guidance for people facing serious illness.* New York: Oxford University Press.

McKnight's career guide. (2008). Retrieved June 20, 2008 from http://media.haymarketmedia.com/Documents/1/CareerGuide%202008_467.pdf

Mace, N. L., & Rabins, P. V. (2006). *The 36 hour day: A family guide to caring for persons with alzheimer disease, related dementing illnesses, and memory loss in later life* (3rd Ed.). Baltimore: Johns Hopkins University Press.

Mehr, J. (2001). *Human services: Concepts and intervention strategies.* New York: Allyn and Bacon.

Mittelman, M. S., Haley, W. E., Clay, O. J., & Roth, D. L. (2006). Improving caregiver well-being delays nursing home placement of patients with Alzheimer disease. *Neurology, 67,* 1592–1599.

Moody, H.R. (2000). *Aging: Concepts and controversies* (3rd ed.). Thousand Oaks, CA: Pine Forge Press.

Morris, V. (1996). *How to care for aging parents.* New York: Workman.

Neukrug, E. (2000). *Theory, practice, and trends in human services: An introduction to an emerging profession* (2nd Ed.). Belmont, CA: Brooks/Cole.

Peterson, D. A. (1987). *Career paths in the field of aging: Professional gerontology.* Lexington, MA: Lexington Books.

Robb, C., Chen, H., & Haley, W.E. (2002). Ageism in mental health and health care: A critical review. *Journal of Clinical Geropsychology, 8,* 1–12.

Rowe, J. W., & Kahn, R. L. (1998). *Successful aging.* New York: Pantheon Books.

Saxon, S. V., & Etten, M. J. (2002). *Physical change and aging: A guide for the helping professions* (4th Ed.). New York: Tiresias Press.

Sörensen, S., Pinquart, M., & Duberstein, P. (2002). How effective are interventions with caregivers? An updated meta-analysis. *The Gerontologist, 42*, 356–372.

Wacker, R. R., Roberto, K. A., & Piper, L. E., (1998). *Community resources for older adults: Programs and services in an era of change.* New York: Sage.

Whitehouse, P. J., Bendezu, E., Fallcreek, S., & Whitehouse, C. (2000) Intergenerational community schools: A new practice for a new time. *Educational Gerontology, 26*, 761–770.

Zeiss, A. M., & Steffen, A. M. (1996). Interdisciplinary health care teams: The basic unit of geriatric care. In L. L. Carstensen, B. A. Edelstein, & L. Dornbrand, (Eds.), *The practical handbook of clinical gerontology.* (pp. 423–450). Thousand Oaks: Sage.

American Health Care Association
http://www.ahcancal.org/Pages/Default.aspx

American Psychological Association Division of Adult Development and Aging
http://apadiv20.phhp.ufl.edu/

American Psychological Association Section on Clinical Geropsychology
http://www.geropsych.org/

American Society on Aging
http://www.asaging.org/index.cfm

Association for Gerontology in Higher Education
http://www.aghe.org/site/aghewebsite/

Gerontological Society of America
http://www.geron.org/

National Association of Professional Geriatric Care Managers
http://www.caremanager.org/

WEB ADDRESSES FOR MAJOR PROFESSIONAL ORGANIZATIONS IN AGING

American Association of Homes and Services for the Aging: http://www.aahsa.org/

American Geriatrics Society
http://www.americangeriatrics.org/

Chapter 10

INDUSTRIAL-ORGANIZATIONAL PSYCHOLOGY

Lori Foster Thompson & Paul E. Spector

Industrial-Organizational (I-O) psychology is one of the major applied branches in the field of psychology. It is concerned with people's attitudes, behaviors, cognitions, emotions, needs, and personalities at work. I-O psychologists are involved in research on employees and the application of psychological principles from that research to the workplace. There are many different jobs and settings in which I-O psychologists operate, giving them wide latitude to pursue interesting work. Many I-O psychologists are college or university professors who conduct research and teach. The majority, however, work as practitioners in applied settings, e.g., private companies and consulting firms. Consulting firms provide I-O services to organizations that hire them. In the United States, the most common tasks done in these applied settings include: (a) developing tests and systems to select new employees, thereby helping organizations decide whom to hire; (b) designing training programs for employees; (c) designing systems to assess employee job performance; (d) analyzing the tasks involved in jobs and the attributes people need to accomplish those tasks; and (e) conducting surveys of employee attitudes about their jobs. I-O psychologists often get involved in issues of civil rights for minorities and individuals with disabilities. For example, they devise methods to combat discrimination in hiring. I-O psychologists do many additional types of work that are not mentioned above. Moreover, they work in settings other than universities, private companies and consulting firms. The government and the military, for instance, employ I-O psychologists.

BRIEF HISTORY

The beginnings of I-O psychology date back to the early 1900s when scientists began studying problems related to work and work behavior (Krumm, 2001). In fact, the subdiscipline of I-O is nearly as old as the parent discipline, psychology, which was founded in the late 1870s (Landy, 1997). The fields of experimental psychology and engineering heavily influenced the development of I-O. Within those disciplines, several individuals, including Hugo Münsterberg, Walter Dill Scott, Frederick Winslow Taylor, and Frank and Lillian Gilbreth, were very influential (Spector, 2008).

Münsterberg was an experimental psychologist who was interested in how to select qualified employees for different types of jobs. He developed tests that were administered to applicants for a variety of positions, including that of traveling salesmen for the American Tobacco Company, motormen for the Dallas street railway system, and ship captains (Krumm, 2001). In 1913, Münsterberg published *Psychology and Industrial Efficiency*, considered the first industrial psychology textbook.

Around the same time, another experimental psychologist named Walter Dill Scott was also studying methods of employee selection, in addition to a variety of other workplace problems. He is well known for applying psychological principles to advertising (e.g., helping people understand what makes consumers pay attention to advertisements) (Berry, 1998). Scott even introduced the idea of using incentive pay to motivate employees (Krumm, 2001). In 1903, he published his groundbreaking book titled *The Theory of Advertising.*

Frederick Winslow Taylor was another pioneer within the field of I-O psychology. Unlike Münsterberg and Scott, Taylor was not a psychologist. He was an engineer who studied employee efficiency and productivity in the early 1900s. Taylor's system for applying scientific principles to the analysis and design of work came to be known as *Scientific Management* (Riggio, 2008). Frank Gilbreth (an engineer) and his wife Lillian (a psychologist) were two of Taylor's most notable followers. The Gilbreths refined Taylor's ideas, utilizing procedures known as time-and-motion studies to define the specific movements involved in the performance of a job and record the amount of time each movement required. They used this information to determine the "one best method" or "the most efficient combination of movements" for the task at hand. This enabled employers to teach workers the best methods for doing their jobs, thereby increasing efficiency and productivity (Spector, 2008).

In 1917, the United States entered World War I and faced the problem of deciding the type of job to which each recruit should be assigned. A group of psychologists, led by Robert Yerkes, helped the Army with this placement problem by developing intelligence tests that were administered to recruits. Test scores provided information about individuals which could be compared to job demands so recruits could be matched with jobs for which they were best suited. This was the first time large-scale testing was used to place people into jobs. The visibility of this project boosted the development of I-O psychology by demonstrating to employers how systematic and scientific methods could be used to solve personnel problems (Spector, 2008).

During the decades between WWI and WWII, the science and practice of I-O psychology progressed. Organizations began hiring I-O psychologists to help solve workplace problems, especially those related to productivity. At that point, the field was still known as "Industrial Psychology," which is the part of I-O that tends to take a management perspective of organizational efficiency through the appropriate use of people's talents. In contrast, the organizational side of I-O focuses more on the individual employee and seeks to understand behavior and enhance the well-being of employees (Spector, 2008). The "O" side of the profession was launched in the 1920s, with a group of scientists who were working on a series of studies in the Hawthorne, Illinois plant of the Western Electric Company. These now-famous studies inadvertently introduced what has come to be known as the human relations movement–a perspective that emphasizes the importance of social factors in influencing worker performance (Riggio, 2008).

The World War II effort in the 1940s drew heavily on the skills of I-O psychologists, who again played important roles in the selection and placement of wartime recruits. Tests were developed to separate recruits into categories based on their abilities to learn and perform military duties. Additionally, screening tests were created to select candidates for officer training (Riggio, 2008).

Since World War II, several legal events have shaped the development of I-O. For example, the Civil Rights Act of 1964 and the Americans with Disabilities Act of 1991 made it illegal for U.S. employers to unfairly discriminate against minorities and persons with disabilities when making employment decisions such as who to hire and/or promote. Many I-O psychologists have worked to develop hiring, promotion, and other personnel systems that prevent unfair discrimination against protected classes of people. Most recently, we see the impact of technological change on the field. As the world has been drawn together with the Internet, the way I-O psychologists operate has evolved even more so. In the past, the assessment systems, employee surveys, and other devices developed by I-O psychologists were commonly administered in a paper-and-pencil format; now, many of these tools are electronic, and/or can be accessed online.

MISSION

Why does I-O psychology exist? The mission or objective of I-O psychology is to: (a) help organizations function more effectively; (b) enhance the health, safety, and well-being of employees in the workplace; and (c) understand work behavior. As mentioned previously, I-O psychologists work in a variety of jobs and settings. It is possible to meet two I-O psychologists whose jobs look very dissimilar. Yet, regardless of the specifics of an I-O psychologist's employment, he or she is doing that job in order to accomplish one or more of the three objectives listed above.

TYPICAL CONSUMER PROFILE–"WHO YOU WORK WITH"

I-O professionals have four types of clients: organizations, workers, other I-O psychologists, and students. Consider the following example, which illustrates the manner in which organizations and their departments benefit from I-O. Suppose an I-O practitioner designs a system to assess nurses' performance within a hospital department. Both the department and the hospital benefit by obtaining accurate information on the proficiency with which each employee does his or her job. Such information is very valuable. The department and the organization can use it to promote and reward the best performers. Moreover, they can draw on it to determine who needs supplementary job training, thereby using training resources wisely and enhancing performance within the department. There are many additional uses for the performance information as well. In short, almost any department and organization could be key clients and would have much to gain from I-O psychology.

Importantly, the organization and the department are not the only ones who would benefit from the performance appraisal system described above. Many nurses could personally gain from the accuracy and fairness of a valid evaluation and reward system. Indeed, workers within organizations are also primary consumers of I-O psychology. As noted earlier, one of the goals of the profession is to enhance the health, safety, and well-being of employees. I-O interventions benefit workers both directly and indirectly. An I-O psychologist who recommends a program to help employees cope with job stress may directly affect the quality of employees' work lives. An I-O psychologist who designs a valid system for selecting employees may indirectly enhance employee well-being by helping to ensure that individuals are well-suited to the jobs they're asked to perform. Thus, workers within organizations are important consumers of I-O psychology.

Other I-O professionals serve as a third type of consumer. Many I-O psychologists spend time conducting research and making it available to others in the profession. As practitioners helping workers and organizations, I-O psychologists base their advice and their methods on research that has been presented at conferences and published in journals.[1] Unsolved problems within organizations drive the work of researchers, who also base their methods on empirical work conducted by others. I-O psychologists rely heavily on each other's insights; therefore, they too are consumers within the field.

Finally, I-O professors and practitioners work with students both inside and outside of the classroom. Of course, professors teach classes, advise students, and mentor them in conducting research studies. Practicing I-O psychologists often work with students as well. Some teach at colleges and universities as adjunct professors. Others supervise student interns in off-campus settings, such as consulting firms or corporations.

TYPICAL NEEDS OF CLIENTS

In general, most clients desire the same basic things: people who are well-suited to their jobs; good job performance (productive employees, whether they're working as individuals, groups, or teams); a healthy, safe, and high-quality workplace; high work motivation; high job satisfaction; low absenteeism; and low turnover. These are the typical needs of I-O clients.

PHILOSOPHICAL ASSUMPTIONS

The field of I-O psychology is driven by an ideal called the scientist-practitioner model. This means that the I-O profession values both theory and the application of that theory to the workplace. As scientists, I-O psychologists direct their research toward problems that are important to the people working in organizations. As practitioners, they base their interventions on evidence-based methods that have been supported by research. In other words, they implement approaches that have worked or produced the intended result during prior research trials.

The Guidelines for Education and Training at the Doctoral Level in I-O Psychology provided by the Society for Industrial and Organizational Psychology (SIOP, 1999) emphasize the scientist-practitioner model, noting that I-O professionals are often both the generators of knowledge and the consumers of such knowledge. This dual emphasis on theory and practice is valuable regardless of whether one works primarily as an I-O researcher or practitioner. As noted by the SIOP Guidelines, "Those interested in academic careers need to understand both theory and practice to develop sound research. Academicians will also be charged with teaching new generations of I-O psychologists about the theory and applications associated with each content area . . . Thus, students not only need to know each topic in a theoretical sense, they also need to know 'how to' develop and implement associated products" (p. 3).

Thus, the scientist-practitioner model is a philosophy that drives I-O students and pro-

---

1 A more in-depth understanding of research and practice within the field of I-O psychology can be attained by examining the content of the journals and publications from which I-O psychologists draw and to which they contribute. See page 36 (i.e., the Appendix) of Zickar and Highhouse (2001) for a list of 23 scientific journals that publish I-O psychology research findings.

fessionals. In the role of the scientist, I-O psychologists research topics related to organizational problems. Professors who work for universities often spend their time on such research. In the role of the practitioner, I-O psychologists apply research findings to organizational problems. Professionals who work for companies and consulting firms, usually spend a good deal of time in the practitioner mode. Importantly, there are many I-O psychologists in universities, companies, consulting firms and other places who strive to balance the "scientist" and "practitioner" roles. For example, if they work for universities, they do private consulting on the side. Or if they work as consultants, they obtain permission to do research within the organizations where they work. In fact, research and practice settings frequently overlap, with researchers testing their methods "in the field" and practitioners engaging in research before they implement new techniques.

MAJOR THEORETICAL ASSUMPTION

There are numerous theories pertaining to the science and practice of I-O psychology. Most are designed to describe, explain, and/or predict people's attitudes, behaviors, cognitions, emotions, needs, and personalities in the context of work. The I-O psychology profession is driven by profession-specific theories, along with some overarching theoretical assumptions. "Person-job fit" is an example of a major theoretical assumption that underlies most applied work. The concept of "person-job fit" is based on the premise that each person has a particular combination of talents, known as Knowledge, Skills, Abilities, and Other characteristics (KSAOs). It is further assumed that each job has specific requirements, and good

fit occurs when workers have the KSAOs required for their jobs. Much I-O work is geared toward the attainment of person-job fit. In general, this fit can be achieved by: (a) *Measuring the Job.* Determine which characteristics are necessary to perform the job successfully. This process is known as job analysis; (b) *Measuring the Person.* Measure the extent to which applicants or incumbents possess the job-related characteristics identified during job analysis; (c) *Matching the Person to the Job.* This can be accomplished by hiring only those applicants who possess the necessary job-related characteristics identified during job analysis. It can also be accomplished via training, i.e., teaching employees who do not have them the essential job knowledge and skills.

It is assumed that both employers and employees are better off when people are well-suited to their jobs. From the employer's perspective, workers who do not possess the necessary KSAOs are not likely to be productive. From the employee's perspective, a poor fit between the resources/demands of a work environment and the needs, goals, and KSAOs of the worker can lead to stress, strain, illness, and low job satisfaction, among other things (Edwards & Van Harrison, 1993; French & Caplan, 1972; Riggio, 2008). Consequently, I-O psychologists spend a good deal of time assessing the extent to which person-job fit occurs and reducing the gap between job requirements and worker KSAOs.

AREAS OF APPLICATION

I-O professionals apply psychology to a variety of workplace problems. Major areas of application include: selection and placement, training and development, performance measurement, organizational development, and quality of worklife (SIOP, 2001).[2]

2 In addition, some I-O psychologists also work in other areas of psychology, such as consumer psychology and engineering psychology, which is also known as human factos or ergonomics (Riggio, 2008; SIOP, 2001).

In the area of selection, I-O psychologists help organizations determine procedures for deciding which applicants to hire. This often involves developing tests to identify those most qualified. With regard to placement, I-O professionals design systems that allow organizations to determine the jobs for which new hires are best suited. In the area of training and development, I-O psychologists help organizations design programs that effectively teach people what they need to know to do their jobs, while encouraging them to use their newly acquired knowledge and skills on the job. I-O professionals who work in the domain of performance measurement, develop and implement tools and procedures for accurately evaluating employees' job performance.

Many I-O psychologists specialize in organizational development–a family of techniques used to improve the functioning of organizations overall. At its core, an organizational development effort strives for positive change (Cascio, 1995). The goal is to improve how people do their work, how they communicate with each other and how they coordinate their efforts (Spector, 2008).

Over the years, organizations and I-O psychologists have devoted great effort toward the improvement of worklife. Quality of worklife is the condition of all aspects of life at work. It is determined by many factors, including the compensation and benefits workers receive, their chances to participate and advance within the organization, job security, the meaningfulness of work, the quality of interactions among various organizational members, and so forth (Riggio, 1990). Employee health and safety also are topics of notable concern. In fact, *occupational health psychology* (OHP) is a rapidly emerging subarea of I-O psychology, which focuses exclusively on health-and-safety-related topics in an attempt to ensure that employees have the opportunity to operate in a safe and healthy work environment.

PREPARATION AND DEVELOPMENT TO WORK IN THE FIELD[3]

It requires a graduate (master's or Ph.D.) degree to be considered an I-O psychologist. In the U.S., these two degrees can be found among practitioners (those who work in organizations); however, salaries and opportunities are generally higher for Ph.D.-level psychologists. Professors almost always have a Ph.D. In other countries (e.g., some in Western Europe) the situation is more defined by terminal degree, with the master's being the degree of practitioners and the Ph.D. being the degree of professors and researchers.

In the U.S., there are approximately 125 graduate programs, about half of which offer only the master's degree and about half of which offer Ph.D.s. Programs that offer only the master's degree are called "terminal master's programs," whereas those that offer Ph.D.s are called "Ph.D. programs." Ph.D. programs typically allow students to acquire their master's en route to the Ph.D., and therefore it is therefore possible for a student to enter a Ph.D. program directly after earning a bachelor's degree. It is also possible for a student to enter a Ph.D. program after getting a master's degree from a terminal master's program. In this case, the Ph.D. program will often recognize the master's degree earned elsewhere and require less coursework than what is required for someone entering the Ph.D. program without a prior master's degree.

In the U.S., admission is very competitive to most Ph.D. programs. It is based largely but not entirely on grade-point average (GPA–sometimes only junior and senior years) and graduate record exam (GRE–quantitative plus verbal scores at most schools). Letters of recommendation are typically required, but hold less weight than do GPA and GRE scores. Relevant background, such as employment in an I-O relat-

---

3 The following is reprinted, with permission, from Spector (2000).

ed setting or research experience may also be considered during the admissions process. In general, master's programs are easier to get into than Ph.D. programs. Those Ph.D. programs considered the most prestigious are among the most difficult to get into for graduate programs in any field. Solid "A" averages approaching 4.0 and GRE quantitative plus verbal scores of 1200 and often significantly higher are required by the most competitive programs. Most of these programs accept a small number of students each year, and often have over 100 applicants, so they can be very selective. Over the past 10 years, as the popularity of I-O psychology has increased, entry requirements have increased as well. Information about I-O graduate programs in English-speaking countries, including Canada and the U.S., can be found on the Society for Industrial and Organizational Psychology (SIOP) website (www.siop.org). Details about most programs, including entrance requirements can also be located at this site. More details can be obtained from the universities themselves. A good place to start is the individual program websites (the SIOP site has links to most of them).

Most I-O graduate students were undergraduate psychology majors, but many were majors in other fields. Nonetheless, the undergraduate psychology major is helpful as the basic psychology principles and terminology will be familiar. This makes the first year of graduate school easier, but people from other backgrounds can do well with extra effort. Graduate school is far more difficult than undergraduate as the workload is much heavier, and students are expected to work more independently. A master's degree takes about two years to complete; a Ph.D. takes at least four (starting from the B.A.) but the average is around six. As with most difficult endeavors, not everyone who begins a program will complete it. Determination and self-discipline are required, over and above intellectual ability.

The following steps are recommended to students contemplating an I-O career: (a) Take an undergraduate I-O psychology course. If your university doesn't offer one, read an I-O textbook. (b) Get to know three professors—you will need letters of recommendation. The best way to do this is by volunteering to help with research. They don't have to be I-O professors or even psychology professors. (c) Get a good psychology background. Courses most relevant are social and cognitive psychology. (d) Take all the research methods and statistics courses your psychology department offers. (e) Be sure you have a solid background in basic mathematics (i.e., college algebra). Be familiar with computers, as you will have to learn how to use statistical software. Be familiar with word processing, PowerPoint, Excel, and e-mail, and know how to navigate the Internet. (f) Be sure you can communicate well in both spoken and written English. These skills will be needed in graduate school and later in your career. (g) Be sure to get good grades. A solid "A" average will be needed for most programs. (h) Begin investigating graduate programs no later than early in your senior year. Consider a program's emphasis and quality, as well as entry requirements. Most American programs are relatively similar, but there are some that have a specific emphasis, often due to the interests of their faculty. Programs also vary in quality; however, determining program quality is not always easy. SIOP (2006a) offers some criteria against which to judge the quality of graduate programs. These criteria are posted online at the following website: http://www.siop.org/gtp/GTPchoose. aspx. A good way to begin assessing potential programs is to ask professors who are familiar with the I-O field. Look also at the numbers of faculty and students in a program. When evaluating faculty, it is important to look at their research accomplishments. Consider opportunities for practicum experiences and internships, which are important aspects of practitioner training. You also may find it helpful to talk to faculty and graduate students at programs you are considering. (i) Early in your senior year, take stock–compute your GPA and project what it will likely be when your application is considered. Most programs have admission deadlines in early January and make their decisions around March 1st for the following fall semester. Take the GRE early enough so that you can retake it (if necessary) and have your scores submitted before the application deadline. This usually means you should take the GRE around September of your senior year. Once you know your GPA and GRE, you can figure out where to apply. If you have a 3.95 GPA and a 1400 (quantitative plus verbal) GRE score, any program is a possibility. If you have a 3.2 GPA and a 1020 GRE, your possibilities are more limited, but don't give up your career goals yet! Perhaps you can retake some classes, take a GRE prep course and/or try a program with lower entry requirements. Our advice is to go to the best program that will accept you, but don't feel that your career is over before it has begun because you didn't get into one of the "top" programs. There are many great programs from which to choose, even among those that aren't on anyone's top 10 list (Spector, 2000).

WORK SETTINGS

I-O psychologists work in a variety of settings. A recent survey of I-O psychologists asked respondents to indicate the kind of employment setting in which they work (SIOP, 2006b). Overall, 17 percent reported working in the private sector. IBM, JCPenney, and Microsoft are a few examples of private sector organizations that employ I-O psychologists. Meanwhile, 41 percent of the survey respondents said they work in

academic settings, mostly as college professors; whereas 22 percent were employed by consulting firms (Development Dimensions International is an example of a consulting firm); and 9 percent reported working in the public sector, which includes settings such as the U.S. Navy or the City of St. Petersburg. Finally, the remaining 11 percent of the survey sample said they work in some other type of employment setting (SIOP, 2006b).

To some extent, the setting shapes the nature of an I-O psychologist's job. Consequently, the tasks performed by an I-O professor often look quite different from those performed by a practitioner. Spector (1999) provides details regarding the types of tasks commonly performed by professors and practitioners in the field of I-O psychology.

Regardless of the setting, I-O professionals may or may not hold the job title "I-O psychologist." Alternative job titles, such as Management Consultant and Research Scientist, are not uncommon. Other job titles held by I-O psychologists working in industry include Corporate Vice-President, Director, Manager, or Staff Member of Organizational Development, Talent Management, Management Development, Human Resources Research, Employee Relations, Training and Development, and Leadership Development. I-O psychologists working in private research or consulting companies are sometimes titled President, Principal, Vice-President, Director, or Consultant. Meanwhile, those who work in academic settings may have titles such as Assistant, Associate, or Full Professor of: Psychology, Management, Organizational Behavior, or Industrial Relations (SIOP, 2008).

PURPOSES AND INTERVENTIONS

Types of Interventions

The nature of an I-O psychologist's interventions depends upon the area in which he or she is working. Several areas of application (selection, training, etc.) were described previously. I-O professionals working in the area of selection and placement often intervene by developing tests or assessment tools and administering them to help organizations decide whom to hire, whom to promote, and/or which types of jobs different employees should be assigned to. For example, an I-O psychologist might develop a test to measure word processing skills in order to help an organization decide whom to hire for unfilled word processing positions. Prior to administering these tests, however, I-O psychologists spend time validating the test instruments to verify that they measure the intended KSAOs. It is important to ensure that the tests administered to applicants measure knowledge, skills, etc. that are relevant to the job–I-O professionals analyze jobs to determine the essential responsibilities involved and the KSAOs necessary to complete each job successfully. Finally, they develop and implement comprehensive selection, placement, and promotion programs which guide employers in the administration, scoring, and interpretation of tests for applicants and/or current employees.

Those involved in the area of training and development work to identify which employees need training and in what areas. They formulate and implement both technical training programs (e.g., teaching employees how to use a piece of software) and/or programs to improve nontechnical skills (e.g., management and leadership skills). Most I-O psychologists don't actually deliver the training themselves; this is often done by people who specialize in training delivery. I-O psychologists evaluate the effectiveness of training by assessing the degree to which employees like training programs, learn from them, and use their newly acquired knowledge and skills on the job. They also measure the degree to which organizations profit from training. Furthermore, they assist employees to better plan their career efforts. They design career development systems that help people reach their full potential (Campion, 1996).

Performance measurement interventions often begin with criterion development. For example, I-O psychologists might analyze jobs and subsequently specify the requirements for "good performance" within those positions. Afterwards, they may create performance rating forms, which require raters to assess how well employees are doing various aspects of their jobs. I-O psychologists might even help determine which people would be the most appropriate raters and show the raters how to use performance rating forms properly. After developing valid criteria and performance measurement tools, I-O professionals often use performance data to help evaluate overall organizational effectiveness and/or assess the usefulness of training programs and other organizational interventions that are designed to improve productivity.

An I-O psychologist working in organizational development uses a variety of interventions, including team building and survey feedback. Team building requires work teams to complete exercises designed to improve their joint task performance (e.g., smooth coordination of effort) and/or their interpersonal cooperation (e.g., reducing interpersonal conflict). Survey feedback is an organizational development technique that involves conducting a survey of employee attitudes and opinions concerning, for example, job satisfaction, perceptions of job conditions, and opinions regarding problems at work. After survey results are compiled into a report, they are presented to employees. Next, there is a presentation of the results and potential solutions to problems uncovered by the survey are discussed, followed by an effort to implement these solutions (Spector, 2008). There are many other organizational development interventions, in addition to team building and survey feedback. Some involve the analysis of an organization's structure. Most are designed to facilitate organizational change in order to maximize the satisfaction and effectiveness of individuals and work groups.

As previously suggested, quality of work-life is a broad area that involves the conditions of all aspects of life at work. *Occupational health psychology* is a subarea, that focuses on the development of a safe and healthy work environment. I-O professionals who assist in these areas spend time assessing the quality of work life within an organization. Such an assessment may involve measuring absenteeism, turnover, accident rates, employee satisfaction levels, job stress, and so forth. I-O psychologists use a variety of strategies to enhance health, safety, and worklife quality. For example, they may implement programs that increase employee participation in organizational processes or they may redesign jobs to make them safer or more meaningful (Riggio, 1990). Simultaneously, they use research methods to assess whether their interventions improve the quality of worklife as intended.

Goals of Interventions

In short, I-O psychologists employ a variety of interventions. As diverse as these interventions appear, they are all executed in order to achieve a common set of goals. The purpose of each intervention is to: (a) help organizations function effectively; (b) enhance the health, safety, and well-being of employees; and/or (c) understand work behavior.

HOW SERVICES ARE UTILIZED

Organizations in the private and public sectors use the services of I-O psychologists who work either directly for the organizations or for consulting firms that are hired by the organizations. Services are used to improve the workplace; thus, both organizations and their workers are I-O psychologists' clients. As noted, many I-O psychologists work as researchers/professors in colleges and universities. Their clients are students who use their services to learn about things like psychology, business, research methods, and statistics. In a sense, an I-O psychologist's services also are used by other I-O professionals, who base their research and practice on previous I-O work.

PROFESSIONAL ORGANIZATIONS

The Society for Industrial and Organizational Psychology (SIOP) is the major professional organization for the field of I-O Psychology. It is the I-O division of the American Psychological Association (APA). Members of SIOP are also members of either the APA or the Association for Psychological Science (APS). Many I-O psychologists also belong to the Academy of Management (AOM), the International Association of Applied Psychologists (IAAP), the Society for Occupational Health Psychology (SOHP), and/or smaller regional and state associations.

CAREER ADVANCEMENT, OPPORTUNITIES, AND SALARY

Within the field of I-O, career advancement opportunities are generally quite good. Salaries vary widely according to the type of job and organization. A recent survey conducted by Khanna and Medsker (2007) notes that in the year 2006, the median salary for master's-level SIOP members was $72,000. (In other words, half of the master's-level survey respondents earned less than $72,000, and half earned more than $72,000.) The median salary for Ph.D.-level SIOP members was $98,500. The median starting salary for professors was $55,600, whereas median starting salary in applied settings (e.g., corporations and consulting firms) was $73,750. Overall, the range of salaries is large, depending upon the specific job setting and region of the country, with many I-O psychologists earning over $100,000 per year.

OUTLOOK

The I-O job market has traditionally been strong, and as of this writing it is perhaps the best it has ever been in both the academic and applied areas. In the academic realm, many universities have been starting or expanding their graduate programs, and an academic job can be found for individuals with reasonably strong records (for a new Ph.D., this means a few publications and some teaching experience). In the applied area, jobs are plentiful; however, there can be spot shortages in applied jobs, especially in places that have I-O programs turning out people who compete with one another. Applied jobs are found mainly in large cities, so it can be difficult to have a career as an I-O practitioner in a small town. Layoffs sometimes occur, but we know of no one who has left the field because he or she was unable to find an I-O job, and those who lose jobs typically find new ones rapidly. The future for the field looks bright, although during economic slow-downs, jobs become more difficult to find. It does not seem that the existing programs will turn out

too many I-O psychologists, so the job market should remain good in the foreseeable future (Spector, 2001).

SUMMARY

Most employers and employees desire the same things: people who are well-suited to their jobs; good job performance; a healthy, safe, and high-quality workplace; high work motivation; high job satisfaction; low absenteeism; and low turnover. The field of I-O psychology, which dates back to the early 1900s, is concerned with achieving these ideals. It requires a graduate degree to be considered an I-O psychologist. Once that degree is obtained, career opportunities are quite good. I-O professionals offer their services to organizations, employees, other I-O psychologists and students. They work in many areas, including selection (hiring), training, and organizational development, to name just a few. In general, I-O psychologists spend their time researching jobs and employees and subsequently applying psychological principles from that research to the workplace in order to understand work behavior; help organizations function more effectively; and enhance the health, safety, and well-being of employees. Much applied work is carried out in order to achieve a good fit between workers and the jobs they are asked to do.

REFERENCES

Berry, L. M. (1998). *Psychology at work: An introduction to industrial and organizationalpsychology* (2nd ed.). Boston: McGraw-Hill.

Campion, M., (1996). Why I'm proud to be an I-O psychologist. *The Industrial Organizational Psychologist, 34* (1), 27–29.

Cascio, W. F. (1995). Whither industrial and organizational psychology in a changing world of work? *The American Psychologist, 50,* 928–939.

Edwards, J. R., & Van Harrison, R. (1993). Job demands and worker health: Three-dimensional reexamination of the relationships between person-environment fit and strain. *Journal of Applied Psychology, 78,* 628–648.

French, J. R. P., & Caplan, R. D. (1972). Organizational stress and individual strain. In A. J. Marrow (Ed.), *The failure of success* (pp. 30–66). New York: AMACOM.

Khanna, C., & Medsker, G. J. (2007). 2006 income and employment survey results for the Society for Industrial and Organizational Psychology. *The Industrial-Organizational Psychologist, 45*(1), 17–32.

Krumm, D. J. (2001). *Psychology at work.* New York: Worth.

Landy, F. J. (1997). Early influences on the development of industrial and organizational psychology. *Journal of Applied Psychology, 82,* 467–477.

Riggio, R. E. (1990). *Introduction to industrial / organizational psychology.* Glenview, IL: Scott, Foresman and Company.

Riggio, R. E. (2008). *Introduction to industrial / organizational psychology* (5th ed.). Upper Saddle River, NJ: Pearson Prentice-Hall.

SIOP (1999). *Guidelines for education and training at the doctoral level in industrial/organizational psychology.* Bowling Green, OH: Society for Industrial and Organizational Psychology, Inc.

SIOP (2001). *Who are industrial-organizational psychologists?* [Online] Available November 10, 2001: http://www.siop.org/TIP/SIOP/brochure.html. Available May 6, 2008: http://www.psychology.uwaterloo.ca/gradprog/programs/phd/ind_org/io_field_desc.html.

SIOP (2006a). *How to choose a graduate training program.* [Online] Available May 16, 2008: http://www.siop.org/gtp/GTPchoose.aspx.

SIOP (2006b). *Member survey: Overall report.* [Online] Available May 6, 2008: http://www.siop.org/reportsandminutes/survey_results06.aspx.

SIOP (2008). *Maximizing human potential within organizations: Learning the science behind talent management* [Online] Available May 7, 2008: http://www.siop.org/visibilitybrochure/complete.pdf.

Spector, P. E. (1999). *What's an I-O job like?* [Online] Available May 16, 2008: http://shell.cas.usf.edu/~spector/iojob.html.

Spector, P. E. (2000). *Pursuing an I-O psychology career.* [Online] Available May 7, 2008: http://chuma.cas.usf.edu/~spector/pursuingio.html.

Spector, P. E. (2001). *Industrial/organizational psychology: Frequently asked questions, FAQ.* [Online] Available May 7, 2008: http://chuma.cas.usf.edu/~spector/iofaq.html.

Spector, P. E. (2008). *Industrial and organizational psychology: Research and practice* (5th ed.). New York: John Wiley & Sons.

Zickar, M. J., & Highhouse, S. (2001). Measuring prestige of journals in industrial-organizational psychology. *The Industrial-Organizational Psychologist, 38* (4), 29–36.

ADDITIONAL SOURCES AND THEIR WEBSITES

Academy of Management
http://www.aom.pace.edu

American Psychological Association (APA)
http://www.apa.org

Association for Psychological Science (APS)
http://www.psychologicalscience.org/

European Association of Work and Organizational Psychology (EAWOP) http://www.eawop.org/web/

Human Factors and Ergonomics Society
http://www.hfes.org

International Association of Applied Psychology Organizational Psychology Division http://allserv.rug.ac.be/~pcoets/div/home.htm.

Occupational Information Network, O*NET
http://online.onetcenter.org/

Occupational Outlook Handbook (For all "I'm A People Person" occupations) http://www.bls.gov/OCO/

The Professional I-O Psychologist Network
http://www.piop.net/

Research on the Net Page
http://psych.hanover.edu/Research/exponnet.html

Society for Industrial and Organizational Psychology http://www.siop.org

Society for Occupational Health Psychology (SOHP) http://www.sohp-online.org/

Chapter 11

MARRIAGE AND FAMILY THERAPY

SCOTT JOHNSON

The field of marriage and family therapy comprises a wide range of activities and approaches to the problems of human behavior and relationships. Although like other helping professions, it has roots extending back to the nineteenth century, it is one of the more recently established mental health fields.

Its signature feature, the practice of seeing not just individuals in psychotherapy, but couples and family members, or even roommates and coworkers, initially helped distinguish it in outward appearance from other mental health professions. Yet beyond the number of people in the room with the therapist, marriage and family therapy is unique for its premise that the behavior of individuals cannot be separated from the context of their relationships. Further, what we often call dysfunctional behavior in individuals is in many cases influenced or caused by basic problems in those relationships themselves. Thus treating human mental health problems requires addressing and understanding people's intimate connections.

Not all couple or family therapy involves multiple people in the therapy room. But all good family and couple therapists, whether working with individuals, partners or spouses, families or other constellations, organize their thinking around how clients' relationships impact their problems. Family therapy concepts have even been applied to relationships that imitate family structures, but are not actual families, including business groups and other organizations.

Marriage and family therapy aims to enhance couple and family relationships as well as individual functioning (Gurman & Kniskern, 1981; Gurman & Jacobson, 2002), and has been used to ameliorate domestic violence (Stith, Williams, & Rosen, 1990), child and sexual abuse (Busby, Glenn, Steggell, & Adamson, 1993), substance abuse (Haley, 1987), eating disorders (Haley, 1984), chronic illness (Minuchin & Fishman, 1981), and mental illnesses such as schizophrenia (Bowen, 1988), and major depression (Keitner, 2005). Increasingly, it is used to help solve problems in businesses and other organizations (Staub, 1997), and even occasionally employed to examine relationships between nations in conflict (Morris, 2006).

HISTORY AND DEVELOPMENT

Like other human service fields, marriage and family therapy developed from the conjunction of several influences, including new theories in clinical mental health, frustrations with individual psychotherapy, and larger social forces in the early and middle 1900s. Two of the most powerful theories were Ludwig von Bertalanffy's (1968) *General System Theory*, which argued that many forms of human experience and social and scientific problems could be thought of as *systems*, and Murray Bowen's (1988) *transgenerational* theory of families, which held that the ways we relate to others in our marriages and families are largely learned from the relationships of our forbearers.

General System Theory

General System Theory basically contended that it was important to try to see a variety of phenomena in the context of larger structures. Whether it was physicists studying atoms or social scientists looking at communities, "it is necessary," Bertalanffy wrote, "to study not only parts and processes in isolation, but also to solve the decisive problems found in the organization and order unifying them" (1968, p. 31).

To relationally oriented therapists looking for better ways to understand how people functioned in relationships, Bertalanffy's ideas were electric, because they gave them a firm basis to stop thinking of human behavior in isolation—looking solely at an individual's unconscious thoughts or her instinctual responses to stimuli as was common at the time—and instead focus on the ways that people interacted with each other, how they argued or agreed, how easy or difficult it was for them to share their feelings with one another, whether both became agitated if one was upset, and how they felt when other people—in-laws, coworkers, friends—attempted to join their family or couple activities. To early family therapists, write the scholars Irene and Herbert Goldenberg (2004), Bertalanffy's "systems concepts became a useful *language* for conceptualizing a family's interactive process" (p. 71; italics in original). Marriage and family therapists in fact often refer to the major theories and perspectives of the field as *systemic* or *systems* concepts because of Bertalanffy's influence.

Bowen Family Systems Theory

The second theoretical development central to the growth of marriage and family therapy was Murray Bowen's (1988) vision of how family behaviors were passed down over generations, an idea he called the *intergenerational transmission process*. Bowen's argument was that many of the actions we commonly think of as solely under the control of individuals—the choice of whom to marry (or not), of whether or not to have children, and even seemingly nonvolitional things like symptoms of depression or anxiety, often had their roots in learned behaviors established by our progenitors. Thus, for example, the widely commented on pattern associated with John F. Kennedy, or his brothers Joe and Robert, of engaging in extramarital affairs is, in transgenerational terms, less a reflection of their own personal failings or even the marriages they were in per se, than their affairs and marriages were reflections of the kinds of relationships and interactions they had learned from their parents, and that their parents had learned from their mothers and fathers before them. Such patterns are maintained, in Bowen's view, because they serve a variety of practical purposes, and also merge sympathetically with behaviors that have been transmitted to spouses during their development.

Scholars have noted, for example, that, while the Kennedy men's extramarital involvements made them appear as "cads" and "cheats," they also made them look masculine and powerful (McGoldrick & Gerson,1985). And being wed to a man whom some of the world's most beautiful and famous women clearly were attracted to inevitably enhanced a wife's own aura of desirability. He might have an affair with a movie star, but he had married *her*. Both husbands and wives, from such a perspective, clearly derived benefits from what otherwise looked simply like "infidelity," but in reality was far more complex.

Further, patterns of "cheating" husbands and "betrayed" wives–or vice versa–often can go back several generations, as was true of the Kennedys (McGoldrick & Gerson, 1985). Bowen's central idea was that understanding such factors–how by and large our relationships are shaped by the relationship patterns of our progenitors–can give us sufficient information to consciously choose alternative behaviors. In Bowen's view, such knowledge allows us to "differentiate" ourselves from our ancestors, rather than simply mindlessly following in their footsteps–or mindlessly rejecting them.

Unlike Bertalanffy's General System Theory, in which the concept of "system" was largely a metaphor, Bowen claimed that all families actually *are* systems. Thinking of families systemically for Bowen was a recognition of the true nature of families' basic structure, even in the animal world. Scholars (Johnson, 1996) in fact have examined intergenerational patterns in chimpanzee families such as those studied by the renowned primatologist, Jane Goodall, which has helped validate Bowen's point.

Frustration with Orthodox Psychotherapeutic Approaches

Apart from their novelty and insight, the ideas of Bertalanffy, Bowen, and other early marriage and family therapists gained followers because of many clinicians' frustrations with traditional individual psychotherapy. Carl Whitaker (1972), one of the most influential figures in the early years of the field, wrote about his disillusionment with trying to treat clients with schizophrenia through individual and later group sessions. It simply wasn't, he felt, getting anywhere. "Dissatisfied with each of these as a method of understanding or treating schizophrenia," he said, "we moved on to treating couples and then entire families" (p. 97). Many were frustrated that the dominant psychological and psychoanalytic concepts still had not moved beyond individual treatment. "Psychoanalytic concepts," David Chabot (1983) wrote, "continue to err in the direction of focusing too much on the individual's internal representation of an internal experience" (p. 331)–thus ignoring the impact of people's relationships on behavior.

Social Forces

A number of converging social forces also played important roles in the development of the marriage and family therapy profession. These include the work of sex researchers such as Magnus Hirschfeld and Alfred Kinsey in the early and middle twentieth century, and the family life education and marriage guidance movements of the mid-1900s (Broderick & Schrader, 1981).

Sex Research and Education

Studies in this previously forbidden area of human sexuality had obvious impacts on intimate couples and families. Just as today people write or phone to ask advice from genuine sex scholars such as Ruth Westheimer (the well known "Dr. Ruth") or, less reliably, "teletherapists" such as Phil McGraw ("Dr. Phil"), people in the early 1900s were hungry for knowledge about sexual intimacy (Broderick & Schrader, 1981)–a time when contraception was still illegal in much of the U.S. Childbirth was particularly hazardous, and was a common cause of death among women. As Margaret Sanger (2004), founder of Planned Parenthood, noted the "blessed event" was, for many women in the early 1900s, a highway to the grave. These developments helped give people permission to discuss what had previously been taboo, opening up the possibility of one day actually consulting experts on marital and family matters.

Family Life Education and Marriage Guidance

Family life education and marriage guidance had similar effects. Family life education, begun as an effort to improve parenting in the 1880s, led in the middle 1900s to courses and workshops in mate selection, sexual ethics, sex education for children, and improving the process of divorce (Broderick & Schrader, 1981). Many of the central figures in family life education, such as Ernest Groves and Paul Popenoe, not surprisingly, became leaders in the early development of marriage counseling, since their students invariably sought premarital and marital guidance from them. "If one raised pragmatic, immediate, significant life questions with people," the scholars Calfred Broderick and Sandra Schrader wrote, "it was inevitable that they would wish to discuss them further with their instructor" (p. 11).

Marriage guidance, which in the early twentieth century had been the province of clergy, physicians, attorneys, teachers, and social workers (Broderick & Schrader, 1981), gradually came to take on the organization, scholarship and standards which would lead to its development as part of the regulated field of marriage and family therapy. In the spring of 1945, at the close of World War II, Groves and several colleagues officially founded the American Association of Mar-

riage Counselors, forerunner of the American Association for Marriage and Family Therapy, with the specific intention to "establish and maintain professional standards in marriage counseling" (Broderick & Schrader, 1981, p. 13).

Specialized training for clinicians who wished to practice in this new field, as well as the creation of a code of ethics specifying acceptable standards of behavior for marriage and family therapists soon followed (Broderick & Schrader, 1981). State legislatures began officially to recognize the unique nature of therapy with couples and families, and the special dangers to the public of practitioners who lacked advanced training, and passed laws regulating marital and family therapy practice, first in California in 1964, followed quickly by Michigan in 1966, and New Jersey in 1968 (Nichols, 1992).

Resistance to Marriage and Family Therapy

No profession develops without resistance. Some of the first clinicians to work with families did so in secret, fearful their colleagues might view them as violating psychotherapy's traditional resistance to therapist contact with a client's relatives (Chabot, 1983). Members of other mental health communities sometimes attempted to argue that marriage and family therapy was simply another technique, rather than a genuinely new way of understanding human behavior (Nichols, 1992). Yet such obstacles have, over time, been overcome, largely through efforts to continuously improve training and clinical services, and to demonstrate to regulatory agencies and others in the U.S., Canada, and other nations the singular nature of marriage and family therapy practice, and its clear therapeutic benefits.

The primary force in much of this success has been the American Association for Marriage and Family Therapy, which developed specialized graduate training and credentialing standards, along with scholarly periodicals and conferences, and has lobbied extensively for state regulation to protect the general public. In 1978, the U.S. Department of Education (then called the Department of Health, Education and Welfare) recognized the Association's accrediting arm, the Commission on Accreditation for Marriage and Family Therapy Education, as the official accrediting body for marriage and family therapy, making its standards for training family and couple clinicians the touchstone for the field (Nichols, 1992). At present, the Commission oversees over one hundred masters, doctoral and post-graduate training programs. Marriage and Family therapy also became one of, if not the first mental health discipline to require specific training for clinical supervisors, creating the Approved Supervisor designation to assure trainees that their clinical mentors in fact were qualified to oversee their work (Nichols, 1992).

As of this writing, the practice of marriage and family therapy is regulated in 49 U.S. and two Canadian jurisdictions, and the field itself is recognized by the U.S. federal government as one of five "core" mental health disciplines, along with psychiatry, psychology, social work, and psychiatric nursing (Substance Abuse and Mental Health Services Administration, 2007).

MISSION AND OBJECTIVES

The most general definition of the mission and objectives of the field of marriage and family therapy is the improvement of both individual well-being and intimate relationships through a better understanding of the emotional connections that influence our lives. And while this mission is mainly accomplished through clinical interventions –working with people in therapy–family therapy also has the potential to help us all better understand the role relationships play in shaping human behavior.

Scholars have noted that family systems concepts help us comprehend many aspects of human behavior apart from clinical problems. Some of the greatest works of art and literature, from *Hamlet* (Lidz, 1975) to Arthur Miller's *Death of a Salesman* (Lipton, 1984) to classic works of sculpture (Johnson, 1992) are reborn in the light of family systems analysis. Lipton in particular noted how relational themes such as parent child alliances and parentified children–children asked to take on the role of a parent–are notable throughout Miller's masterpiece. One recent author (Morris, 2006) has used systems concepts to examine the current relationship between the United States and Iraq, while Jacob Weisberg (2008), editor of *Slate* magazine, has undertaken what can only be called a family systems exploration of President George W. Bush, studying how his family relationships influenced the vast majority of his political decisions, from tax cuts to the invasion of Iraq.

CLIENTS TYPICALLY SERVED

In the early days of family therapy, many of its clients were children and families from the inner cities (Minuchin, Montalvo, Guerney, Rosman & Schumer, 1967). Family therapists and their progenitors also founded a number of child and marriage guidance centers around the U.S. and Canada (Broderick & Schrader, 1981), including the Council for Relationships (formerly the Marriage Council of Philadelphia), Child and Family Guidance Centers, in Dallas, Texas, and Woods Homes in Calgary, Alberta. Many, like Woods Homes, were specifically intended for the underprivileged or indigent.

By and large, family therapists serve the range of people found in modern society. Victims of kidnappings (Molina, Agudelo, de los Réos, Builes, Ospina, Arroyave, Lopez, Vásquez & Navia, 2005); family business owners (Staub, 1997); people of color, immigrants, gay and lesbian families, couples, and individuals (McGoldrick, 1998); substance abusers and their relatives (Haley, 1987); sexual assault survivors, people with eating disorders, families with young children, couples experiencing divorce (Gurman & Kniskern, 1981); individuals and families struggling with major mental illnesses (Keitner, 2005), people dealing with the deaths of children or other loved ones (De-Frain, 1991); adoptive families (Friedlander, 1999); blended families (Shalay & Brownlee, 2007); elderly clients (Faber, 2003); rural couples and families (Bagarozzi, 1982); couples seeking premarital help or marital enrichment (Gurman & Kniskern, 1981); wealthy families or poor; healthy individuals, couples and families; or individuals, couples and families in distress—there is no end to a list such as this. Family therapists have even worked with the British comic actor John Cleese (Skynner & Cleese, 1984) and the fictional prime-time television family, the Simpsons (Pipkin, 1989).

PREEMINENT THEORIES AND PRACTICAL APPLICATIONS

Over the years, therapists have classified theories about marriage and family therapy in a number of ways (Gurman & Kniskern, 1981; Goldenberg & Goldenberg, 2004). Most are commonly regarded as either *psychodynamic, transgenerational* (which we have discussed earlier), *structural, strategic, experiential, behavioral,* or *postmodern.* No theory or model has thus far been shown to be objectively preferable to another, though the field is filled with many debates. There are even arguments that it is not the *differences* in models but their *similarities* which are most important to therapeutic progress, a perspective called *common factors.*

Psychodynamic Theory

Psychodynamic family therapy can be seen as a way to use the concepts and symbols of traditional Freudian psychoanalysis as a means to conceptualize roles and patterns in the relationships of couples and families. The family therapist Nathan Ackerman (1982), for example, wrote about a family consisting of a mother and father in their middle forties, a 16-year-old daughter and the mother's mother, who have come for therapy because the daughter has shown signs of psychosis—a state of being divorced from reality.

Ackerman described the family relationship in classic Freudian terms. The parents, he surmised, were unready to become parents when the daughter was born, and thus project onto her their own negative feelings, seeing her as the cause of their unhappiness. She symbolizes, he wrote, "the alien and dangerous elements in the family" (p. 429)—Freud's *id*, while the grandmother, who wants to send her to boarding school and thus literally get rid of her, takes on the role of the *superego*—the rigid, moralizing part of ourselves which is often singularly harsh and critical. The mother allies with her own mother against her offspring, while the father is the ineffectual *ego*, or self of the system, unable to help the id and superego—the daughter and the mother and grandmother, learn to live with and accept each other.

With this perspective on the family established, treatment became relatively straightforward: helping the mother differentiate from the grandmother and lessening the grandmother's influence, supporting the father, who, in Ackerman's view, wanted to be both a good husband and father, but was thwarted by the mother-grandmother alliance, and removing the daughter from her role as holder of all things bad in the family, helping both parents to gradually accept and appreciate her presence as a positive addition to, rather than a detraction from, their household.

Ackerman does not tell us if this approach was successful—presumably it was—but what he does clearly show us is how a Freudian analytic perspective can be used to help understand and attempt to cure the dysfunctions in a troubled family.

Structural Theory

A structural approach to marriage and family therapy, as the name implies, looks for problems in the nominal structure of relationships. This can take any number of forms, but among the more common is the "parentification" of children, in which children are forced to take on adult responsibilities.

A common instance occurs, for example, when parents struggle with alcoholism, and children of necessity become responsible for things such as making meals, cleaning the house, and ensuring they all get to and from school. In structural terms, the *executive* subsystem—the parental structure, is broken, forcing the children to take over. Parentification also can happen if a parent dies and a child takes on the role of the missing parent, or if a parent is habitually immature or irresponsible, forcing children into parental duties.

The aim of structural family therapy is to help reestablish proper boundaries between the roles of children and those of parents, placing the children back into what structural therapists call the *sibling subsystem*, dependent on and subordinate to the parents—not the other way around (Minuchin & Fishman, 1981).

Strategic Family Therapy

The term "strategic" implies many things, but largely it connotes that the therapist, rather than the client, is responsible for bringing about change in the client system (Haley, 1987). Rather than focus on insight, as classical psychoanalysis and many of its derivatives had, strategic therapy was meant to solve problems. "If successful therapy," wrote Haley (1987), "is defined as solving the problems of a client, the therapist must know how to formulate a problem and how to solve it. And if he or she is to solve a variety of problems, the therapist must not take a rigid and stereotyped approach to therapy" (p. 8).

Strategic therapy, therefore, was to be flexible, problem focused, and above all, economical. If classical psychoanalysis might last months or years and be held as often as two or three times a week, strategic therapy should be as efficient as possible. When the client or clients thought the problem was solved, therapy should end, regardless of the therapist's own view of the situation. Whereas in psychodynamic or structural family therapy, the problem that clients identified—such as the teenage daughter—was seen simply as a mask to cover the "real" issue—the parents' ambivalence about having a child in the first place—in strategic therapy relieving the symptom was sufficient. The therapist was not to substitute her or his judgment of what the clients needed for the clients' opinion (Haley, 1987).

These ideas were seen by many as radical, and by some as unethical (Gurman & Kniskern, 1981)—but they had great impact and appeal. Strategic therapists became well known—sometimes infamous—for creating unorthodox tasks and ordeals for clients in order to foment change, a practice that became enshrined as "ordeal therapy" or *paradoxical interventions* (Haley, 1984).

A family whose five-year-old still was not toilet trained might be warned, for example, of the "consequences" of having this problem corrected–did they think they could adjust to a "normal" life? They were used to cleaning up after their son. All that would change if he used the toilet (Haley, 1984).

This approach is known as *restraining change* in order to increase the clients' unconscious motivation to behave differently. Yet many therapists found such methods unacceptable. "Critics have argued," noted the Goldenbergs (2004), "that strategic methods are too manipulative and authoritarian, and that many of their paradoxical efforts are simplistic and transparent" (p. 264). Nevertheless, they have had widespread influence.

Strategic therapy also gave rise to *brief family therapy*, sometimes called *solution-focused therapy* (de Shazer, 1988), and the *Milan model* of family therapy (Boscolo, Cecchin, Hoffman & Penn, 1987). Like strategic therapy, both approaches aim for short treatments periods, often only a handful of sessions. Both approaches also look for large changes developing from seeming small or ambiguous interventions.

Experiential Approaches

The two best known exemplars of experiential family therapy are Carl Whitaker (Whitaker & Bumberry, 1988) and Virginia Satir (1968). Both developed approaches that often have been seen as idiosyncratic to themselves, and thus difficult to teach others, yet both had important impacts in the field. For both Whitaker and Satir, the "genuineness" of the therapist was critical and was a means of modeling behavior for clients. Satir saw the goal of therapy as helping clients learn to "level" with each other, to talk frankly and clearly from their own perspectives. Like Bowen, she encouraged clients to make "I" statements rather than speak for others or trying to "mind read." "I'd like to go to the movies. How about you?," clearly was preferable to "Would you like to go to

the movies?" which tells nothing of the speakers' feelings.

Equally critical to good therapy was what she and others called the *self of the therapist* – the willingness to be personally engaged in the therapeutic process (Whitaker & Bumberry, 1988). "As a professional therapist," Whitaker stated, "you must care enough to get in and get involved, while retaining enough love of self to withstand the cultural mandate of sacrificing yourself to save the family" (p. 35). Whitaker also insisted that all the relevant members of an emotional system be present in therapy. If a couple came in complaining that one or both had had an affair, the therapist must insist that the paramours attend as well, strange as that might seem to others. His point, of course, was that the *system* involved not just those related by blood or law, but by *emotional connections*, good or bad. Whitaker called this the *battle for structure*, and it was a central part of his work (Whitaker & Bumberry, 1988).

Behavioral Approaches

Behavioral approaches to marriage and family therapy, as the name implies, tend to stress the importance of practicing healthy behaviors and ways of relating (Gurman & Kniskern, 1981). Much behavioral family and couple therapy involves having parents or couples practice clearer communication and effective interactions in session and at home, on the theory that what is practiced repeatedly will ultimately change the nature of our habits of thinking, a process known as *cognitive restructuring* (Goldenberg & Goldenberg, 2004).

Early work in behavioral marital and family therapy focused on a number of classic behavioral conditioning concepts. Couples in behavioral marital therapy are encouraged to develop positive expectations of change and to practice desirable behaviors in order to reinforce them (Jacobson, 1981).

Behavioral parent training focuses similarly on restructuring parent responses and examining the patterns of actions and consequences in families (Gordon & Davidson, 1981). Recent work in this area has resulted in what are called "Integrated" behavioral approaches. These are said to more fully look at the feelings of clients in therapy, rather than simply at behavior, and give greater room for feelings as part of the course of treatment (Goldenberg & Goldenberg, 2004).

Postmodern Therapy

"Postmodern" approaches to marital and family therapy primarily revolves around uses of and ideas about language and the nature of reality. ". . . Beyond language," wrote the Chilean scholars Carlos Mendez, Fernando Coddou and Humberto Maturana (1988), "there are no things" (p. 168). Others have likewise asserted that there is no reality except in language and that it is the language we use which creates our sense of problems in our lives (Anderson, 1996).

Many scholars have challenged such assertions, arguing that they distort the meaning of terms like language and reality, and defy common sense (Held, 1995; Koertge, 1998). Others have said the term "postmodern" itself has no real meaning and note that there are few if any commonly accepted definitions of the term (Miller, 1994).

As a rule, postmodern therapists tend to eschew ideas like "expertise" and "therapeutic knowledge" (Hoffman, 1992), and argue that the client must be the "expert" and involved in *coconstructing* the course of treatment with the therapist. The central element in postmodern therapy is the idea that simple conversation, as opposed to rehearsals or ordeals, examinations of family history or the genuineness of the encounter, is the critical element in helping clients change.

Postmodern therapists thus ask questions designed to elicit information both for themselves and the client's understanding (Anderson, 1996). As conversation develops, new formulations of the problem and potential solutions emerge (Anderson, 1996; McNamee & Gergen, 1993).

It is arguable, of course, that this approach simply takes us back to insight as the basis for change–more talk equals greater client understanding. *Narrative therapy* (White & Epston, 1990) attempts to offer specific kinds of conversations in order to facilitate change.

Narrative therapists, for example, argue that therapists should specifically encourage clients to see problems as existing *outside* themselves, rather than being part of who they are. Thus a child who is plagued by encopresis–defecating involuntarily in one's pants–is told not that he "poops his drawers" but that he is being attacked by "sneaky poo," and that in order to improve, he doesn't need to change *himself,* only to "fight harder" against the "poo" that "sneaks up on him" (White & Epston, 1990). This is called *externalizing the symptom*–making clear to the client that the problem is not *in* him or her, not a part of his or her identity, but something external she or he can do something about. This is similar to the tendency in the helping professions generally to avoid, for example, calling someone "paranoid" and instead saying that the person *suffers from paranoia,* a phenomenon external to the person. Narrative therapists further encourage their clients to *restory* their problems. Rather than saying, "I've tried everything and failed," clients are encouraged to think of what they haven't tried, and thus see themselves, for example, as "persistent" rather than unsuccessful (White & Epston, 1990). Again, however, it is unclear how this differs from the technique of *reframing,* or providing an alternative perspective on an experience, which is common to nearly all therapies.

PROFESSIONAL PREPARATION AND DEVELOPMENT

Training in marriage and family therapy in order to practice independently requires a master's degree in marriage and family or equivalent coursework, supervised clinical experience, and passing a licensing examination, typically the Association of Marital and Family Therapy Regulatory Boards' (AMFTRB) Examination in Marital and Family Therapy (amftrb.org).

Courses typically cover systems theory, clinical models, individual and systemic psychopathology and assessment, human development, and research methods. In programs accredited by the Commission on Accreditation for Marriage and Family Therapy Education, masters' students typically receive 500 hours of supervised face-to- face client contact, half of which is therapy with couples or families. Students also commonly receive at least one hour of supervision for every five hours of therapy they conduct, and at least half their supervision usually involves two supervisees or fewer with one supervisor. Half or more of supervision typically is conducted via live observation through one-way mirrors, video monitors, or reviews of videotaped therapy sessions. This ensures that supervision is immediate, and actually focuses on what has occurred in the clinical session.

Doctoral training expands on this base, involving advanced work in theory and models, additional training in human development, and intensive work in research methods. It also requires coursework and experience in the supervision of marriage and family therapy trainees, and additional supervised clinical training along similar lines as master's-level work, including a nine- to 12-month off campus clinical internship. Students serve internships at presti-

gious centers in the U.S. and Canada, including the Houston Galveston Institute, the Chicago Center for Family Health, and the University of Nebraska Medical Center.

Doctoral students also must produce a dissertation exploring a previously unexamined aspect of the marital and family therapy world. Articles from such dissertations frequently find their way into some of the fields most important journals, including the *Journal of Marital and Family Therapy, Family Process,* and *Contemporary Family Therapy.*

Once licensed, clinicians also may train to become Approved Supervisors. To do so, they must complete a course in supervision, provide 180 hours of supervision to at least two trainees and undergo 36 hours of face-to-face work with her or his training supervisor–the person who oversees preparation for this credential.

Beyond a master's degree in the field, states' licensing boards typically require an additional two years of supervised clinical work beyond graduate training and successful completion of the licensure exam. Compared with other master's-level licensed mental health fields, training in marriage and family therapy can be somewhat more time consuming and expensive. Yet it also is clearly the best training available for those who genuinely wish to work with individuals, couples, and families from a family systems perspective.

WORK SETTINGS

Just as family therapists treat people from all walks of life and in a wide variety of contexts, so the work settings of family therapists are extremely varied. Many work in traditional independent practice, as psychotherapists have done for years, while others may serve in group settings with a collection of helping professionals–physicians, psychiatrists, psychologists, counselors (Goldenberg & Goldenberg, 2004). Still others practice in churches and community agencies, social service departments, medical schools, college counseling centers, or are professors at major research universities. Some have practiced in the military, as chaplains, social workers, and psychologists, including some who have served in combat, and aboard naval aircraft carriers (D. Fennell & E. Boyette, personal communications, 1995 & 2007).

As previously mentioned, an increasing number of marital and family therapists are turning their skills toward the problems of businesses and organizations, since the ability of well-trained, systemic thinkers to see orders and patterns of relationships is not limited to family connections. In such settings, their skills in sorting out role conflicts and confused patterns of communication often are highly valued (Staub, 1997). Salaries for consultants in this area can easily range into six figures (personal communication, J. Paul, 2002).

PROFESSIONAL ORGANIZATIONS

Marriage and family therapists are represented in a variety of settings by several important organizations. The American Association for Marriage and Family Therapy (aamft.org) represents over 25,000 practitioners in the United States and Canada, advancing the protection of clients, the progress of research and study, the improvement of graduate and postgraduate training, of governmental regulations, and the general education of the public in systemic concepts and practice.

This work is complemented by the Association of Marital and Family Therapy Regulatory Boards (amftrb.org), a collection of delegates from state licensure boards around the U.S., which, as noted earlier, develops and oversees the administration of the Examination in Marital and Family Therapy, reviews standards, as well as ensures that clinicians disciplined for malpractice or other violations do not simply move to new jurisdictions to avoid censure or forfeiture of their right to practice.

The American Family Therapy Academy (afta.org), is a group of scholars and researchers dedicated to advancements in the knowledge and understanding of marriage and family therapy theory and practice (Nichols, 1992). Not a credentialing or lobbying organization, they instead hold conferences and other activities intended to improve knowledge in the field.

The International Family Therapy Academy is similar to The American Family Therapy Academy but functions on an international scale. Both groups often coordinate conferences, especially those held in the United States.

Other mental health professions also have subgroups which offer membership for those interested in marriage and family therapy. The American Psychological Association (apa.org) has a division devoted to family psychology, Division 43, while professional counselors interested in marriage and family therapy may join the International Association of Marriage and Family Counselors (iamfc.com).

FUTURE OUTLOOK

There seems little question that the demand for family-based services will only continue to grow. Trends in society such as the recent "family values" movement and interest by legislators, policy makers, scholars, and the public in the critical nature of family functioning seem to ensure a healthy demand far into the future for a variety of marriage and family services, as well as for the vital insights of systemically trained thinkers. Given the relative newness of the profession itself, it is a field where young professionals often are able to quickly make important contributions. This seems especially true in the search for collaborations with medical and other professionals, including the emerging interest in clinical practices based on sound empirical evidence (Denton, Walsh & Daniels, 2002).

Family therapy, wrote Gus Napier (1972) nearly forty years ago, "is part of the movement toward greater openness" (p. 40) in society, part of a trend toward fuller and clearer examination of what it means to be human, to live life fully, passionately, hopefully. It was seen as a new window into human understanding, one that offered families, couples, and individuals the hope of better relationships, of fuller and happier lives.

Much has changed since that time, but family therapy still offers such hope today. Those hopes will be realized by those with the courage to explore the sometimes frightening, often perplexing, sometimes amusing, and always fascinating bonds that are the fabric of our lives. It will require new pioneers in research, in practice, in education, and in advocacy for the field. That is the future and the challenge before us.

SUMMARY

"'Far more human activity,'" wrote Murray Bowen in 1975, "'is governed by man's emotional system than he has been willing to admit'" (*Psychotherapy Networker*, 2007). Far more of our lives, in other words, are controlled by our relationships than we have heretofore recognized. Just as Freud's discovery of the unconscious revolutionized our understanding of individuals, so the discovery of systemic concepts has changed forever the ways we see ourselves. The theories and models of family therapy help us reexamine, explore, and ultimately fix the challenges and difficulties of human relationships. For "none of us," as the master family therapist Nathan Ackerman (1958) noted, "lives his life alone" (p. 15).

REFERENCES

Ackerman, N. W. (1958). *The psychodynamics of family life.* New York: Basic Books.

Ackerman, N.W. (1982). In D. Bloch, R. Simon & N.W. Ackerman (Eds.), *The strength of family therapy.* New York: Taylor & Francis/Routledge.

Anderson, H. (1996). *Conversation language and possibilities: A postmodern approach to therapy.* New York: Basic Books.

Bagarozzi, D. (1982). The family therapist's role in treating families in rural communities: A general systems approach. *Journal of Marital and Family Therapy, 8,* 51–58.

Bertalanffy, L. von. (1968) *General system theory* (Rev.). New York: George Braziller.

Boscolo, L., Cecchin, G., Hoffman, L., & Penn, P. (1987). *Milan systemic family therapy.* New York: Basic Books.

Bowen, M. (1988). *Family therapy in clinical practice.* Northvale, NJ: Jason Aronson.

Broderick, C.B., & Schrader, S.S. (1981). The history of professional marriage and family therapy. In A.S. Gurman & D.P. Kniskern (Eds.), *Handbook of family therapy* (pp. 5–35). New York: Brunner/Mazel.

Busby, D.M., Glenn, E., Steggell, G.L., & Adamson, D.W. (1993). Treatment issues for survivors of physical and sexual abuse. *Journal of Marital and Family Therapy, 19,* 377–392.

Chabot, D.R. (1983). Historical perspective on working with the individual in family therapy. In E.G. Pendagast (Ed.), *Compendium II: The best of the Family 1978–1983* (pp. 40-44). New Rochelle, NY: The Center for Family Learning.

de Shazer, S. (1988). *Clues: Investigating solutions in brief therapy.* New York: W.W. Norton.

DeFrain, J. (1991). Learning about grief from normal families: SIDS, stillbirth, and miscarriage. *Journal of Marital and Family Therapy, 17,* 215–232.

Denton, W.H., Walsh, S.R., & Daniel, S.S. (2002). Evidence-based practice in family therapy: Adolescent depression as an example. *Journal of Marital and Family Therapy, 28,* 39–45.

Faber, A.J. (2003). Therapy with the elderly: A collaborative approach. *Journal of Family Psychotherapy, 14,* 1–14.

Friedlander, M.L. (1999). Ethnic identity development of internationally adopted children and adolescents: Implication for family therapists. *Journal of Marital and Family Therapy, 25,* 43–60.

Goldenberg, I., & Goldenberg, H. (2004). *Family therapy: An overview* (6th ed.). Pacific Grove, CA: Books/Cole–Thomson Learning.

Gordon, S.B., & Davidson, N. (1981). Behavioral parent training. In A.S. Gurman & D.P. Kniskern (Eds.), *Handbook of family therapy* (pp. 517–555). New York: Brunner/Mazel.

Gurman, N.S., & Jacobson, A.S. (Eds.). (2002). *Clinical handbook of couple therapy.* New York: Guilford.

Gurman, A.S., & Kniskern, D.P. (Eds.). (1981). *Handbook of family therapy.* New York: Brunner/Mazel.

Haley, J. (1984). *Ordeal therapy.* San Francisco: Jossey-Bass.

Haley, J. (1987). *Problem solving therapy* (2nd ed.). San Francisco: Jossey-Bass.

Held, B.S. (1995). *Back to reality: A critique of postmodern theory in psychotherapy.* New York: W.W. Norton.

Hoffman, L. (1992). A reflexive stance for family therapy. In S. McNamee, & K. Gergen (Eds.), *Therapy as social construction* (pp. 7–24). London: Sage.

Jacobson, N.S. (1981). Behavioral marital therapy. In A.S. Gurman & D.P. Kniskern, (Eds.), *Handbook of family therapy* (pp. 556–591). New York: Brunner/Mazel, Inc.

Johnson, S. (1992). The *Laocoon*: Systemic concepts in a work of art. *Journal of Marital and Family Therapy, 18*(2), 113–124.

Johnson, S. (1996). Family of the forest: Fatal enmeshment and other systems issues in the animal world. *Contemporary Family Therapy: An International Journal, 18*(3), 447–461.

Keitner, G.I. (2005). Family therapy in the treatment of depression. *Psychiatric Times.* Available online at http://www.psychiatrictimes.com/display/article/10168/52636.

Koertge, N. (Ed.). (1998). *A house built on sand: Exposing postmodern myths about science.* New York: Oxford University Press.

Lidz, T. (1975). *Hamlet's enemy.* New York: Basic Books.

Lipton, A. (1984). "Death of a Salesman": A family systems point of view. *The Family, 11,* 55–67.

McGoldrick, M. (1998). *Re-Visioning family therapy: Race, culture, and gender in clinical practice.* New York: Guilford Press.

McGoldrick, M., & Gerson, R. (1985). *Genograms in family assessment.* New York: W.W. Norton.

McNamee, S., & Gergen, K. (eds.) (1992). *Therapy as social construction.* London: Sage.

Mendez, C.L., Coddou, F., & Maturana, H.R. (1988). The bringing forth of pathology. *The Irish Journal of Psychology, 9,* 144–172.

Miller, Stephen. (1994, January). A postmodern age: What is it? *Current.*

Minuchin S., & Fishman, H.C. (1981). *Family therapy techniques.* Cambridge, MA: Harvard University Press.

Minuchin, S., Montalvo, B., Guerney, B.G. Jr., Rosman, B.L., & Schumer, F. (1967). *Families of the slums: An exploration of their structure and treatment.* New York: Basic Books.

Molina, B., Agudelo, M.A., de los Réos, A., Builes, M.V., Ospina, A., Arroyave, R., Lopez, O.L., Vásquez, M., & Navia, C.E. (2005). Kidnapping: Its effects on the beliefs and the structure of relationships in a group of families in Antioquia. *Journal of Family Psychotherapy, 16,* 39–55.

Morris, M. (2006). *A cybernetic analysis of the United States of America's relationship with Iraq* [electronic resource]. Available at: http://scholar.lib.vt.edu/theses/available/etd-12232006-234249/.

Nichols, W. (1992). *Fifty years of marital & family therapy.* Alexandria, VA: American Association for Marriage and Family Therapy.

Pipkin, M. (Producer). (1989). Family therapy [television episode]. *The Simpsons.* Century City, CA: Twentieth Century Fox Broadcasting.

Psychotherapy Networker. (2007). The most influential therapists of the past quarter century. Retrieved on 29 June 2008 from http://www.psychotherapynetworker.com/index.php?category=magazine&sub_cat=articles&type=article&id=The%20Top%2010&page=6.

Sanger, M. (2004). *The autobiography of Margaret Sanger.* Mineola, NY: Dover Publications.

Satir, V. (1968). *Conjoint family therapy.* Palo Alto, CA: Science and Behavior Books.

Shalay, N., & Brownlee, K. (2007). Narrative family therapy with blended families. *Journal of Family Psychotherapy, 18,* 17–30.

Skynner, R., & Cleese, J. (1984). *Families and how to survive them.* New York: Oxford University Press.

Substance Abuse and Mental Health Services Administration (SAMSHA). (2007). Minority fellowship program. Washington, DC: Author.

Staub, D. (1997). *The heart of leadership: 12 practices of courageous leaders.* West Valley City, Utah: Covey Leadership Center.

Stith, S.M., Williams, M.B., & Rosen, K.H. (Eds.) (1990). *Violence hits home: Comprehensive treatment approaches to domestic violence.* New York: Springer.

Weisberg, J. (2008). *The Bush tragedy.* New York: Random House.

Whitaker, C. (1972). We became family therapists. In A. Ferber, M. Mendelsohn & A. Napier (Eds.), *The book of family therapy* (pp. 83–133). Boston: Houghton-Mifflin.

Whitaker, C., & Bumberry, W.A. (1988). *Dancing with the family: A symbolic-experiential approach.* New York: Brunner-Mazel.

White, M., & Epston, D. (1990). *Narrative means to therapeutic ends.* New York: W.W. Norton.

Chapter 12

MEDIATION: A COLLABORATIVE APPROACH TO DISPUTE RESOLUTION

William A. Lambos

Mediation is one of many methods, or approaches, that parties may choose to use when they have a disagreement, problem, or issue to solve. Specifically, mediation involves the hiring of a specially trained person—the mediator—to help the parties communicate and negotiate, and hopefully achieve a resolution of their problem or dispute. Unlike many other forms of dispute resolution, such as litigation (i.e., lawsuits), the parties to mediation agree to enter the process on a voluntary basis; furthermore, the mediator has no authority to impose any form of settlement. Rather, the mediator plays the role of peacemaker, strenuously avoiding taking sides and using his or her skills to assist the parties in reaching a mutually acceptable resolution to the dispute.

Mediation is often referred to as a form of *alternative dispute resolution*, or ADR. But to what is it an alternative? Alternative dispute resolution refers to methods of dispute resolution that are an alternative to adversarial litigation where the parties present their arguments to a judge or jury who ultimately decides the dispute. ADR evolved because litigation typically is very expensive, takes a long time, and usually results in at least one side being the loser. Most people involved in the field of mediation contrast their approach not only with litigation but with other approaches to settling conflicts or disputes as well. Some of the other ADR approaches include negotiation, arbitration (which may be binding or nonbinding), and neutral evaluation. Each of these approaches differs in at least one or more important ways from mediation. For example, in arbitration, the neutral decides the matter, like a judge would do, but arbitration is typically less formal and less expensive than litigation.

Mediation is often seen as highly desirable relative to its alternatives. Not only is it far less expensive than litigation, it also takes a fraction of the time in most cases. While litigation tends to create or increase rancor between the parties, mediation tends to generate goodwill (or at least not increase ill will). In fact, most participants surveyed after mediation report mediation was greatly preferred to the known alternatives (Friends Conflict Resolution Programs of Philadelphia [FCRPP], 2007). Perhaps most telling, mediation, both as a process and as a profession, tends to be greatly enjoyed by *mediators* themselves. Forrest Mosten, in his 2001 edition of *Mediation Career Guide*, wrote:

You can visit any conference of mediators, mediation Web site, or local mediation firm or group, and you will be impressed by the mediators as people and by their positive outlook toward themselves as professionals and their lives outside the office. The spring in the step of mediators is in contrast to the burnout of and stress that many lawyers experience with the legal system (and often with their adversarial colleagues), the frustration that mental health professionals feel toward the intrusive stranglehold of managed care, the depression of public school teachers, and the unhappiness and lack of control that pervade so many in corporate life. (p. 3)

Surely, if ever there were a process and a profession that was deemed "win-win-win" by every party involved (including the mediator), it would be mediation. Fortunately, the occupation of Professional Mediator may be just this. For the right individual, few professions can match the rewards, both intrinsic and extrinsic, of professional mediation (Bowling & Hoffman, 2003).

STATE OF THE ART OF PROFESSIONAL MEDIATION

What then, makes mediation unique? The section on "Philosophical Assumptions and Theories" later in the chapter addresses the distinguishing characteristics of mediation in detail. For the present, nonetheless, it can be asserted that mediation differs from other approaches to dispute resolution by virtue of its adherence to the following set of principles, each summarized as follows:

1. *Voluntary Participation.* Parties to mediation agree to participate. While a governing body such as a court may compel participants to appear at mediation, any party, at any time, can leave mediation without reaching an agreement.
2. *Self-Determination.* This is a fundamental principle of mediation. The media-

tor can assist the parties in arriving at a solution but can never *impose* one. The parties are the ones who self-determine the outcome to their dispute or problem.
3. *Impartiality and neutrality.* Ethical standards typically provide that a mediator must be impartial—must act even-handedly with all parties. The mediator also must be neutral—disengaged from the outcome and not seek to decide the matter for the parties. If any circumstance arises that threatens or impacts the mediator's ability to act impartially or to remain neutral, he or she must withdraw from the process.
4. *Confidentiality.* Communications by the parties in a mediation session are generally confidential and may not be revealed or discussed outside of the mediation session.
5. *Empowerment.* One of the mediator's objectives is to *empower* the participants to participate in the mediation process. The mediator seeks to promote a process where all parties feel they have a voice and an opportunity to be heard.
6. *Facilitation.* Another of the goals of mediation is to *facilitate* or help the parties to communicate and negotiate with one another. The mediator uses a variety of strategies, tools, and techniques in order to facilitate the *resolution* of the dispute at hand.
7. *Consensus.* The ultimate goal of mediation is to arrive at a consensus or an agreement that effectively settles the dispute in the most desirable manner that can be achieved under the circumstances. In mediation, consensus is achieved when all involved in mediation reach an agreement. This is different from most meetings where it may only take a majority (51%) to determine the outcome.

The above assumptions and basic principles describe the mediation process, but they do not define it. We will defer a more detailed level of description on the section on "Theories and Assumptions" later in the chapter. For the present, it can be stated that if any approach to negotiating a dispute embodies the above principles it would likely qualify as mediation and in all likelihood would *not* qualify as any other approach to dispute resolution (including nonbinding arbitration).

HISTORY AND DEVELOPMENT OF THE MEDIATION PROFESSION

Unlike some of the other professions described in this book, the historical development of mediation is difficult to discern and describe. There are several reasons this is so. For one thing, although mediators have existed since at least the beginning of civilization, they have been called different names and ascribed different functions. It is not taking much of an anthropological risk to propose that human beings have been experiencing and resolving disputes for as long as we have existed as a species. Cultural anthropologists such as Laura Nader and P.H. Gulliver, beginning in 1969 and 1973 respectively, studied the development of so-called alternative dispute resolution (ADR) and provided research for later application of its principles. But there has been precious little in the way of agreement as to definitions of both mediation and ADR, and definitions have changed as quickly as has history. Evan R. Seamone (2000) noted:

> Anyone with the ambition to accurately chart the development of mediation step-by-step and program-by-program would face a number of uphill battles, to say the

least. First, mediation is a relative term. A number of articles describe the current scenario in which even the most noted mediation scholars have problems agreeing on the definition of mediation. See, e.g., LINDA R. SINGER, SETTLING DISPUTES: CONFLICT RESOLUTION IN BUSINESS, FAMILIES, AND THE LEGAL SYSTEM 15 (2d ed. 1994) ("unfortunately, even professional dispute resolvers do not always refer to the same process when they use a particular word to describe it (referencing confusion over the term "mediation"). The second major problem is the fact that a proper inquiry into the development of mediation would require a science for categorizing programs into different stages and then drawing a precise line to delineate exactly which programs, against the advice of the experts, would not qualify. (Downloaded on 4/14/2008 from http://www.uiowa.edu/~cyberlaw/elp00/Evan/mediation/origin.html.)

Thus we can track only the modern history of mediation as it is known today. Some authors (i.e., FCRPP, 2007) trace modern approaches to mediation in the United States to the Quakers. Seamone (2000) preferred to look more immediately backward to the 1970s, where he sited the importance of the Roscoe Pound Conference of 1976. Roscoe Pound had been an influential force in critiquing the legal system early on in American history. In 1976, legal scholars met to continue his legacy by brainstorming possible improvements for the American legal system. As technological change began to accelerate and the industrial revolution gave way to the information age, the courts began to be overwhelmed by litigation involving concepts for which no precedents existed. Copywriting software, patents for firmware, the switch to shipping containers from bulk carriers, intellectual property issues, digital rights protection, and many other similar issues began to emerge that courts were ill-equipped to deal with. Moreover, as the courts ramped up to address these new complex issues, less complex and more routine disputes backed up and the court system became nearly overwhelmed. The urgent need for alternatives to litigation in these as well as other areas resulted in the concept of the Multi-door Courthouse (Sander, 1979), where the court would offer a number of dispute resolution options such as mediation and arbitration as well as the Neighborhood Justice Center (Seamone, 2000). In both cases, alternatives to litigation arose that were more efficient and resulted in faster resolution, one of which was mediation as it is currently practiced. Even so, by 1997, only 7 percent of civil cases were being addressed by private mediation (Mosten, 2001). Today it is closer to 20 percent.

Other countries experienced similar trends and adopted analogous approaches. Australia in particular led the way for the exponential growth of mediation by declaring mediation, conciliation, and negotiation to be the central tenets of its *primary dispute resolution* (PDR) system. Litigation is considered the alternative system and increasingly is invoked only as a last resort. Mosten (2001) believed that similar circumstances will force this pattern to appear in most other industrialized countries. Regardless of whether or when his prediction comes to pass, there remains an increasing need for mediators in the United States.

PREDOMINANT PROFILES OF MEDIATION CLIENTS

There is almost no limit to the types of disputes with which mediators may provide assistance. For example, some issues that social workers or mental health counselors might be interested in mediating include divorce, healthcare, child and elder abuse, and almost any other issue that falls within the realm of social work. In some states, mediators are certified or otherwise qualified to be mediators whereas in other states there is no official process for qualifying as a mediator. Florida is an example of a state where mediators are certified by the Florida Supreme Court in four distinct areas: (a) family, (b) dependency, (c) circuit civil, and (d) county court mediation. Presently a social worker or mental health counselor with a master's degree would be eligible for certification in each of these four areas. Of course, specialized mediation training and relevant mentorship experiences are also required.

Family mediators mediate mostly marital and divorce issues. Families and couples have many other issues to resolve besides divorce; in fact, mediation of a family dispute can be employed to *prevent* divorce (even if this was not the intent of the mediation). Other issues brought into family mediation involve disputes over a family business entity, creating or restructuring pre- and postnuptial agreements, issues regarding child-rearing, and many others in which the goal of the mediation is not to arrive a postmarital settlement agreement, but rather to resolve an ongoing family problem or conflict.

It must be pointed out that even though many family mediators are in fact also licensed mental health counselors or licensed marriage and family therapists, *mediators do not practice therapy with mediation clients.* Not only is it a violation of many ethical codes, it doesn't make much sense. The mediator must be a *neutral* and *impartial* party who assists two (or more) parties in reaching an agreement with regard to some dispute or disagreement. A family or couples therapist's job is to counsel the couple on repairing or strengthening their relationship(s). The therapist in such situations often cannot remain impartial or neutral. The therapist's job is to show how the behavior and assumptions of each member of the couple contribute to the difficulties in getting along or maintaining a mutually satisfying relationship, including identifying and correcting behavior deemed as destructive or even pathological. One cannot do this and remain impartial and neutral (or at least be perceived as impartial and neutral). Thus although the lines of work of family mediator and family therapist seem to have much in common, they also are characterized by important differences, and a family mediator must make it clear that they cannot provide therapy, either in their role as mediator or separately.

A second area where mediators work is *dependency mediation*. Dependency mediators (also called child protection mediators) attempt to settle disputes related to the living and care arrangements of minor children who have been abused, neglected, or abandoned. The parties to these mediations typically include the parents other family members, court-appointed guardians ad litem, child protection caseworkers, and prosecutors, and in some cases the child as well. Dependency mediation typically requires, as noted, separate training and certification from family mediation.

A third area in which mediators practice in Florida is *circuit civil mediation*. As the name implies, circuit civil mediation is more closely associated with the state circuit (rather than the county) court system. It is increasingly being used as a means to resolve disputes such as contract, real estate, medical malpractice, product liability, personal injury, and other types of disputes more quickly and more effectively than via litigation in the circuit court system. Sometimes, these cases are complex and involve multiple parties in mediation.

In some jurisdictions, only attorneys who are licensed to practice law in their state may be certified as circuit civil mediators. This was the case in Florida until just recently when the attorney or former judge require-

ment was removed by the Florida Supreme Court. The Court's decision reflected both (a) the growing need for a diverse group of qualified mediators and the recognition that being an attorney is not a necessary prerequisite to being a good mediator, and (b) that properly trained and certified mediators who are not attorneys may bring skill sets to the table that actually may enhance their ability to properly mediate even complex legal disputes.

MISSIONS AND OBJECTIVES OF THE MEDIATION PROFESSION

There is a continuing need for qualified and professional mediators. Today, professional organizations and state governments are grappling with how to determine the minimum qualifications for entry into the profession and how to promote mediation. Even so, the missions and objectives of the profession are reasonably clear.

The Association for Conflict Resolution (ACR) is a national professional organization dedicated to enhancing the practice and public understanding of conflict resolution. Their stated mission is "promoting peaceful, effective conflict resolution." This association serves a membership that includes more than 6000 mediators, arbitrators, facilitators, educators, and others involved in the field of conflict resolution and collaborative decision-making. Anyone interested in the field of conflict resolution is welcome to join (http://www.acrnet.org/membership/index.htm).

Mediation is not the only type of alternative (or collaborative) dispute resolution (again, ADR). Mediation holds a special niche within the ADR space, however, in that it aims to maximally empower those it serves and be minimally restrictive with regard to the imposition of a solution to any dispute. As stated above, a mediator never imposes a solution, but rather plays the role of facilitator and peacemaker to assist his or her clients in reaching a mutually agreeable settlement.

Professional organizations often help to set standards and requirements for mediator training and certification that are sufficient to protect the public and the profession. Mosten (2001) addressed this problem succinctly by point out that:

> Quality pays off in every product and service. It is no less true in the field of mediation—and perhaps even more so.
>
> One of the reasons that so many rush into the field of mediation and then exit just as quickly is that there is no regulation or licensing monitoring minimal competency for entry into the field. Although there are certification programs that reward competency, mediators, unlike lawyers, mental health practitioners or housing contractors, do not need a license to practice. This can lead to consumer abuse that hurts the entire field. (pp. 12–13)

This chapter's author's opinion, however, is that the drawbacks of increased bureaucracy and costs are more than offset by the benefits and protections of mediator licensing at the state and federal levels. In many jurisdictions, the certification requirements already approach those of licensure. One notable exception is the absence of standardized testing of mediator skills and knowledge—in Florida for example, one can become a certified mediator without having to sit for any type of examination. This situation is difficult to defend, and the hope is that sooner rather than later mediators will be required to pass a rigorous examination in their area of expertise in order to become qualified as a mediator.

PHILOSOPHICAL ASSUMPTIONS AND PREEMINENT THEORIES

Earlier in the chapter, the core values and principles of mediation were described as being characterized by *Voluntary Participation, Self-Determination, Impartiality and Neutrality, Confidentiality, Empowerment, Facilitation and Consensus.* Collectively, these are what differentiate mediation from other approaches to dispute resolution, and even other forms of ADR. But as noted earlier, these assumptions and principles describe the mediation process, but they do not define it. Next, it is necessary to carefully describe that process in terms of various theoretical approaches adopted by skilled mediators. Given the limitations of available space, the following briefly examines two such approaches.

Principled Negotiation

Much mediation practice is based on an approach referred to as Principled Negotiation. This approach was described in a now famous text, *Getting to Yes: Negotiating Agreement Without Giving In*, by Roger Fisher and William Ury, the first edition which was published in 1981. Their approach revolves around reaching consensus through a principled negotiation process based on building a foundation for mutual problem solving. Principled negotiation has many interesting, even fascinating aspects. First, it aims to separate the individuals involved with the dispute from the dispute itself. Separating the people from the problem takes feelings and egos out of the equation, and this is often half the battle in reaching an acceptable compromise or solution. We are reminded of a funny scene in the movie "My Big Fat Greek Wedding" in which a mother and daughter get the husband/father to agree to something he would otherwise object to by getting him to believe he proposed the solution. Although this may be seen as manipulation, mediators do not manipulate their clients. Merely making clear the difference between the problem (the dispute) from the people involved allows the participants the opportunity to rationally consider alternatives instead of defending themselves or attacking the other side. It is hard to overstate the power of this simple distinction until one has seen it work in practice.

A second aspect to principled negotiation is to guide the focus away from "positions" and toward each party's "interests." The following table lists the differences between Positions and Interests:

Table 12-1.

Positions	Interests
Based on *Wants*	Defined by *Needs*
Specific, and often rigidly so	General and flexible
Based on *Demands*	Based on *Preferences*
Often incompatible with interests and therefore, the goals of negotiation	Obviously compatible with the goal of mediation (reaching a settlement)

To any individual who has read even a single book by the late Albert Ellis (cf. Ellis, 2000), these two columns overlap to substantial degree with his distinctions between rational and irrational thinking. In fact, as we shall see below, being an effective mediator and encouraging rational thinking share much in common.

Third in the list of "to do" items associated with conducting any principled negotiation is to generate options for mutual gain.

This notion overlaps with another principle, which is the difference between so-called *distributive* vs. *integrative* negotiations. In a distributive negotiation, it is assumed that (a) what is desired is a resource of fixed value, and (b) the negotiation involves splitting up this fixed-sized "pie" in the fairest way possible. But what if we could rearrange things so as to *make the pie bigger*! This would obviously result in more value for everyone and increase the chances of a win-win result. Many readers will be surprised to discover that this is exactly what skilled mediators are able to do by applying the principle of integrative negotiation. Mediators are trained to recognize that anything that impacts value can, and usually does, affects the size of the pie. These include transaction costs, goodwill, tax consequences, feelings of empowerment, time and timing-sensitive variables, stress, and even guilt reduction, as well as many others.

Fourth, and finally, a skilled professional mediator creates or lists objective criteria for evaluating alternatives and options. As long as both or all parties to the negotiation (or mediation) agree to the criteria, achieving success then becomes a matter of simple arithmetic.

Rational Mediation

Another aspect of a theoretical approach to mediation is what the author refers to as *Rational Mediation*. Rational Emotional Behavior Therapy (REBT) and its philosophical parent, Rational Theory (RT), are approaches to the reduction of emotional disturbance based on the assumption that individuals are, through the irrational beliefs they hold, responsible for their own emotional disturbance and can be empowered to learn how to cease disturbing themselves. Their irrational beliefs are often deep-seated and largely unconscious to the individual, and those who study RT are taught to recognize and dispute such beliefs, both in themselves and in their clients. Successfully disputing and reframing one's irrational beliefs and replacing them with rational cognitions instead generally leads to a significant reduction of emotional disturbance.

Mediation and RT rarely have been viewed as related approaches to the reduction of human discord. Here it is argued that they should be. The application of some of the techniques of REBT to the process of mediation seems like a very natural and potentially productive area of intersection. The author of this chapter was trained in Rational Theory at The Albert Ellis Institute prior to becoming a certified mediator, and the overlap between the two approaches is simply too compelling to overlook.

As noted above, mediation typically does not proceed well until each party is shown the importance of focusing on the problem at hand, instead of on their (usually) negative and emotionally charged perceptions of one another. Parties engaging in mediation are very often quite disturbed by their belief that the other side is selfish, wrong, or evil and that they therefore "deserve" something in return. Although it is certainly not the mediator's purpose or goal to practice therapy during a mediation session, Rational Theory nonetheless can provide mediators with an exceptionally powerful set of tools to quickly reduce the level of emotional disturbance in the parties in a mediation session. Doing so can greatly facilitate the parties in reaching a mutually acceptable agreement. Additionally, the tools of REBT and RT can be used: (a) to assist the negotiation process by enabling the parties to find creative solutions to their disagreements; (b) to focus upon their interests as opposed to their needs and demands (i.e., their "positions"); (c) to widen the solution set of available options (enlarging "the pie" rather than dividing it); (d) to adopt a cooperative, rather than competitive style of negotiating; and (e) to rationally con-

sider the alternatives to reaching a mediated agreement (i.e., being forced to live with a court-imposed settlement).

It is quite interesting that many of the core concepts behind mediation overlap to a large degree with the core concepts of REBT and RT: self-determination, empowerment, facilitation, personal responsibility, and peaceful coexistence. By this point the reader should be well aware that when a mediator sits with the parties who are in negotiation, he or she is in control of the process but not the agreement, which must be determined by the parties. Nevertheless, the mediator's role as facilitator is often the deciding factor in whether an agreement will be reached. The mediator is responsible for setting the tone of the session and for facilitating principled negotiation, that is, for structuring the negotiation so that parties are likely to reach agreement. As described above, principled negotiation revolves around separating the individuals (and their perceptions of one another) from the issues to be resolved, to lead the parties to focus on their interests as opposed to their positions (which are typically stated as demands), to assist the parties in inventing options for mutual gain, and to develop objective criteria for measuring the outcome. In affecting this, the mediator has a wide variety of tools to choose from. Once again, tools based on the tradition of Rational Theory seem especially effective in this regard.

Consider, for example, the first goal of the mediator in structuring the negotiation: *separate the people from the problem.* RT teaches the value of rating behaviors as opposed to other people. It is undoubtedly helpful for a mediator to encourage parties not to think of each other as bad, nasty, or evil people, but rather as another whose behavior with which they have an issue. The former stance leads to blame of others, instead of accepting personal responsibility for situations, which is far more amenable to cooperative interchange going forward. Similarly, RT encourages individuals to flag and dispute their demands and focus instead in preferences and interests. Effective mediators know that negotiation proceeds more effectively when parties focus on their interests as opposed to their positions.

Table 12.2 summarizes the overlap between the goals of mediation through principle negotiation and the advice given by RT and REBT for reducing discord:

Table 12.2

Component of Principled Negotiation	Corresponding Concept from Rational Theory
Cooperation Trumps Competition	Be Accountable to Self and Others
Separate the Parties from the Problems	Don't Rate Others (or Self)–Focus on Issues
Focus on Interests, not Positions	Replace Demands with Preferences or Desires
Invent Options for Mutual Gain	Substitute Taking Responsibility for Blaming
Develop Objective Criteria for Evaluating Agreements	Dispute Demands and Irrational Beliefs on the Basis of Evidence, Logic and Pragmatic Value

Thus, Mediation and Rational Theory share many underlying assumptions and strategies in terms of achieving their stated goals of reducing discord. Mediation focuses on resolving disputes among two or more parties, whereas Rational Theory is aimed at reducing discord within individuals, but the two approaches adopt methods and guidelines that show a surprising degree of overlap.

Mediation as a career choice is not appropriate for everyone. Individuals who possess a low tolerance for confrontation will not be happy, as mediation often involves some level of confrontation, at least in the early stages. Individuals who think very concretely may not be suited to mediation–creativity and the ability to reframe and reevaluate situations and perspectives are vital to achieving success as a mediator. Finally, mediators need to possess or acquire many of the same skills as those of experienced and competent mental health counselors or psychotherapists: perceptions must be managed, nonverbal cues need to be recognized and acted upon, and the participants must be assessed as to their communicative styles. Both participant comfort level *and* a disciplined environment must be maintained (which can be a fine line to walk).

REAL WORLD APPLICATIONS AND SALARIES

Application Example

A good example of a real-world application of mediation is demonstrated by the following illustrative case. Amy and Jeff are divorcing. They disagree about many issues including how to create a parenting plan for their children which spells out the time their children, Alice and Billy, will each spend with Amy and Jeff after they separate. If they are not able to reach agreement on their own, they have different paths they can choose to resolve their dispute. One option is to go to court and have the judge decide how they should raise their children. Another option is to go to mediation. In mediation, the mediator will help them to decide upon a parenting plan that they can customize to their own situation. They can consider what their children's needs are and how to best meet those needs. The mediator would encourage them to consider a number of different parenting plan options and then assist the parents in mutually resolving in a manner that is acceptable to both. The family mediator would be likely to use the "PEACE" model in this mediation. PEACE, an acronym that family mediators often use to guide and structure family mediation sessions, is made up of the following terms:

P–Parenting
E–Equitable Distribution of Assets
A–Alimony
C–Child Support
E–Everything Else

In addition to the obvious appeal of the acronym, the process helps to structure the activities and issues discussed in the course of a typical mediation for a settlement concerning the dissolution of a marriage (i.e., divorce mediation). Space limitations prohibit examining each step in detail, but the reader can readily see how as each area is resolved, the couple moves closer to reaching an overall agreement.

Each of the other areas of specialty in mediation (i.e., dependency, circuit civil, etc.) has similar applications and tools to provide structure to the process of reaching an agreement. Because of the complexity of some cases in circuit civil mediation, however, there is no single overarching template but rather a collection of approaches that are combined as necessary depending on the particulars of the cases involved.

Salary and Earnings

Mediators can work either on a salaried or hourly basis for the family, county, or civil court system, or in private practice. In both cases, payment is typically based on per hour of mediation work, and the cost is borne by the participants. Hourly remunera-

tion rates can range from $50 to as high as $500 or more, depending on the mediator's qualifications, experience level, reputation, and other factors. Typical rates in Florida range from $50 to $250 per hour. Compared to the costs of alternatives, mediation, when successful, is less expensive because it typically requires less attorney, custody evaluator, and accounting assistance.

One note of caution should be added. Many mediation training programs do an excellent job of marketing their programs and provide credible training for the budding mediator but offer little assistance in guiding the student in finding work after training. As Mosen (2001) pointedly stated in his *Mediation Career Guide*, "after luring training participants into expensive programs by feeding on the glow of a lucrative future as a professional mediator, the reality is that after the training (perhaps many trainings), there are few jobs and realistic practice building opportunities. Mediators are dressed up with nowhere to go" (pp. 4–5).

The point is not that mediation training programs are unethical, but that they should include more practice-building skills in their training programs. We live in a competitive economy in which perseverance and self-promotion are rewarded, and would-be mediators need to understand the business side of the profession.

PROFESSIONAL PREPARATION, DEVELOPMENT AND WORK SETTINGS

Training and Education Requirements

States and municipalities differ in the exact set of requirements for mediator certification (and eventually, it is hoped, licensure), but a general set of standards can be described. In many jurisdictions, certified mediators must hold a master's degree in an area that is relevant to the type of mediation for which they seek certification. As noted above, for example, many family and dependency mediators are also mental health counselors, who possess a master's degree in that field. Because many mediations deal with issues of monetary and economic value, many mediators have a background in accounting, including certification as public accountants. Also as noted above, many mediators are trained as attorneys.

The master's or required degree, however, is only the first of many entry requirements. Next, the aspiring mediator must take certification training courses specific to the area in which they intend to practice. Such courses are typically 30 to 50 hours in length, are offered at both universities and mediation training centers, and must be certified by their state as such. Separate courses exist for each of the various areas in mediation, and a would-be mediator who wishes to practice in more than one area should count on taking a separate training course in each area in which they intend to become certified to practice.

Following the training course(s), it often is necessary that graduates of these training courses attend some number of actual mediations, first as observer and then as comediator, before they can attain certification. Certainly this is the case in the state of Florida. Other states vary in their requirements.

Upon meeting all the requirements, the new mediator is then issued his or her certificate. In Florida, the certificates are issues by the State Supreme Court, but the certifying body, if it exists, in other states may differ.

Finally, there now exist undergraduate programs specializing in mediation training and in many jurisdictions; these plus a one-year internship meet the minimal require-

ments for mediator certification (Mosten, 2001). The interested reader is referred to one of the professional associations listed in the next section for more specific information related to their state and desired area of practice.

Work Settings

Mediators work in both public and private settings. The most common public settings are public courthouse buildings, most of which have set aside or created rooms and areas dedicated to mediation. Otherwise, mediations are conducted in the private offices of mediators. In larger cities, private centers dedicated to mediation are found (e.g., The Mosten Mediation Center in Los Angeles, CA), but these are the exception. Most private mediators practice out of their offices, either in a conference room or similar setting. A flip chart and pad are usually to be found at hand, and notes are taken as issues are listed and mediated.

PROFESSIONAL ORGANIZATIONS

There are many local, state, and national professional organizations that represent the interests of both mediators and their clients. In the United States, the largest interdisciplinary organization for mediators is the Association for Conflict Resolution (www. acrnet.org). It was formed by the merger of three smaller organizations, The Academy of Family Mediators, The Conflict Resolution Education Network, and The Society of Professionals in Dispute Resolution.

Another nationally recognized professional organization that represents mediators is the Association of Family and Conciliation Courts (AFCC)–an interdisciplinary and international association of professionals dedicated to the resolution of family conflict. Its members include mediators, judges, lawyers, psychologists, researchers, academicians, counselors, court commissioners, custody evaluators, parenting coordinators, court administrators, social workers, parent educators, and financial planners.

FUTURE OUTLOOK

Mediation has a bright future, and, for the reasons explained in the introduction to this chapter, the exponential growth that the field has experienced can only be expected to continue for some time to come. This optimistic assessment reflects simple economics–our society can no longer afford to support litigation as the answer to every dispute. Court systems are overwhelmed and underfinanced. Most individuals cannot afford litigation, and at the corporate level, global competition makes it harder if not impossible for most companies to pass on the costs of multimillion dollar lawsuits to their customers. This author believes that sooner or later, the United States will be forced by economic realities to follow Australia's lead in placing mediation and related forms of ADR as the *primary* approach to dispute resolution, and that litigation will become an avenue of final resort rather than the *de facto* standard it now enjoys.

In addition to the economic factors, the fact is that society as a whole benefits from approaches to dispute resolution based on peacemaking rather than adversarial conduct. The author sees a parallel to the near future of health care in our society. It is no longer economically viable or ethically defensible to sustain an approach to health care that profits from keeping people sick and managing their symptoms rather by making them well–the underlying philosophy of the wellness movement towards preventive medicine. Mediation offers an alternative to conflict resolution that is based on a similar philosophy. The reader can expect to hear much more about mediation as a profession in the near future.

REFERENCES

Bowling, D., & Hoffman, D.A. (2003). *Bringing peace into the room: How the personal qualities of the mediator impact the process of conflict resolution.* San Francisco: Jossey-Bass.

Ellis, A. (2000). *How to stubbornly refuse to upset yourself about anything, yes anything.* New York: Carol Publishing Group

Fischer, R., & Ury, W. (1981). *Getting to yes: Negotiating agreement without giving in.* Detroit, MI: Houghton-Mifflin.

Friends Conflict Resolution Programs of Philadelphia (2007). *The mediator's handbook.* Victoria, Canada: New Society.

Lenski, T. J. (2008). *Making mediation your day job: How to market your ADR business using mediation principles you already know.* Lincoln, NE: iUniverse.

Mosten, F. S. (2001). *Mediation career guide.* San Francisco: John Wiley & Sons.

Sander, F. E. A. (1979). Varieties of Dispute Processing. In A. Levin & R. Wheeler (Eds.), The pound conference: Perspectives on justice in the future. St. Paul, MN: West.

Seamone, E. R. (2000). *Bringing a smile to mediation's two faces.* University of Iowa College of Law Website. Downloaded on 4/14/2008 from http://www.uiowa.edu/~cyberlaw/elp00/Evan/mediation/origin.html.

The USF Conflict Resolution Collaborative (2005). *Family mediation training program.* Tampa, FL: Author.

Chapter 13

MENTAL HEALTH COUNSELING

GARY G. GINTNER & GAIL MEARS

Mental health problems are more prevalent than most people believe and appear to be on the rise (Keyes, 2007). By the age of 55, half of all adults will have had at least one significant psychiatric disorder, and in any given year one in four report some kind of a serious psychiatric episode (U.S. Public Health Services, 1999). Keyes and Lopez (2002) noted that depression is becoming more prevalent and appearing at earlier ages. By the year 2020, depression is expected to be the second most costly health problem, eclipsed only by heart disease (Murray & Lopez, 1996). To address this growing health burden, mental health professionals in the twenty-first century will need to step out of the current box of simply treating symptoms and dysfunction (World Health Organization [WHO], 2004). They will need to expand their efforts to bolster positive mental health which has been shown to prevent the occurrence and lessen the severity of psychiatric problems.

Mental health counselors are uniquely poised to meet this challenge. Mental health counseling is considered one of the core mental health professions with its own distinctive standards of education, training, and practice (American Mental Health Counsel-ors Association [AMHCA], 2004). The scope of practice ranges from diagnosing and treating psychiatric disorders to helping people cope with normal stressful events and life transitions. An underlying orientation in all of these efforts is one of promoting both development and wellness. In this chapter we will: (a) provide a history and overview of the profession; (b) describe training and professional practice standards; (c) profile services delivered and populations served; and (d) discuss the occupational outlook for the profession.

HISTORY OF MENTAL HEALTH COUNSELING

Mental health counseling emerged as a new profession in the 1970s. Several pieces of legislation were instrumental in the growth of this new group of mental health practitioners. Responding to national worry that we would lose the space race, the National Defense Education Act (NDEA) of 1958 authorized funding for counselor education programs. This funding was provided with the hope of improving school guidance programs so students with math and science potential could be identified early and encouraged to go to college. This increased funding resulted in a proliferation of Counselor Education Programs and ultimately in a large group of trained counselors.

A second important piece of early legislation was the Community Mental Health Act of 1963 which spawned the development of community mental health centers across the United States. Suddenly, there were unprecedented job opportunities for mental health professionals. This occurred at about the same time when there was an overabundance of trained school guidance counselors relative to the positions available. As a result, many of these counselors, trained initially in school guidance, found work in clinical settings and brought counseling's developmental and wellness perspective to their work. These early mental health counselors provided clinical services similar to psychologists and social workers but, at that point in time, lacked a clear professional identity and a professional organization. The American Mental Health Counselors Association was founded in 1976 to meet the needs of this group (Brooks & Weikel, 1996; Mears, 2006; Smith & Robinson, 1996). Mental health counselors have made great strides since the 1970s and their early school guidance roots have evolved into a rigorous mental health profession. They are currently licensed in 49 states and are able to receive third-party reimbursement for diagnosis, assessment and psychotherapy services in most states.

PHILOSOPHICAL ASSUMPTIONS AND THEORIES

Philosophical Assumptions

Mental health counselors have three basic beliefs about the best ways to help people change (Remley & Herlihy, 2007). The first belief is that individuals need to be understood in terms of their developmental context. From this perspective, many issues can be conceptualized as either responses to normal developmental issues or difficulty in moving through a life phase. For example, an adolescent's highly argumentative and oppositional behavior may be best understood as reflecting difficulty in dealing with developmental issues like autonomy and establishing personal identity. These types of difficulties are often due to underdeveloped life skills that are needed to negotiate the particular developmental challenge. As such, intervention efforts might target building necessary life skills such as assertion, problem solving, communication, and relationship skills (Darden, Gazda & Ginter, 1996). In this way, counseling is seen as an avenue to promote the individual's personal development.

A second basic belief is that counseling efforts should strive to enhance overall wellness. Meyers, Sweeney, and Witmer (2000) defined wellness as, "A way of life oriented toward optimal health and well-being in which the mind, body and spirit are integrated by the individual to live life more fully within the human and natural community" (p. 252). Counselors move beyond simply treating "problems" to helping people flourish and function more optimally. Counselors are involved not only in ameliorating symptoms but also in building positive aspects of mental health such as life satisfaction, autonomy, resilience, and interpersonal intimacy. They may also encourage healthy lifestyle behaviors such as regular exercise and healthy eating habits in order to promote overall health.

A third basic belief is that people need to be understood in the context of their personal, social, and cultural environments. These life systems play a major role in shaping the person's personal identity, belief systems, and coping style (Herr, 1989). What at first glance may seem like a maladaptive response may actually be an understandable reaction to living in a dysfunctional social situation. For example, a child who grows up in a home with parental alcoholism may cope by becoming overly self-reliant and consequently have difficulty with intimacy and interpersonal trust. Similarly, lack of meaningful employment opportunities may predispose an individual to hopelessness which can spawn depression or substance abuse (WHO, 2004). Mental health counselors not only help clients liberate themselves from these limiting types of life conditions, but also advocate for social change that impact the population at large. For example, they may work toward improving local schools, reducing the stigma associated with seeking mental health care, and supporting legislation that promotes a just society.

Major Theories

The common theories that mental health counselors draw upon today reflect the basic assumptions discussed above regarding personal growth (person-centered theory), developing skills and capacities (behavioral and cognitive theories) and understanding individuals in the context of the systems in which they live (systems theory). Surveys of mental health counselors indicate that most endorse an eclectic approach (Prochaska & Norcross, 2007). This means that they use a variety of theories and therapeutic techniques depending upon what the counselor thinks is most helpful with a particular client with their set of characteristics. Empirical research, professional experience, and the client's preferences all inform the counselor's decision about what approach to use. In this section, we will discuss each of these major theories in terms of basic assumptions, theory of change and major therapeutic techniques.

Person-Centered Theory. Carl Rogers is considered the originator of person-centered therapy (Prochaska & Norcross, 2007). His theory is based upon on a positive view of human nature in which people are seen as basically trustworthy, capable of self-direction, and growth-oriented (Rogers, 1961). He believed that people have an inherent tendency or drive to become all that they can become. We are born with an internal compass of sorts that helps us recognize experiences that are growth enhancing versus those that are impediments. People also have a strong need for positive regard or love from others. Difficulties can arise when individuals begin to value the conditions which they perceive will bring them love over those of their internal valuing system. When this occurs, experiences which do not fit with these conditions of worth are distorted or put out of awareness resulting in an individual becoming alienated from his or her internal valuing system. Instead they strive to do those things that will bring acceptance, such as pleasing others or achieving success. The result is an unstable sense of self-worth that vacillates as a function of meeting these external standards. This can lead to problems such as anxiety, depression, and low self-esteem.

The goal of therapy is to help individuals unshackle themselves from these conditions of worth so that they can become fully functioning individuals. According to the theory, this occurs in the context of a special type of therapeutic relationship in which the counselor is empathic, genuine, and is perceived as having unconditional positive regard for the client. Empathy helps clients perceive and integrate parts of themselves that they may have distorted. Unconditional positive regard provides an atmosphere in which clients feel prized for whom they are, rather than what they do as far as meeting any condition of worth. Finally, counselors have to be perceived as real or genuine in the relationship and not simply playing a role. According to Rogers, these conditions are necessary and sufficient to bring about change and to activate an individual's inherent growth tendencies. Some theorists, however, consider Rogers' conditions necessary but not always sufficient.

Because the relationship is seen as the curative mechanism, person-centered therapy does not have a set of specialized techniques. What is more important is the counselor's ability to be accepting and to listen to and accurately reflect what the client is experiencing. Two therapeutic skills are important in this regard. *Reflective listening* is an interviewing skill in which counselors feedback the content, feeling and/or meaning of the client's verbal and nonverbal communication. Counselors also use *immediacy responses* which are comments about what is occurring in the here and now with the client. Both of these skills help clients to become more aware and to experience their emotions more readily and accurately. Interestingly, research reports that the person-centered approach may be especially important to use in the earlier stages of counseling when relationship building and consciousness-raising are more critical therapeutic tasks (Prochaska & Norcross, 2007).

Behavior Therapy. Behavior therapy is based upon the principle that maladaptive behaviors are acquired and modified by the same learning principles as everyday behavior. Involuntary behaviors like crying or fear are controlled by antecedents or events that precede it. For example, the sight of a snake evokes an immediate strong fear response. Voluntary behaviors like studying are controlled by expected consequences such as rewards or punishments. For example, individuals with bulimia may purge after eating a large quantity of food because they expect that they will feel better afterwards. Most behavior therapists today ascribe to social learning theory which states that behavior is

a function of the person-environment interaction. As a result, it is important to assess person factors such as thinking, feeling, and behavior as well as the environment or context in which the behavior occurs. To understand what is controlling a behavior, behavior therapists attempt to delineate the antecedents or cues, the responses themselves, and the consequences of the behavior.

Once a behavioral problem has been analyzed in this way, change can occur by modifying relevant antecedents, responses, and/or consequences. Antecedent control is a set of techniques designed to either limit exposure to problem cues or increase exposure to cues that would encourage the person to respond more adaptively. For example, a client with bulimia might be asked to eliminate binge foods from the house and replace them with healthier options. Responses can be modified by developing a better coping option. Instead of bingeing to deal with loneliness, the client might be encouraged to call a friend or engage in pleasant activity. Finally, consequences can be modified so that they will encourage adaptive responses. For example, a child with school conduct problems might only be given access to privileges like video games on days when the parents receive a positive behavior report from the teacher. Behavioral interventions are especially helpful with problems such as anxiety, eating disorders, child behavior problems, and compulsive behaviors (Roth & Fonagy, 2004).

Cognitive Therapies. Cognitive therapies postulate that events themselves are not the cause of our distress but rather the way we interpret them (Prochaska & Norcross, 2007). For example, two students may respond very differently to the same exam grade depending upon how they construe the event (e.g., a hard test versus a sign of personal failure). There are two major brands of cognitive therapy: (1) Albert Ellis developed Rational Emotive Behavior Therapy which is based upon the principle that irrational beliefs cause emotional upset; and (2) Aaron Beck's Cognitive Therapy widens the problem thinking net to include an assortment of dysfunctional modes of thinking (e.g., overgeneralizing, personalizing, dichotomous thinking). Both approaches rest on the premise that emotional well-being ultimately depends upon individuals being able to think more realistically and logically.

We can either think our way into a new way of thinking or we can act our way into a new way of thinking. The former approach relies on helping the clients challenge their distorted thinking using a variety of cognitive techniques that essentially help clients generate evidence for and against the thought. Based upon these "facts," the client then makes a decision whether to accept the thought or to modify it based upon the "evidence." The second general approach is to ask the client to carry out behavioral exercises that are designed to test out the thought. For example, a client might be asked to solicit feedback from friends regarding his or her behavior in a social situation. Both general approaches have been shown to be effective ways to modify dysfunctional thinking. Research findings indicate the cognitive therapies are particularly useful in the treatment of anxiety disorders, depression, and eating disorders (Roth & Fonagy, 2004).

Systems Therapies. While there are a number of different systems therapies, all share the belief that individuals are best understood in the context of the life systems in which they function (Prochaska & Norcross, 2007). Systems like the family have rules and roles which dictate how members relate to one another (e.g., parent versus children subsystems). From this perspective, maladaptive behavior is seen as a way of maintaining the family system's current pattern of relating. For example, a marital problem may be deflected by focusing on a child's misbehavior, thereby maintaining the current family

homeostasis. As a result, the target of treatment is the systemic dysfunction in the family or other relevant life system (e.g., the school).

The goal of treatment in the case of a family is to improve the family's overall functioning and communication. Early in treatment the counselor would observe how the family members relate in order to understand family system dynamics. *Reframing* is a technique used to help the family understand the role of a problem behavior from a systemic perspective. For example, an adolescent's oppositional behavior may be reframed as an attempt toward independence in a highly enmeshed family system. Another intervention would be to have the parent subsystem work together rather than play out their problem by involving another family member. Research has found that family therapy is an effective modality of treatment especially for child and adolescent problems and substance abuse (Roth & Fonagy, 2004).

PROFESSIONAL ISSUES

Having discussed the professional orientation of mental health counselors, in this section we examine professional issues such as education, licensing and credentialing, and professional organizations. Current and emerging trends are then discussed in terms of how they may impact the field.

Educational and Training Standards

Licensing. Educational standards for licensure as a mental health counselor are dictated by state law. The majority of states require that practitioners graduate from a 60-credit hour graduate program in mental health counseling or its equivalent in order to be license eligible. In addition to graduate studies, clinical mental health counselors need to meet postgraduate requirements that include supervised field work and a passing grade on either the National Counselors Exam (NCE) and/or the National Clinical Mental Health Counselors Exam (NCMH CE). These exams are regulated by the National Board for Certified Counselors (NB CC). Each state that licenses clinical mental health counselors has a licensing board that approves applications for licensure and oversees adherence to the law and rules that regulate the practice of mental health counseling. Links to state licensing boards can be found on the website for the American Association of State Counseling Boards (AAS CB): www.aascb.com. Licensed mental health counselors have different practice titles depending on the sate in which they are licensed. The following is a list of titles used:

Licensed Professional Counselor (LPC)
Licensed Professional Mental Health Counselor (LPMHC)
Licensed Clinical Professional Counselor (LCPC)
Licensed Professional Counselor of Mental Health (LPCMH)
Licensed Clinical Mental Health Counselor (LCMHC)
Licensed Mental Health Practitioner (LMHP) (ACA, 2008; pg. 3)

In states with licensing laws, it is typically illegal to present oneself as a licensed psychotherapist and to provide psychotherapy (diagnosis, assessment and treatment of mental disorders) without a license.

Program Accreditation. The accrediting body for counselor education programs is the Council for the Accreditation of Counseling and Related Education Programs (CACREP). CACREP accredits counselor education programs in mental health counseling; community counseling, marital, couple and family counseling; gerontological counseling; career counseling; college counseling; and school counseling. At this time, nonetheless, CACREP is undergoing standards revisions and it is likely that the mental health and community specializations will be merged into one specialty in clinical mental health counseling. Other likely changes include the discontinuation of the gerontological specialization and the addition of a new program specialty in addictions counseling.

CACREP accredited programs need to cover core counseling content areas as well as specialization coursework in addition to a supervised practicum and internship in the area of specialization. Programs accredited in mental health counseling have core counselor education course work in helping relationships, theories of counseling, human development, group counseling, family counseling, professional orientation, social and cultural foundations, career development, research design and program evaluation, and assessment. Specialty coursework includes the history of mental health counseling, and the roles and functions of the mental health counselors; legal, ethical, and cultural issues; mental health service delivery systems, program evaluation and management of clinical services; mental health consultation and advocacy; biopsychosocial assessment and diagnosis; prevention; treatment planning; and clinical interventions. Most states require that counselors seeking mental health licensure come for a CAC REP accredited program or have completed required coursework and field experiences that are consistent with CACREP requirements. Information on CACREP can be found at www.CACREP.org.

PROFESSIONAL ORGANIZATIONS

National Board for Certified Counselors

Individual practitioners can be credentialed at the state and national levels. The National Board for Certified Counselors is the organization that credentials counselors at the national level. Counselors of all specializations can be credentialed as National Certified Counselors (NCC). This certification requires that counselors pass the National Counselors Exam (NCE) and complete a graduate counseling program of at least 48 credits hours with courses in specific counseling content areas. Postgraduate requirements include 3,000 hours supervised work experience with at least 100 hours of supervision.

Counselors can be credentialed as a Certified Clinical Mental Health Counselor (CCMHC) if they: (a) hold the NCC credential; (b) complete a graduate counseling program of at least 60 credits that includes course work in counseling theories and psychotherapy, psychopathology, human growth and development, career development, professional orientation and ethics, research, appraisal, social/cultural foundations, and clinical field-based experience of at least nine credit hours; (c) pass either the Examination of Clinical Counselor Practice (ECCP) or the National Clinical Mental Health Counseling Examination (NCMHCE); and (d) provide NBCC with an audio or video-taped critiqued work sample.

Other types of certification are also available. Counselors who are credentialed as NCEs can become Master Addictions Counselors (MAC) by the addition of 12 semester hours of graduate study in addictions (up to six of these hours may be in group and family), three years of experience in the addictions field (two of which must be postgradu-

ate) and passing the Examination for Master Addictions Counselors (EMAC). The Center for Credentialing and Education (CCE) is a corporate affiliate of the NBCC that offers credentialing in clinical supervision, technology-assisted counseling, and career facilitation. Information on the NBCC and the CCE can be found at www.nbcc.org.

American Counseling Association

The American Counseling Association (ACA) is an umbrella professional organization that serves the interests of a number of counseling professionals (e.g., school counselors, marriage and family counselors, mental health counselors, career counselors, etc.). With approximately 40,000 members, the ACA provides practice resources, professional development opportunities, and advocacy for counseling practitioners and consumers. ACA was originally incorporated in 1952 under the name of the American Personnel and Guidance Association. The name was later changed to the American Association for Counseling and Development, and renamed the American Counseling Association in 1992 (Sheely, 2002). Currently the ACA has 19 divisions that address different areas of counseling specialty and interest. ACA publishes a monthly trade newspaper, *Counseling Today*, and a quarterly scholarly journal, *The Journal of Counseling and Development.* Information on ACA can be found at www.counseling.org.

American Mental Health Counselors Association

The American Mental Health Counselors Association focuses exclusively on the needs and interests of mental health counselors. Incorporated in 1976, it was founded to meet the needs of a growing number of trained counselors working in clinical mental health settings who were not represented by the existing professional organizations. In 1978, it opted to join as a Division of ACA (then called the American Personnel and Guidance Association). Currently the American Mental Health Counselors Association is a division of ACA but operates as an independent organization. With a membership of approximately 6,000 members, it lobbies for legislation that will expand the practice rights of mental health counselors and increase access to services for mental health counseling consumers. This organization also originated the training standards ultimately adopted by CACREP and the CCMHC credential now regulated by NBCC (Smith & Robinson, 1996). It has two publications, a monthly trade newspaper, *The Advocate*, and a quarterly scholarly journal, *The Journal of Mental Health Counseling*. Information about the American Mental Health Counselors Association can be found at www.amhca.org.

CURRENT TRENDS

Mental health counseling is being influenced by trends in the health care field as well as in society at large. These current trends include managed care, practice guidelines, the promotion of positive mental health, and social justice.

Managed Care

Over the past 20 years, health care costs have soared. As a result, private insurance companies, employers, and governmental agencies have looked for ways to lower the overall cost of providing their services. One such cost containing effort has been the emergence of managed care organizations (MCO). Basically, MCOs monitor requests for healthcare services and determine

whether these services are necessary and appropriate. MCOs have developed specific guidelines and criteria for most types of healthcare services that must be met before these services are approved for reimbursement. MCOs are now a staple of most private and governmental health care plans. To be an approved provider in these MCOs, a healthcare professional must meet particular professional standards (usually state licensing) and agree to abide by the MCO's guidelines and payment schedules. Nationally, mental health counselors are approved providers for most managed care companies (American Mental Health Counselors Association, 2004). Managed care has changed the landscape of mental health care in the United States. Gone are the days of extended hospital stays and long-term outpatient therapy. Rather, MCO guidelines encourage brief therapy and the use of treatments that have an empirical track record of success. As a result, mental health professionals who currently practice need to know how to work in a managed care environment so that they can provide the services that their clients require.

Practice Guidelines

The growth of managed care has also fueled greater interest in identifying treatments that work. In recent years, there has been an explosion of research activity looking at which types of treatments work best with which types of disorders. These efforts have led to the development of practice guidelines by professional organizations like the American Psychological Association and the American Psychiatric Association. To date, guidelines have been developed for most of the common psychiatric disorders including mood disorders, anxiety disorders, many child and adolescent disorders, and eating disorders (Roth & Fonagy, 2004).

Clinically, these guidelines are recommendations that clinicians can refer to in order to select treatments. For example, a cognitive-behavioral treatment for panic disorder is about 85 percent effective in comparison to other standards treatments that may be less than 20 percent effective (see Roth & Fonagy, 2004). Thus, these types of findings serve to inform clinical decision-making. However, they are not intended to be a cookbook or regimented standard of care. The evidence base is simply not that developed. While there is still much of the "art" of counseling that is drawn upon to craft these interventions, in the twenty-first century, practioners will increasingly use more science to inform their practice of mental health counseling.

Positive Mental Health. The burgeoning research on treatment efficacy indicates that even our best treatments are only partially effective and, too often, are short-lived (Keyes, 2007). For example, our best psychotherapies and psychotropic medications are about 60 to 80 percent effective in reducing symptoms. Typically, the efficacy is closer to the lower number. As a result, researchers have looked at other ways to improve treatment outcome. One such effort has been the positive psychology movement which focuses on improving indices of positive mental health (Seligman, 2002). Interventions that have been developed out of this approach are designed to increase positive emotions and to help individuals live a more engaged and meaningful life. These techniques include exercises such as identifying your signature strengths, focusing on daily pleasant emotions, expressing gratitude to significant others, and using a signature-strength to help someone else. Interventions based on these techniques have been shown to reduce residual depression and anxiety symptoms, prevent future depressive episodes, improve overall outcome of standard treatment packages, and enhance life satisfaction (Keyes, 2007). In the future they will become an ever-growing part of the types of services that mental health professionals provide.

Social Justice. Over the past decade or so, there has been increasing interest in developing cultural competencies for counselors that are responsive to the diversity in our society. The counseling profession has taken the lead in this regard and Kiselica and Robinson (2001) noted that there is a long history of social action in the field of counseling. In fact, the counseling codes of ethics require counselors to practice culturally competent counseling (American Counseling Association [ACA], 2005; American Mental Health Counselors Association, 2000). Further, in 2003 the ACA adopted advocacy competencies that outline the skills that counselors need for effective advocacy at the individual, community, and social/political levels (Lewis, Arnold, House & Toporek, 2008). Mental health counselors help clients understand the relationship between social oppression and individuals' emotional responses to disempowerment. They also advocate for social justice and help clients advocate for themselves.

EMPLOYMENT

Services Provided

According to statistics from the United Stated Department of Labor (2008), there are about 100,000 mental health counselors in the United States. The services they offer include individual, group, couple, and family therapy as well as crisis intervention, case management, and consultation. They provide a range of assessment services for emotional, behavioral, educational, career, and diagnostic issues. They also frequently offer psychoeducational programs in life skills such as parenting, couple communication skills, stress management, and social skills. The actual mix of these services, however, is largely determined by the particular practice setting in which they work.

Work Settings

Mental health counselors work in a variety of settings that range from those offering intensive psychiatric care to those that provide primarily preventive and educational services (American Mental Health Counselors Association, 2004). At the more intensive end of the continuum, they may work in inpatient psychiatric hospitals, residential treatment centers, and day treatment programs, all of which provide services for individuals who have significant and sometimes chronic mental health problems. In the midrange, they also work in outpatient mental health centers, university counseling centers, schools, family counseling agencies, substance abuse clinics, and employee assistance programs. A number of mental health counselors also work in private practice either by themselves or as part of a practice group. Finally, they are employed in a variety of local, state, and federally funded social service agencies that offer counseling services as well as prevention programs.

POPULATIONS SERVED

There is no typical consumer profile for mental health counseling services. Clients served reflect the diversity of the community in which counselors work. The types of consumer problems, however, often reflect the particular practice settings. In the more intensive psychiatric settings, clients typically have significant psychiatric disorders like schizophrenia, severe depression, and bipolar disorder. In outpatient settings, the clients

have problems ranging from depression, anxiety, trauma, substance abuse, and child behavior problems to phase of life problems like beginning a new career, changing schools, marital or parenting problems, and retirement.

OCCUPATIONAL OUTLOOK

As noted earlier, mental health counselors have made remarkable gains over the past 30 years. These gains are, in large part, due to the lobbying efforts of the AMHCA, ACA, and NBCC. At this point in time, mental health counselors are licensed in every state but California. Active efforts to get licensure in California are underway. In 2006, mental health counselors were recognized as providers by the Veterans Administration. This opened up practice venues for mental health counselors and increased access to mental health care for veterans. Mental health counselors are not yet recognized as core providers under Medicare and Tricare (though CCMHCs are recognized as Tricare providers), but significant lobbying efforts continue to obtain recognition.

The outlook for mental health counseling is very good. The 2008–2009 Occupational Outlook Handbook (U.S. Department of Labor, 2008) predicts a 30 percent increase in job growth for mental health counselors. Addictions counselors and behavioral disorders specialists have a predicted job growth rate of 34 percent. Though there was a significant range across work settings and location, the median salary for mental health counselors in 2006 was $34,380 and counselors in private established practice typically made more than those working in agencies. Given the predicted growth in jobs and the expected expansion of practice rights, mental health counseling is a promising specialization in the mental health field.

SUMMARY

Mental health counseling is a core mental health profession that is uniquely poised to meet the health care demands of the twenty-first century. It distinguishes itself from other mental health professions by its training, traditions and professional organizations. Mental health counselors treat the mental health continuum, spanning from significant psychopathology to life adjustment and life transition problems. In all these efforts, they move beyond simply remediating symptoms. Rather, their ultimate goal is to help consumers live a more satisfying, meaningful, and productive life.

REFERENCES

American Counseling Association. (2008). *Licensure requirements for professional counselors: A state by state report.* Alexandria, VA: Author.

American Counseling Association. (2005). *American Counseling Association code of ethics* (3rd ed.). Alexandria, VA: Author.

American Mental Health Counselors Association. (2000). *American Mental Health Counseling Association code of ethics* (2nd ed.). Alexandria, VA: Author.

American Mental Health Counselors Association. (2004). *Why use a mental health counselor?* Retrieved May 21, 2008 from http://www.amhca.org/why/.

Brooks, D. K., & Weikel, W. J. (1996). Mental Health Counseling: The first twenty years. In W.J. Weikel & A. J. Palmo (Eds.), *Foundations of mental health counseling* (2nd ed., pp. 5–29). Springfield, IL: Charles C Thomas.

Darden, C., Gazda, G., & Ginter, E. (1996). Life skills and mental health counseling. *Journal of Mental Health Counseling, 18,* 134–141.

Herr E. L. (1989). *Counseling in a dynamic society: Opportunities and challenges.* Alexandria, VA: American Counseling Association.

Keyes, C. L. (2007). Promoting and protecting mental health as flourishing: A complementary strategy for improving national mental health. *American Psychologist, 62*(2), 95–108.

Keyes, C. L., & Lopez, S. J. (2002). Toward a science of mental health: Positive directions in diagnosis and treatment. In C. R. Snyder & J. Lopez (Eds.), *Handbook of positive psychology* (pp. 45–59). New York: Oxford University Press.

Kiselica, M. S., & Robinson, M. (2001). Bringing advocacy counseling to life: The history, issues, and human dramas of social justice work in counseling. *Journal of Counseling & Development, 79,* 387–397.

Lewis, J., Arnold, M. S., House, R., & Toporek, R. (2003). *Advocacy competencies* [Electronic version]. Retrieved June 11, 2008, from http://www.counseling.org/Resources/

Mears, G. (2006). Highlight section: American Mental Health Counselors Association: Taking the Profession into the 21st Century. In W.J. Weikel, A. J. Palmo, & D. P. Borsos (Eds.), *Foundations of mental health counseling* (3rd ed., pp. 49-54). Springfield, IL: Charles C Thomas.

Meyers, J. E., Sweeney, T. J., & Witmer, J. M. (2000). The wheel of wellness: Counseling for wellness. *Journal of Counseling and Development, 78,* 251–266.

Prochaska, J. O., & Norcross, J. C. (2007). *Systems of psychotherapy: A transtheoretical analysis* (6th ed.). Pacific Grove, CA: Thomson Brooks/Cole.

Remley, T. P., & Herlihy, B. (2007). *Ethical, legal, and professional issues in counseling.* Upper Saddle River, NJ: Pearson Merrill Prentice Hall.

Rogers, C. R. (1961). *On becoming a person.* Boston: Houghton Mifflin.

Roth, A., & Fonagy, P. (2004). *What work for whom? A critical review of psychotherapy research* (2nd ed.). New York: Guilford.

Seligman, M. E. P. (2002). *Authentic happiness: Using the new positive psychology to realize your potential for lasting fulfillment.* New York: Free Press.

Sheely, V. L. (2002). American Counseling Association: The 50th year celebration of excellence. *Journal of Counseling and Development, 80,* 387–393.

Smith, H.B., & Robinson, G. P. (1996). Highlight section: Mental health counseling: Past, present, and future. In W.J. Weikel & A. J. Palmo

(Eds.), *Foundations of mental health counseling* (2nd ed., pp. 38–50). Springfield, Il: Charles C Thomas.

United States Department of Labor. (2008). *Occupational Outlook Handbook 2008–2009.* Indianapolis, IN: IST Publishing.

U.S. Public Health Service. (1999). *Mental health: A report of the Surgeon General.* Rockville, MD: Author.

World Health Organization. (2004). *Promoting mental health: Concepts, emerging evidence, practice* (Summary report). Geneva: Author.

WEB SITES

American Association of State Counseling Boards
    http://www.aascb.com
American Counseling Association
    http://www.counseling.org
American Mental Health Counselors Association
    http://amhca.org
Council for the Accreditation of Counseling and
    Related Education Programs http://cacrep.org
National Board of Certified Counselors
    http://nbcc.org

Chapter 14

PUBLIC ADMINISTRATION

JOHN L. DALY

Catastrophic events like Hurricane Katrina provide vivid images of the critical need for professionally trained public service. Hurricane Katrina will long be remembered first because of the damage and suffering it caused coastal residents in proximity to its wrath. However, closely following this fact, many citizens will remember the failure of government to intervene quickly and effectively in its rescue efforts. Often we fail to realize the importance of public servants until their intervention is required. Thankfully, not all interventions are as poorly managed as was the case with Hurricane Katrina.

The public's perception of government and those serving in it has fallen substantially over the past half-century. Since President John F. Kennedy's assassination in 1963, it has become increasingly fashionable for elected officials and the media to bash public servants (i.e., public administrators). Public servants are frequently referred to as inefficient, ineffective, and self-serving bureaucrats. As with any occupation, failures do occur and when related to these negative characteristics should be exposed as a means of protecting the public's interest. However, less frequently do citizens read about or hear praises for service effectiveness afforded through the hard work and dedication of the public servant. It may surprise many that survey feedback from those receiving public service generally indicates high satisfaction with assistance received. Thus, the negative "bureaucrat" stereotype portraying government employees may be more the exception than the rule (Goodsell, 1994). This disapproving label is unfortunate, because it portrays public service as something to be avoided–almost at all costs! In reality, serving the public is a noble cause as well as both professionally enriching and personally rewarding. Many public administrators choose to serve even when other professions provide significantly higher monetary rewards–primarily because they receive significant satisfaction knowing they are helping to create better, safer and more enjoyable "quality of life" outcomes for those living in their community.

HISTORICAL ROOTS OF PUBLIC ADMINISTRATION IN AMERICA

Origins of "Modern" Public Administration in America (1880–1930)

Public service exists to provide better, safer and more enjoyable communities for our citizens. This noble goal is not new; efforts to improve community well-being have been ongoing for thousands of years. Nevertheless, the origins of "modern" American public administration can be traced to the writings of a young political scientist in the late 1880s. This young scholar, Woodrow Wilson, would eventually serve as our nation's 28th President (1913-1921). In his influential work, *The Study of Administration*, published in 1887 Wilson called for improved government based on professional administrative precepts and practices. He demanded government to be more "business-like" in its actions. Grover Starling noted that:

> In Wilson's view, the size and complexity of modern society had grown to a point at which the "science of administration" was essential. The time had come, he argued, to make the execution of government policy more businesslike. "The field of administration is a field of business. It is removed from the hurry and strife of politics." (Starling, 2002, p. 53)

Woodrow Wilson set the stage for the development of modern government, which began shifting away from the then-customary practice of selecting public employees based on patronage principles. His efforts, along with the passage of the Pendleton Act of 1883 establishing the U.S. Civil Service Commission, placed increased emphasis on the concept of government employment determined through merit principles, that is

based on "what one knew" rather than "whom one knew."

Certainly a number of other early public administration theorists significantly influenced the development of public administration theory and practice during this period. Among some of the other notable theorists making seminal contributions include:

- Frederick Taylor (1900), whose *The Principles of Scientific Management* focused on improved management practices through task and process research;
- Frank Goodnow (1900), author of *Politics and Administration*, the first published book on public administration theories and practices;
- Max Weber (1922), whose work delineated the benefits of bureaucratic form to organizations;
- Elton Mayo (1927), whose research identified the "social nature" of organizations that led to the development of human relations school of management; and
- Mary Parker Follett (1930) whose research on individual and group motivation would serve as the forerunner to participatory management theories and practices.

Growth of the Administrative State (1930-1980)

Administrative involvement and increased government participation in citizens' lives fundamentally grew during this period because of two key world events: the Great Depression of 1929 and America's entry into World War II in 1941. America's business sector's economic collapse during the Great Depression created a vacuum of leadership. Out of desperation, citizens turned to government as the mechanism for ensuring social calm and economic stability. Fundamentally, these events reshaped America's philosophic perspective of "government by exception" to "government as the rule."

America's leadership during World War II and its industrial infrastructure being spared from most of the war's destruction propelled it into an economic dominant position during the 1950s and 1960s. Other nations' economic capacities, transportation infrastructures, and investment capacities were destroyed, allowing American industry to develop into its world leading economic position. Such growth increased income in the pockets of Americans and led to their demands for increased public goods and services.

These increased service demands resulted in a rapid growth of government employment opportunity for professional public servants to manage federal, state, and local government agencies. The growth of American government employment was particularly pronounced within state and local governments between 1950 and 1975. On average, one of every nine Americans is employed directly by some branch of government. But the number of individuals whose employment is reliant on public funds is substantially more - with up to one out of every three jobs today influenced by the expenditure of public resources.

Public Administration in the Era of Retrenchment, Reinvention and Globalization (1980–present)

As previously mentioned, America's self-confidence and trust in government began to crumble shortly following the assassination of John Kennedy in 1963. Confidence in governmental institutions, and secondarily for those who served in government, was further shaken with the outcome of the Vietnam conflict. Other events (e.g., the gasoline shortages of the early 1970s, Nixon's Watergate and his eventual forced resigna-

tion in 1974, and Jimmy Carter's perceived mishandling of the American economy and the Iran hostages in 1979–1980) also created citizenry doubts about government.

In 1980, Ronald Reagan was elected as America's fortieth president. A major thrust of his campaign was that government does not solve public problems; rather that "government is the problem." Change and cutbacks in government became vogue. Public perception had come full circle, casting doubt over the ability of public servants and public administration to solve pressing public policy problems. Calls for reform were common, even to the point that some communities mobilized to curb, and in some instances limit, the taxing authority of public leaders through state and local referenda. Specific examples of successful tax revolutions occurred in the states of California, Ohio, and Texas. In the case of California, local governments were mandated to cut rates of taxation on property by as much as 25 percent. In a matter of days, California governments were placed in the position of managing public services with substantially lower revenue bases (Osborne & Grabler, 1992). Reinventing government became a necessity in these cases; not unexpectedly, government survived as public administrators learned to do more for their citizenry with stable or reduced (as opposed increasing) revenue bases (Hammer & Champy, 1993).

In the new millennium, our citizens remain concerned about government's ability to aid all in achieving the American dream. We now live in a global society where our jobs are exported to China, to India, or to other low labor cost developing nations. We worry about our government's ability (and willingness) to stabilize energy and petroleum prices, which presently appear to have no meaningful relationship to market reality. We hate war but fear the potential of terrorist acts in our homeland.

Most of these acts are more in the control of national elected officials and out of the control of the average public servant. Ironically, we view bad times as being the fault of our government and our public servants yet frequently we fail to credit them during periods of economic growth and prosperity.

THE MISSION OF PUBLIC ADMINISTRATION AND PUBLIC ADMINISTRATORS

The American Society of Public Administration's Code of Ethics best encapsulates the primary mission for those serving in public administration:

- Serve the public good by using discretionary authority that promotes the public's interest;
- Respect the law and the constitutional rights of the individual by understanding its contents and by avoiding unlawful application of governmental laws and policies;
- Demonstrate personal integrity that inspires confidence and trust in public service;
- Promote open, honest, and ethical communication and behavior that maintains accountability of conduct; and
- Strive continually for the highest of professional excellence and competence. (Paraphrased from ASPA's Code of Ethics-for a fuller delineation of this policy go to http://www.aspanet.org/scriptcontent/index_codeofethics.cfm).

PUBLIC ADMINISTRATORS: WHO THEY SERVE AND CLIENT NEEDS THEY ADDRESS

In business, the relationship between the seller and buyer is easily understood based on the exchange of money for a good or service. This economic exchange is not so easily defined in public service because public administrators often serve multiple, and at times conflicting, clients. The "customers" whom public administrators serve, often simultaneously, include:

End-Customers: Citizens and organizations receiving public services, such as police and fire dispatches for assistance, social service assistance, requests for building permits, and refuge/garbage collection;

Internal-Customers: Staff providing support within public organizations to other units to ensure better end-customer service outcomes, such as human resources specialists providing selection and training assistance to other departments, procurement/purchasing agents securing supplies and equipment for operational departments, and maintenance/fleet services personnel keeping motorized vehicles in operation;

Elected Officials: Public servants frequently respond to information queries from their superiors—elected officials, such as the president, state governors, and local commissioners/council members—who are directly accountable to the public; and,

Taxpayers: Public administrators and unit personnel are also accountable to the citizens who provide the revenues to run government. In this case, public servants have an ethical obligation, within reasonable parameters, in the execution of their duties.

Government agencies at all levels require skilled personnel to meet varied needs for running and overseeing organizational programs and activities. The broad-based client needs that public administrators address include the following:

Program Management/Administration– administrators who serve in executive capacities, strategically planning for the organization's future needs as well as overseeing ongoing operations;

Management/Policy Analysis–individuals who act in problem solving capacities seeking to facilitate the effective implementation of policy and program initiatives;

Policy/Program Evaluation–evaluators who serve to monitor program initiatives as well as evaluating policy outcomes and impacts; and,

Target Group Advocacy/Ombudsmen Role–public servants who serve to protect the interests of individuals who are politically disenfranchised or incapable of promoting their own group's needs. Examples of groups needing assistance include the homeless, indigent people, and persons with disabilities, and other politically powerless groups with special needs.

PHILOSOPHICAL ASSUMPTIONS DRIVING THE ACTIONS OF PUBLIC ADMINISTRATORS

Stephen K. Bailey's research identifies the philosophic assumptions that define what public administration is concerned with through the development of four theories (Bailey, 1968). He suggests that public administration is concerned with:

1. *Descriptive theory*–identifying and describing effective hierarchical structures, systems, and relationships with its task environment;
2. *Normative theory*–understanding the "value goals" of the field, what public administrators should do once policies have been legislated and what administrative scholars should recommend to practitioners relating to public policy;
3. *Assumptive theory*–cognition of the administrative realities of public administration, a theory that balances objectively the demands that face public servants; and,
4. *Instrumental theory*–striving to improve managerial techniques with the goal of enhancing the effective and efficient attainment of public objective.

MAJOR PUBLIC ADMINISTRATION THEORIES

Public administration as a professional discipline focuses much of its attention on Bailey's four theoretical approaches. This is particularly so with regards to the need for reflecting on public administrative assumptive and instrumental practices. Four management theories that have had a major influence on the study and practice of public administration are identified and briefly discussed below. They have been selected because of the dominance they have had and continue to have in this discipline.

Scientific Management Approach (1900–1940)

This early theory of organizational management (1900–1940) was based largely on the works of Frederick W. Taylor. Scientific

Management principles call for the application of a systematic approach for managing tasks in order to identify the "one best way" with which to design work and work relationships. The goal of this theory was to identify the fastest, most efficient, and least fatiguing production methods, thereby improving desired organizational outcomes.

Human Relations Movement (1930–1970)

The Human Relations Movement grew out of the research conducted at the Western Electric's Hawthorne Works plant in Chicago in the late 1920s and early 1930s. Harvard University researcher Elton Mayo and his associates' findings led to the questioning of "scientific approaches" as the only means for management and administration oversight. Through their research, it was discovered that social relationships and social groups' needs among workers were often more powerful inducements to productivity outcomes. This led to an increased emphasis on social and psychological aspects of work and opened the field of public administration to increased utilization of behavioral sciences as a tool to achieve higher quality work outcomes as well as improved cooperation among staff.

Total Quality Management (TQM) (1980–present)

TQM found its origins during World War II, but its understanding and application are linked to W. Edwards Deming and his work in Japan during the early 1950s. Deming, a New York University professor, had sought to put his "quality" tenets to work in American organizations, but his ideas were rejected. Japan, however, in the midst of rebuilding its war-torn economy, willingly accepted his "quality" approach. American organizational interest belatedly began developing in the late 1970s, with fuller acceptance occurring in the decade of the 1980s. TQM, which expands on the concepts of quality control, places heavy emphasis on the continuous improvement of goods and services, with the goal of exceeding the expectations of those customers receiving the goods or services.

Reinvention/Reengineering Movement (1980–present)

The Reinvention/Reengineering Movement couples two lines of recent research in the field of Public Administration. The concept of "reinventing government" stems from the necessity of finding coping mechanisms for "doing more with fewer resources" following the tax revolts in the early 1980s. One predominant work that was highly influential in the process of change was David Osborne and Ted Grabler's *Reinventing Government*, published in 1992. It called for allowing greater monetary flexibility in the uses of governmental resources in order to maximize effective expenditures of limited fiscal resources.

Business Process Reengineering (BPR), referred to here as "reengineering," also focuses on identifying methods to maximize productive outcomes. In this instance, it calls for a reexamination of the processes used to accomplish work. It is seen as being more radical as one of its themes with regard to the design of work processes is "if it isn't broke, break it," thereby forcing the reexamination of task designs in order to identify more efficient methods for accomplishing work. Influenced by the work of Michael Hammer and James Champy, in their book, *Reengineering the Corporation*, published in 1993, the "reengineering" movement's goal of increasing workforce efficiency continues to be of interest to public leaders. It is less favorably received by others, who perceive *reengineering* to be synonymous with organizational downsizing.

Elements and application of both reinventing and business process reengineering continue in practice today, but with the growth in outsourcing of American industry, many private organizations have scrapped their application in favor of shifting their workforces to other "out-of-country" facilities. This is particularly true for industries heavily involved in the manufacturing of goods. Ironically, public organizations and their public administrators may be forced to increase reinvention/reengineering practices as a result of the revenue shortfalls associated with recent economic downturns. Citizens expect to continue to receive services even though funding cuts have occurred in the monies allocated to provide these services. This relationship (that is, the continued expectation of services with fewer resources to provide them) will force governments, especially local municipalities, to find ways of doing more with less. Reengineering may be the only trick up the sleeve of the public administrator to successfully achieve this formidable outcome.

CAREERS IN PUBLIC ADMINISTRATION AND PUBLIC SERVICE

Opportunities for talented and professionally trained individuals abound in the field of public administration. Entry into public service is attainable from virtually all academic disciplines. For example, an individual with a background in chemical engineering might well be qualified for a number of positions in government. This person will find opportunities at all levels of government in such agencies as the U.S. Department of Agriculture, the Environmental Protection Agency, Department of Homeland Security, as well as in state and local departments of health

and numerous other agencies where this specialized knowledge is valued.

Providing complete lists of occupations that exist for those seeking careers in the public administration is impractical for this chapter. Nonetheless, there are occupational categories where training in public administration facilitates the professional development and career advancement of those employed in public service. Eight categories are identified below as "areas of opportunity" for those seeking to identify positions as future public servants. Briefly, the fields (and a description of the primary duties) are identified:

1. *Management and Administration*–Individuals in these areas oversee program operations to ensure that the unit's mission, goals, and objectives are met. Examples of occupations include city managers, county administrators, executive directors, and cabinet secretaries in government agencies.

2. *Financial Administration*–Individuals in this area act as watch guards over the fiscal integrity of resources expended by government. They help hold decision makers accountable for where they allocate resources to maintain and ensure fiscal transparency. Examples of occupations include directors of finance, budget analysts, and governmental accountants.

3. *Human Resource Management*–Professionals serving in this field focus on the attainment, retention, development, and equitable treatment of the organization's workforce. Examples of occupations include human resource directors and managers and personnel specialist in the subfields of compensation/benefits, labor relations, training, and equal employment.

4. *Planning/GIS*–Planners serve their communities by creating convenient, equi-

table, healthful, efficient, and attractive environments for present and future generations (American Planning Association, Internet Citation, go to www. planning.org). Examples of occupations in this area include urban planner, transportation planner, land use/ real estate management, and GIS technicians.

5. *Law Enforcement/Fire Service/Emergency Service*–The public safety professionals seek to secure safer communities through the enforcement of laws, by preventive education (e.g., fire and crime prevention), and through containment efforts when crises arise. Examples of occupations include police chiefs, secret service, FBI and ATF investigators, state troopers, crime labor specialists, fire chief, firefighters, arson specialists, and emergency medical technicians.

6. *Policy Analysis and Evaluation*–People in this subfield determine the best strategies for the implementation of new public policies as well as determining the effectiveness of existing programs and policy. Examples of occupations include General Accountancy Office (GAO) and Office of Management and Budget (OMB) evaluators and policy analysts for numerous other federal, state, and local agencies.

7. *Social Service*–These professionals ensure the health and safety of children and adults who cannot protect themselves as well as help parents and caregivers in need of financial assistance in order to reach higher level of social and economic self-sufficiency. Examples of occupations include human services coordinators, human services specialists, social workers, adult/child abuse counselors, and probate/parole agents.

8. *Economic and International Development*– These specialists identify means for enhancing the factors of productive capacity–land, labor, capital and technology-of a national, state, or local economy. Examples of occupations include economic development coordinator positions with international organizations (e.g., United Nations Development Program, US Agency for International Development) and within federal, state and local governments (e.g., U.S. and state Department's of Commerce) and frequently with larger county/city government.

Career employment opportunities for professionally trained public administrators also exist in many nonprofit organizations and associations as well as in the field of management consulting.

PREPARING FOR CAREERS IN PUBLIC ADMINISTRATION/ PUBLIC SERVICE

Undergraduate Education– Bachelor of Science in Public Affairs/ Administration

Some colleges and universities offer an undergraduate degree in Public Administration/Public Affairs, frequently referred to as the B.S.P.A. degree. However, public service entry level employment does not necessarily require specialized public administration training, as often is the case in many other professions. Because the breadth and depth of opportunities is so wide in government, it often recruits talented undergraduate degree recipients from a number of academic disciplines. Nevertheless, as the need for public administration generalists has increased over time so have opportunities to acquire training in this field. The typical route that many students take is to gain an undergraduate degree in an area where they desire specialized skills development and training (e.g., fields of engineering, economics, political science, business management, psychology, social work). Individuals seeking specialized undergraduate training in the field of public administration (that is, the B.S.P.A.) should consult the National Association of Schools of Public Affairs and Administration (NASPAA) website (see http://www.naspaa.org) for universities offering this degree.

Graduate Professional Training– The Master of Public Administration (MPA)

Following completion of the undergraduate degree, and often with work experience in public service, individuals will return to gain a master's degree in Public Administration/ Public Affairs (referred to here jointly as MPA), Master of Public Policy or Master of Urban Affairs degree. Typically, applicants maintaining an undergraduate grade point average (GPA) of 3.0 or higher (on a 4.0 scale) and who's Graduate Records Examination (GRE) scores for the verbal and quantitative index combined average 1000 or higher will gain admission in most MPA graduate school programs. However, competition for university scholarship funding tends to require higher GPA and GRE scores. This is significantly the case for the highest nationally ranked MPA programs.

The most recognized graduate degree is the MPA. As of September 1, 2007, there were 259 institutions (that is, colleges and universities across America) that are members of NASPAA. Of these programs, the NASPAA 2007-08 Roster of Accredited Programs indicates that 161 programs (from 154 schools) held NASPAA Accreditation (http://www.naspaa.org, n.p.). Thus, approximately 59 percent of NASPAA Institutional

Members also maintain nationally accredited MPA degree programs.

U.S. News & World Report ranks MPA degree offerings across American universities on a biannual basis. For more than a quarter of a century, three programs have consistently ranked among the top three: Syracuse University, Harvard University, and Indiana University, with Syracuse University being the top ranked program as of the March, 2008 ranking, and Indiana University and Harvard University tied as the second best MPA granting schools. The 2008 rankings of Public Affairs (that is, Public Administration) programs can be located at the *U.S. News & World Reports* website (U.S.News & World Report at: http://gradschools.usnews.rankingsandreviews.com/grad/pad/search.)

Doctoral Studies in Public Administration and Public Affairs

Doctoral studies in Public Administration typically flow along two possible routes: the acquisition of a Doctorate of Philosophy in Public Affairs (Ph.D.) or the Doctorate of Public Administration (D.P.A.). According to NASPAA, the choice of degrees pursued is heavily influenced by historical accidents at particular institutions, especially the scope of the formal authority of a graduate school or division that controls the Ph.D. Either name is appropriate for a strong, doctoral-level program of research training. Although not mutually exclusive, a D.P.A. degree tends to be one that prepares individuals for the application of knowledge as a practitioner of public administration. The Ph.D. degree tends to relate more to graduate-level teaching and more in depth research into the theory and practice in the field.

Individuals seeking the doctorate-level Public Administration degree should anticipate a minimum of three years of full-time coursework and one to two years of dissertation preparation beyond the MPA degree. On average, individuals pursuing a doctorate in public administration should anticipate six to eight years of total post-graduate studies.

OCCUPATIONAL WORK SETTINGS FOR THOSE TRAINED IN PUBLIC ADMINISTRATION

Public administration training affords extensive employment variety and occupational flexibility for those entering into public service. Largely, an individual's employment opportunities are also influenced by his/her educational attainment, practitioner experience, and professional network with others in the occupational field of interest.

Working in American Universities and Colleges

For individuals wishing to pursue the academic track of service as professors of American universities, it will be necessary in virtually all cases to hold a doctorate in public administration (or a closely related doctorate degree). This is particular true for those institutions providing graduate level public administration training or seeking NASPAA accreditation.

Working for Government

In May, 2008, 22,808,000 people worked in government (at all levels), with 2,728,000 of these being federal civilian employees (Bureau of Labor Statistics, June 6, 2008). Today, there are over 87,000 governmental units (mostly at the local level) serving distinct constituent needs across the nation (U.S. Census–Statistical Abstract of the United States, 2000, p. 299).

Where one gains employment, is determined more by an individual's occupational interests than by the magnitude of opportunity because the need for talented individuals will continue to exist. Clearly, employment opportunity will be influenced by the general population's desire for sustained public services because the goal of government is to meet some defined service need of identified clients (primarily, but not exclusively, the taxpaying citizenry). Economic conditions also influence demand for public servants; thus, opportunities for employment will be more plentiful in larger hubs of the nation (e.g., New York, Chicago, Atlanta, Los Angles, and Washington, D.C.) especially for individuals wishing to pursue employment in federal government. Likewise, those choosing employment in state government will find greater opportunities in state capitals, where state public employment positions are concentrated. In local government, wealthier and more financially stable governments should also prove to be better places for locating future employment. Employment is most plentiful and most available within municipal (i.e., country and city) and special district (e.g., school, library, water) units of local government. The Bureau of Labor Statistics, for example, estimates that in May, 2008, almost 20 million (19,851,000) people worked in American state and local governments (Bureau of Labor Statistics, June 6, 2008). This is approximately 15 percent (14.34) of all those currently in the American workplace. Clearly, students in undergraduate studies seeking to enhance their potential for employment with public agencies should take advantage of internship and cooperative education employment opportunities. Prior experience, even with short-term internships, often places one at a competitive advantage over others lacking similar experiential backgrounds.

Global Employment in Public Service

It is difficult to find greater opportunities for individuals with a lust to travel and to experience life in different cultural settings than those that exist in government. Numerous opportunities exist to work for national and international governmental organizations. For example, the United Nations offers individuals the opportunity to work toward the goal of global peace and prosperity. Numerous federal cabinet level departments (e.g., U.S. Departments of State, Commerce, Agriculture,) and other independent agencies (e.g., U.S. Environmental Protection Agency, U.S. Agency for International Development) of the U.S. federal government provide "overseas" employment opportunities. In many cases, selection for these opportunities as a Foreign Service Officer is based on a competitive exam process. Information about preparing for the Foreign Service Officer Written Examination and the application process needed to join the Foreign Service is available through most university career placement centers. This information can also be downloaded from the U.S. Department of State website at http://www.careers.state.gov/officer/index.h tml.

Other Areas of Opportunity for Trained Public Administrators

Two additional areas of employment opportunity also deserve mention. Increasing opportunities for employment exist in the nonprofit sector, which in recent years have taken over some of the service provision areas previously provided within local community governments. In many instances, public administration practitioners have

shifted to leadership roles in the nonprofit sector.

A second area where opportunity exists for those trained professionally in public administration is serving as public sector consultants. Frequently, individuals with graduate level degrees in public administration (that is, the M.P.A and/or Ph.D.) gain specialized skills that governments seek to hire on a contractual basis. Examples of contractual services included (but are not limited to): economic development and community planning, information management and technology, compensation and benefits analysis, and organizational training in a wide variety of areas (for example, diversity training, leadership and supervisory skills development, health, and safety).

PROFESSIONAL ORGANIZATIONS IN THE FIELD OF PUBLIC ADMINISTRATION

Many professional associations exist for specific subfields of public administration. Space limitations preclude listing most of these associations. Nevertheless, discussion about the more predominant professional associations affecting public administration is provided below. Among the most predominant American public administration associations are:

1. *American Society for Public Administration* (see www.aspanet.org)–currently AS PA consists of approximately 9,000 Public Administration scholars, practitioners, teachers, and students. It is the largest and most prominent professional association in the field of public administration. ASPA produces a number of public administration journals including the leading journal in

the field of public administration, *Public Administration Review*.

2. *International City/County Management Association* (see ICMA, www.icma.org) —established in 1914, ICMA addresses relevant issues affecting public service in local government (Texas City Management Association, 2008). ICMA provides comprehensive assistance to its membership, including its ICMA University, a training and development resource for its members. It also publishes the monthly journal, *Public Management.*

3. *International Public Management Association for Human Resources* (IPMA-HR, see www.ipma-hr.org)—the IPMA-HR membership is comprised of federal, state, and local government human resource specialists from across the United States and overseas. It is the leading public sector human resource management association. IPMA-HR assists individuals, organizations and agencies involved in the practice of human resource management. In existence since 1973, IPMA-HR formed through the consolidation of the Public Personnel Association, founded in Chicago in 1906, and the Society for Personnel Administration, founded in Washington, D.C. in 1937. IPMA publishes *Public Personnel Management,* a leading journal in the field of public sector human resource management.

4. *National Association of Schools of Public Affairs and Administration* (NASPAA, see www.naspaa.org)—NASPAA is an association of 259 U.S. universities seeking to promote excellence in public service education. NASPAA, in conjunction with the Commission on Peer Review and Accreditation, provide guideline on sustaining and improving public administration education in U.S. colleges and universities.

NASPAA provides an excellent resource for individuals seeking further information about public administration programs across America.

CAREER ADVANCEMENT, EMPLOYMENT OUTLOOK AND COMPENSATION

In most instances government employment provides excellent opportunities for advancement for those willing to continuously develop their skills. Clearly, it has been our experience that individuals willing to seek advanced degrees in the field of public administration studies gain considerable upward mobility in the public sector. This should continue to be the trend as many "Baby Boomers" (individuals born between 1946–1964) begin to retire.

Public Service traditionally has offered more stable employment. It is generally less likely to lay off employees than the private organizations, in part because of the resource base at its disposal. A recent survey conducted by *InfoWorld,* for example, reports that government employment offers the Information Technology (IT) manager strong benefits and solid retirement plans. One respondent's comments reflected the advantage of government employment when he stated,

> While layoffs and firings are certainly possible, they are much less likely than in the private sector. You don't worry too much about whether you'll get your next paycheck, whether you will lose your health insurance, or whether you will have enough money for a decent retirement. (Prencipe & Sanborn, 2001, n.p.)

Opportunities remain strong for protected class members (e.g., African Americans, Hispanic Americans, and women) as most governments strive to set the example of being good employers who apply equal employment and affirmative action standards within their hiring and promotional practices.

The 2008 pay scale for top-level administrators (those in the Senior Executive Service) is capped at $172,200. Lower-level positions that constitute a part of the General Schedule (GS) scale (the scale used for many civilian federal employees) range from approximately $17,046 to $124,010 depending on skills level, time in service in government, and geographic location of employment. The GS scale allows for regional adjustments to this scale based on geographic location of employment. The adjustments range from a low of 13.18 percent up to 32.53 percent for public servants living the San Francisco, California. For additional information, please review the 2008 Base General Schedule Pay Scale–http://www.fedjobs.com/pay/pay.html.

State and local pay is generally competitive with the private sector with one exception. Executives in the private sector–because of stock options, profit sharing, and other prerequisites not generally found in the public sector–often earn substantially more in compensation when compared with executives in public organizations. Nevertheless, many still choose public service because of the non-monetary rewards that they receive from it.

Individuals seeking information regarding salaries in specific state or local government settings can gain this information by contacting a specific agency's human resource/personnel department as, in most cases, the pay scales of public employees is public record.

SUMMARY

Employment within the Public Service provides opportunities for continual professional development, personal gratification, and the knowledge that one is enhancing the achievement of providing better, safer, sustainable, and more enjoyable environments for one's communities. Working in the field of public administration provides the opportunity to interact with interesting people, to travel to distant locales, and to gain personal satisfaction within one's chosen occupation. Contrary to popular perception, the life of public bureaucrats often is an exciting and rewarding experience, one that most would choose over again, if asked to make a choice.

REFERENCES

American Planning Association. *What is planning?* Further information on this topic can be viewed at Internet site http://www.planning.org/careers/field.htm.

American Society for Public Administration. *ASPA's code of ethics*, Information from Internet website: http://www.aspanet.org/scriptcontent/index_codeofethics.cfm.

Bailey, S. K. (1968). Objectives of the Theory of Public Administration. In J. C. Charlesworth (Ed.), *Theory and practice of public administration: Scope, objectives, and methods* (Monograph 8). Philadelphia: American Academy of Political and Social Science (pp. 128–129).

Bureau of Labor Statistics. (2008). *News* (June 6), Department of Labor. Statistic derived from Table B-1). Internet website: http://www.bls.gov/news.release/pdf/empsit.pdf.

Goodsell, C. T. (1994). *The case for bureaucracy* (3rd ed.). Chathan, NJ: Chatham House.

Hammer, M., & Champy, J. (1993). *Reengineering the corporation.* New York: Harper-Business.

National Schools of Public Affairs and Administration (NASPAA). *Search for a graduate school.* Internet website http://www.naspaa.org/students/faq/graduate/schsearch.asp.

Osborne, D., & Grabler, T. (1992). *Reinventing government.* Reading, MA: Addison-Wesley.

Prencipe, L.W., & Sanborn, S. (2001). *What are you worth?* Internet website http://www.itworld.com/Career/1698/IWD010625whatworth/.

Starling, G. (2002). *Managing the public sector* (6th ed.). Fort Worth, TX: Harcourt College Press.

Texas City Management Association (2008). *Development of the city management profession and its related organizations.* Internet website http://www.tcma.org/c-m-history.html,

U.S. Census. (2000). *Statistical abstract of the United States.* p. 299. Internet website http://www.census.gov/prod/2001pubs/statab/sec0 9.pdf.

U.S. Department of Labor-BLS (2000). *State and local government, excluding education and hospitals.* Internet website http://www.bls.gov/ oco/cg/cgs042.htm.

U.S. News & World Report. (2008). Best Graduate Schools-Public Affairs (2008 Ranking), Internet website http://gradschools.usnews.rankingsandreviews.com/grad/pad/search.

Wilson, W. (1887). The study of public administration. *Political Science Quarterly, 2* (June), 197–222.

Chapter 15

REHABILITATION COUNSELING

John D. Rasch & Colleen A. Etzbach

Rehabilitation counseling is a profession dedicated to helping individuals with disabilities achieve productive and independent lives. The discipline is taught and practiced throughout the United States, and training occurs at the master's level. There are also a number of undergraduate rehabilitation services programs around the country, but becoming certified in the discipline requires attending graduate school, earning a master's degree in rehabilitation counseling, and passing a nationally standardized certification examination which is overseen by the Commission on Rehabilitation Counselor Certification (CRCC).

The development of rehabilitation counseling may be traced as far back as the American Charity Organization movement which began in the late nineteenth century (Rubin & Roessler, 2008). Some of the earliest legislation for rehabilitation services was instituted in 1918 through the Soldier's Rehabilitation Act which authorized vocational services for veterans with service related disabilities returning from World War I (Jenkins, Patterson & Syzmanski, 1992). The first comprehensive federal program for individuals with disabilities was the Civilian Vocational Rehabilitation Act of 1920 which

focused on the provision of vocational services for persons with physical disabilities (Obermann, 1965). In 1954, Congress specifically provided funds to train professional rehabilitation counselors for the rapidly expanding state/federal rehabilitation program (Rubin & Roessler, 2008). These training monies went to American universities and served as the financial impetus for the development of the discipline. Presently there are approximately a hundred master's programs nationally accredited by the Council on Rehabilitation Education (CORE).

Rehabilitation counselors currently work in a wide variety of settings extending far beyond the state/federal rehabilitation program. Depending on the agency setting, rehabilitation counselors may work with individuals having physical, mental health, and substance abuse disorders. Disabilities may be congenital, acquired (such as through vehicular accidents, industrial injuries, or other accidents), or caused by chronic illness or disease. The typical consumers of services have a disability that results in barriers that often impede vocational and/or independent living. The role of the rehabilitation counselor is to assist individuals with disabilities to achieve independent, productive, and, above all, personally satisfying lives in their communities.

PHILOSOPHICAL ASSUMPTIONS

Rehabilitation counselors work from the philosophical basis that individuals with disabilities have significant abilities and with appropriate assistance they can achieve productive living and maximize independence. Health problems are inevitable in every society and may strike any person at any time. The rehabilitation profession believes it is in the best interest of society to have services in place that will restore and maintain the independence of any person adversely affected by disability, regardless of time of onset. Moreover, the profession believes society should not isolate or institutionalize (except as a last resort) individuals with disabilities, but should attempt to provide rehabilitation services in the least restrictive environment possible. Furthermore, every effort should be made to provide persons with disabilities life experiences and opportunities that approximate societal norms to the fullest extent reasonably possible (Parker & Szymanski, 1998). The profession of rehabilitation counseling values the individual's right for freedom of choice and maximum community integration.

The profession has attempted to solidify these philosophies and values through legislative efforts. The rights of individuals with disabilities are spelled out in the Individuals with Disabilities Education Act (PL105–17), the Rehabilitation Act of 1973 (PL93–112), including its amendments and reauthorizations, and the Americans with Disabilities Act of 1990 (PL101–336) (Berkowitz, 1987; Bruyere et al., 2006; Carney, 1991; DeJong & Batavia, 1990). The moral basis of this legislation is that it is the principled responsibility of our society to assure and promote the maximum independence of persons with disabilities. Buttressing this moral argument is the fact that effective rehabilitation counseling also has economic justification. To the extent that individuals with disabilities are able to achieve independence, especially as reflected by educational and subsequent vocational success, we reduce the need for public assistance and create tax-paying citizens who would otherwise be dependent on the state (DeJong & Batavia, 1990).

Rehabilitation counseling, unlike many other disciplines, takes a holistic approach to providing services for persons with disabilities (Maki & Riggar, 1997). Its focus is not on just one area of an individual's life, but on all aspects of the person's life where barriers might exist that prevent the individual from becoming as fully integrated as possible into the community (Hahn, 1987). This requires not only attending to "barriers within the individual," but also those that may be present in the family, the community, and society as a whole. It also may mean providing a wide array of services for an individual instead of only one or two.

MAJOR THEORIES

A commitment to what is known as *the rehabilitation process* is the theoretical underpinning of the discipline. Simply stated, this is the step-by-step sequence of activities counselors engage in when working with consumers toward achieving their goals. It generally involves the following steps: (1) identifying individuals needing services, processing applications, and establishing eligibility; (2) evaluation, assessment, and counseling to identify realistic and achievable rehabilitation goals which will become the rehabilitation plan; (3) the provision of physical restoration, vocational education and training, case management, counseling, and any related services necessary to actualize the rehabilitation plan; (4) assistance with locating employment or job placement services; and (5) follow-up and maintenance services as necessary (Roessler & Rubin, 2006; Rubin & Roessler, 2008). Rehabilitation counselors, as well as all human service professionals, work within the mandates of their agencies. However, rehabilitation counselors assure that within those mandates consumers are involved in all aspects of planning and service delivery.

Humanistic psychology has had a very strong impact on the field of rehabilitation counseling, and rehabilitation counselors accordingly encourage and support consumer involvement in their own rehabilitation process to the greatest extent possible. The counseling theories employed by rehabilitation counselors are varied, but many counselors develop an eclectic approach (Cormier, Nurius & Osborn, 2009; Gladding, 2009; Nugent & Jones, 2005; Sharf, 2008) where they attempt to draw from the strengths of different counseling approaches. These include Cognitive-Behavioral, Adlerian, Person-Centered, and Existential approaches. Cognitive-behavioral approaches focus on the connection between thoughts, feelings, and behaviors, and emphasize interventions in dysfunctional thinking processes that lead to distressing emotions and problematic behaviors. Adlerian theory focuses on viewing individuals positively and is based on emphasizing positive qualities and capacities rather than highlighting deficits or inabilities. The education of the rehabilitation counselor emphasizes this as it promotes looking at the person first and then the disability, as presented in the expression, "a person with a disability." Adlerian theory also believes individuals are in control of their lives and are motivated to strive toward their own goals. Rehabilitation counselors encourage their consumers to develop goals and strive to obtain them. Person-Centered

theory emphasizes the importance of empathy for clients, positive regard for them, and genuineness in the counselor's work. Existentialism focuses on the nature of the human condition, which includes freedom of choice, meaning, self-awareness, and responsibility. Rehabilitation counselors assist individuals in exploring various options whether it is for employment, independent living, and/or personal issues. Through this exploration, a rehabilitation plan is developed with goals and responsibilities that are jointly identified.

AREAS OF APPLICATION

Rehabilitation counselors have specific expertise in planning vocational rehabilitation and employment related services; these skills involve: (1) clarifying physical, mental, and emotional strengths and limitations (including prevocational skill deficits); (2) identifying vocational interests, aptitudes, and existing vocational skills (including transferable work skills); (3) relating the above to different job possibilities; and (4) developing and implementing the rehabilitation process (Roessler & Rubin, 2006; Rubin & Roessler, 2008). The training and skills of rehabilitation counselors are applicable to a wide variety of human problems. Although the settings may be varied, the job functions of rehabilitation counselors revolve around the areas of assessing client needs; developing goals and individual plans; and providing case management services, counseling, and guidance. The Council on Rehabilitation Counselor Education Accreditation Manual (2007) defines the needed academic curriculum for master's level programs as follow:

C.1 Professional Identity
Knowledge areas:[1] (a) Rehabilitation counseling scope of practice; (b) History and philosophy of rehabilitation; (c)

Legislation; (d) Ethics; (e) Professional credentialing, certification, licensure and accreditation; (f) Informed consumer choice and consumer empowerment; (g) Independent living; (h) Assistive technology; (i) Public policies; (j) Advocacy; (k) Systems knowledge of healthcare, education and rehabilitation; and (l) The ecological perspective.

C.2 Social and Cultural Diversity

Knowledge areas:[1] (a) Family development and dynamics; (b) Psychological dynamics related to self-identity, self-advocacy, competency, adjustment, and attitude formation; (c) Sociological dynamics related to self-identity, self-advocacy, competency, adjustment, and attitude formation; (d) Multicultural awareness and implications for ethical practice; (e) Diversity issues including cultural, disability, gender, sexual orientation, and aging issues; (f) Current issues and trends in a diverse society; and (g) Personal professional development strategies for self-monitoring

C.3 Human Growth and Development

Knowledge areas:[1] (a) Developmental theories across the life span; (b) Physical development; (c) Emotional development; (d) Cognitive development; (e) Behavioral development; (f) Moral development; (g) Theories of personality development; (h) Human sexuality and disability; (i) Spiritually; (j) Transition issues related to family, school, employment, aging, and disability; (k) Social and learning needs of individuals across the life span; and (l) Ethical and legal issues impacting individuals and families related to adjustment and transition.

C.4 Employment and Career Development

Knowledge areas:[1] (a) Career development; (b) Disability benefits systems including workers compensation, long-term disability, and social security; (c) Career counseling; (d) Job analysis, work site modification and restructuring, including the application of appropriate technology; (e) Transferable skill analysis; (f) Computer-based assessment tools; (g) Vocational planning and assessment; (h) Job and employer development; (i) Employer consultation; (j) Business/corporate human resource concepts and terminology; (k) Workplace culture and environment; (l) Work conditioning/work hardening; (m) Job placement strategies; (n) Computer-based job matching systems; (o) Follow-up/post employment services; (q) Occupational information including labor market trends and the importance of meaningful employment with a career focus; (r) Supported employment, job coaching, and natural supports; and (s) Ethical issues in employment.

C.5 Counseling and Consultation

Knowledge areas:[1] (a) Counseling and personality theory; (b) Mental health counseling; (c) Interviewing and counseling skill development; (d) Theories and models for consultation; (e) Assistive technologies; (f) Vocational consultation; (g) Supervision theories, models, and techniques; (h) Consumer empowerment and rights; (i) Boundaries of confidentiality; (j) Ethics in the counseling relationship; (k) Multicultural issues in counseling; (l) Gender issues in counseling; (m) Conflict resolution strategies; (n) Computer-based counseling tools; and (o) Internet resources for rehabilitation counseling.

C.6 Group Work

Knowledge areas:[1] (a) Group dynamics and counseling theory; (b) Family dynamics and counseling theory; (c) Interdisciplinary teamwork; (d) Group leadership styles and techniques; (e) Group methods, selection criteria, and evaluation strategies; and (f) Group skills development.

C.7 Assessment

Knowledge areas:[1] (a) Assessment resources and methods; (b) Standardization; (c) Measurement and statistical concepts; (d) Selecting and administering the appropriate assessment method (e.g., standardized tests, situational assessment, place-access vs. access-place); (e) Obtaining, interpreting, and synthesizing assessment information; (f) Conducting ecological assessment; (g) Assistive technology; and (h) Ethical, legal, and cultural implications in assessment

C.8 Research and Program Evaluation

Knowledge areas:[1] (a) Review of clinical rehabilitation literature; (b) Library research for rehabilitation related current information; (c) Basic statistics; (d) Research methods; (e) Outcome based research; and (f) Ethical, legal, and cultural issues related to research and evaluation.

C.9 Medical, Functional, and Environmental Aspects of Disability

Knowledge areas:[1] (a) The human body system; (b) Medical terminology; (c) Medical, functional, environmental and psychosocial aspects of physical disabilities, psychiatric rehabilitation, substance abuse, cognitive disability, sensory disability, and developmental disability; (d) Assistive technology; (e) Dual diagnosis and the workplace; (f) The concept of functional capacity; and (g) Wellness and illness prevention concepts and strategies.

C.10 Rehabilitation Services and Resources

Knowledge areas:[1] (a) Case and caseload management; (b) Vocational rehabilitation; (c) Independent living; (d) School to work transition services; (e) Psychiatric rehabilitation practice; (f) Substance abuse treatment and recovery; (g) Disability management; (h) Employer-based and disability case management practices; (i) Design and development of transitional and return-to-work programs; (j) Forensic rehabilitation and vocational expert practices; (k) Managed care; (l) Systems resource information including funding availability; (m) Utilization of community-based rehabilitation and service coordination; (n) Consumer advocacy and empowerment; (o) Marketing rehabilitation services; (p) Life care planning; (q) Strategies to develop rapport/referral network; (r) Case reporting; (s) Professional advocacy; (t) Clinical problem-solving skills; (u) Case recording and documentation; (v) Interdisciplinary consultation; and (w) Computer applications and technology for caseload.

In rehabilitation counseling, the course curriculum focuses on the student obtaining knowledge so as to take a holistic view of individuals and their interactions with their environment and surroundings. The content encompasses information which provides the student the ability to address issues that individuals may face in all areas of their life such as educational, vocational, family, mental health, independent living, and physical health. This differs widely from other counseling professions that traditionally take into consideration fewer aspects of an individual's life (i.e., focusing on classroom behavior or a mental health issue). While vocational counseling is a core and highly important service (Zunker, 2008), rehabilitation counselors must also be able to interpret and utilize medical information, specialized assessments, coordinate services, work with other professionals and the individual's family, and develop rehabilitation plans with clients. This knowledge provides rehabilitation counselors with the skills to advocate for individuals with a disability and ensure they have the ability to integrate into the community with the same opportunities as other individuals in order to reach their maximum potential.

PREPARATION AND DEVELOPMENT TO WORK IN THE FIELD

There is no specific undergraduate major required for graduate studies in rehabilitation counseling, but most students complete an undergraduate major in one of the social or behavioral sciences. Psychology, sociology, and education are fairly typical majors, and as indicated earlier, many universities have undergraduate rehabilitation services programs. Each university has its own admission standards, but a 3.0 undergraduate grade-point average and a combined Verbal and Quantitative score of 1000 on the Graduate Record Examination typically is adequate for admission to most programs.

Master's degree programs in rehabilitation counseling programs range from 48 to 60 semester hours. Specific course titles vary from one university to the next, but the following is fairly typical of required courses: (1) Introduction to Rehabilitation Counseling; (2) Counseling Theories and Techniques; (3) Personality Theories; (4) Psychosocial Aspects of Disability; (5) Medical Aspects of Disability; (6) Evaluation and Assessment; (7) Vocational Aspects of Disability; (8) Rehabilitation Case Management; (9) Research Methods; (10) Practicum; and (11) Internship. Applied clinical experiences are stressed in all accredited rehabilitation programs. Accredited programs have at least one practicum (minimum of 100 field hours) and an Internship (minimum of 600 field hours). If a program is not CORE accredited, the graduate will need a full year of work experience under the supervision of a Certified Rehabilitation Counselor (CRC) before being eligible to sit for the discipline's examination (Certified Rehabilitation Counselor; CRC). Prospective students can identify accredited programs in rehabilitation counseling by contacting CORE or the National Council on Rehabilitation Education (consult the website indicated in the Reference list).

WORK SETTINGS

The most traditional work setting for rehabilitation counselors is the state/federal vocational rehabilitation program and its support agencies. Every U.S. state and territory has this program, which is separately administered by each state and nationally overseen by the Rehabilitation Services Administration of the U.S. Department of Labor. Individuals are eligible for the state/federal program if they have a disability that constitutes a handicap to employment, have a reasonable potential to work as a result of rehabilitation services and cannot obtain needed services from other sources. Employment for persons with a disability is not limited to the competitive sector, and when a more severe disability is present, supported employment, self-employment, or other forms of employment may be more appropriate and achievable rehabilitation goals.

The U.S. Veterans Administration also runs a substantial vocational rehabilitation program that employs many rehabilitation counselors. Rehabilitation counselors also are employed by private-for-profit insurance and rehabilitation companies. In the for-profit sector, clients typically are individuals who sustained industrial injuries covered by state Workers' Compensation laws. Other lines of insurance such as medical malpractice, automobile liability, and long-term disability may also generate referrals for rehabilitation, medical management, life-care planning, and/or vocational expert testimony. These areas require the rehabilitation counselor to focus on the medical issues that the individual will face in his or her remaining years of life, the vocational implications of the disability/illness, how future earning potential may be negatively impacted, and the overall financial impact of his or her disability.

While the above are major employment areas that utilize the vocational expertise of rehabilitation counselors, many graduates work in other human service areas. Emener, Patrick, & Hollingsworth (1984) reported that the traditional areas listed above are far from the only career paths available for rehabilitation counselors; fittingly, many students aspire for and are employed in a variety of areas. The field of rehabilitation counseling provides a vast opportunity to work in many settings and with diverse populations. Settings include rehabilitation facilities, medical hospitals, community corrections and/or prisons, human resources, psychiatric hospitals, independent living centers, mental health agencies, substance abuse treatment facilities, private practice, public schools, vocational schools or colleges, social services, and nursing homes (Koch & Rumrill, 1997; Syzmanski, et al, 1993). Many graduates specialize in areas such as geriatric rehabilitation, pediatric rehabilitation, substance abuse treatment, mental health, employee assistance programs, and disability management (Goodwin, 1992). Although the settings may be diverse, rehabilitation counselors continue to provide services to individuals with various physical and mental disabilities.

PROFESSIONAL ORGANIZATIONS

Rehabilitation counseling is a discipline that spans both the national rehabilitation movement, as represented by the National Rehabilitation Association (NRA), and professional counseling movement, as represented by the American Counseling Association (ACA). It has a professional division within both organizations. The professional division within NRA is the Rehabilitation Counselors and Educators Association (RCEA), and the discipline's division within ACA is the American Rehabilitation Counseling Association (ARCA). There is also a freestanding rehabilitation counseling association, the National Association of Rehabilitation Counselors (NRCA). There are a number of professional journals in the field pub-

lished by the different rehabilitation counseling associations. NRCA publishes the *Journal of Applied Rehabilitation Counseling*, ARCA the *Rehabilitation Counseling Bulletin*, and RCEA the *Rehabilitation Counselors and Educators Journal*. Other major associations in the field are the International Association of Rehabilitation Professionals (IARP) representing the private-for-profit sector of rehabilitation service delivery and the National Council on Rehabilitation Education that focuses on graduate and undergraduate rehabilitation training needs.

CAREER ADVANCEMENT, SALARIES EMPLOYMENT OUTLOOK

The best source of information in this area is the *Occupational Outlook Handbook* (2008–09), which is published by the Bureau of Labor Statistics (U.S. Department of Labor, 2008). It is available in hardcopy from the government and is in most libraries, but foremost readers can easily access it online (consult the list of Additional Sources and their Websites).

Career ladders for rehabilitation counselors most typically lead from the provision of direct services to positions in administration and supervision. Some agency counselors move into private practice, and others go on to become college teachers. Salaries for rehabilitation counselors vary on a state-by-state basis, and depend on what type of setting in which they are employed. The Bureau of Labor Statistics reported mean wages for rehabilitation counselors of $33,350 to $53,170. Starting salaries will naturally be significantly lower.

The online *Occupational Outlook Handbook* (2008–09) describes the future job outlook as follows:

Employment for counselors is expected to grow much faster than average through 2016. The demand for vocational or career counselors will grow due to career and job changes. State and local governments will employ a growing number of counselors to assist beneficiaries of welfare programs who must find employment upon exhausting their eligibility. Job training centers will be employing counselors to assist laid-off workers and others seeking to acquire new skills or careers. Demand is expected to be strong for rehabilitation and mental health counselors. Jobs for rehabilitation counselors are expected to grow 23 percent. Under managed care systems, insurance companies increasingly provide for reimbursement of counselors, enabling many counselors to move from schools and government agencies to private practice. Counselors are also forming group practices to receive expanded insurance coverage. The number of people who need rehabilitation services will rise as advances in medical technology continue to save lives that only a few years ago would have been lost. These individuals will need services to assist with obtaining and maintaining employment as well as live independently. In addition, legislation requiring equal employment rights for people with disabilities will spur demand for counselors. Counselors not only will help individuals with disabilities in their transition into the work force, but also will help companies comply with the law. Employers are also increasingly offering employee assistance programs that provide mental health and alcohol and drug abuse services. A growing number of people are expected to use these services as the elderly population grows, and as society focuses on ways of developing mental wellbeing, such as controlling stress associated with job and family responsibilities. (Occupational Outlook Handbook, Counselors, Job Outlook, paragraph 4; http://stats.bls.gov/oco/ocos067.htm)

SUMMARY

There are a number of different counseling professions that provide exciting career opportunities for those interested in helping others. Rehabilitation counseling is one of the largest and has as its primary focus helping individuals with disabilities achieve productive and independent lives. In the past, rehabilitation counselors mostly worked in traditional government and private settings described above, but graduates of today's programs are employed in a wide variety of human service positions in both the public and commercial sectors.

Endnote: 1. In the Council on Rehabilitation Counselor Education Accreditation Manual (2007), these knowledge areas are "listed." Herein, however, in order to save space, the book's editors have included all of them only as seriated within paragraphs.

REFERENCES

Berkowitz, E. D. (1987). *Disabled policy: American programs for the handicapped.* New York: Cambridge University Press.

Bruyere, S. M., Erickson, W. A., VanLooy, S. A., Hirsch, E. S., Cook, J. A., Burke, J., Farah, L., & Morris, M. (2006). Employment and disability policy: Recommendations for a social science research agenda. In K. J. Hagglund & A. W. Heinemann (Eds.), *Handbook of applied disability and rehabilitation research* (pp. 143–178). New York: Springer.

Carney, N. C. (1991). Disability policy and law: Impact on public sector practices. *Journal of Applied Rehabilitation Counseling, 22,* 24–26.

Cormier, S., Nurius, P. S., & Osborn, C. J. (2009). *Interviewing and change strategies for helpers.* Belmont, CA: Brooks/Cole.

Council on Rehabilitation Education. (2007). *Accreditation Manual.* Retrieved May 14, 2007 from: http://www.core rehab.org.

DeJong, G., & Batavia, A. (1990). The Americans with disabilities act and the current state of

U.S. disability policy. *Journal of Disability Policy Studies, 1,* 65–75.

Emener, W. G., Patrick, A., & Hollingsworth, D. K. (1984). Selected rehabilitation counseling issues: A historical perspective. In W. Emener, A. Patrick & D. Hollingsworth (Eds.), *Critical issues in rehabilitation counseling* (pp. 5–41). Springfield, IL: Charles C Thomas.

Gladding, S. T. (2009). *Counseling: A comprehensive profession* (6th ed.). Columbus, OH: Pearson.

Goodwin, L. R. (1992). Rehabilitation counselor specialization: The promise and the challenge. *Journal of Applied Rehabilitation Counseling, 23,* 5–11.

Hahn, H. (1987). Civil rights for disabled Americans: The foundation of a political agenda. In A. Gartner & T. Joes (Eds.), *Images of the disabled, disabling images* (pp. 181–203). New York: Praeger.

Jenkins, W. M., Patterson, J. B., & Szymanski. (1992). Philosophical, historical, and legislative aspects of the rehabilitation counseling profession. In R. M. Parker & E. M. Syzmanski (Eds.), *Rehabilitation counseling: Basics and beyond* (2nd ed.) (pp. 1–41). Austin, TX: PRO-ED.

Koch, L. C., & Rumrill, P. D., Jr. (1997). Rehabilitation counseling outside the state agency: Settings, roles, and functions for the new millennium. *Journal of Applied Rehabilitation Counseling, 28,* 9–14.

Maki, D.R., & Riggar, T. F. (1997). *Rehabilitation counseling: Profession and practice.* New York: Springer.

Nugent, F. A., & Jones, K. D. (2005). *Introduction to the profession of counseling* (4th ed.). Columbus, OH: Pearson Prentice-Hall.

Obermann, C. E. (1965). *A history of vocational rehabilitation in America.* Minneapolis, MN: Denison.

Parker, R. M., & Szymanski, E. M. (1998). *Rehabilitation counseling: Basics and beyond* (3rd ed.). Austin, TX: PRO-ED.

Roessler, R. T., & Rubin, S. E. (2006). *Case management and rehabilitation counseling: Procedures and techniques* (4th ed.). Austin, TX: PRO-ED.

Rubin, S. E., & Roessler, R. T. (2008). *Foundations of the vocational rehabilitation process* (6th ed.). Austin, TX: PRO-ED.

Sharf, R. T. (2008). *Theories of psychotherapy and counseling: Concepts and cases* (4th ed.). Belmont, CA: Thomson Higher Education.

Szymanski, E. M., Linkowski, D. C., Leahy, M. J., Diamonds, E. E., & Thorson, R. W. (1993). Validation of rehabilitation counseling accreditation and certification knowledge areas: Methodology and initial results. *Rehabilitation Counseling Bulletin, 37,* 109–122.

U.S. Dept. of Labor. (2008). *Occupational outlook handbook 2008-09: Counselors' job outlook.* Retrieved May 14, 2008 from: http://www.bls.gov/oco/ocos067.htm.

Zunker, V.G. (2008). *Career counseling: A holistic approach* (8th ed.). Belmont, CA: Thomson Higher Education.

ADDITIONAL SOURCES AND THEIR WEBSITES

American Counseling Association
    http://www.counseling.org/
American Rehabilitation Counseling Association (ACA Division) http://www.arcaweb.org/
Commission on Rehabilitation Counselor Certification http://www.crccertification.com/
Council on Rehabilitation Education
    http://www.core rehab.org/
International Association of Rehabilitation Professionals http://www.rehabpro.org/
National Council on Rehabilitation Education
    http://www.rehabeducators.org/
National Rehabilitation Association
    http://www.nationalrehab.org/
National Rehabilitation Counseling Association
    http://nrca net.org/
Occupational Outlook Handbook (For all I'm A People Person occupations) http://www.bls.gov/OCO/
Rehabilitation Counselors and Educators Association (NRA Division) http://www.rehabcea.org

Chapter 16

SCHOOL COUNSELING

Dᴇɴɴɪs Pᴇʟsᴍᴀ & Tᴏᴍ S. Kʀɪᴇsʜᴏᴋ

From a historical perspective, school counselors working in the early part of the twenty-first century looks a lot different from the ones you knew when you were in school. Changes in society and legislation that affect education and educational programming, along with the creation of both state and national standards for counselors, have defined new roles for those helping professionals choosing to work in school settings. Counselors must be prepared to adjust and adapt to an ever-changing world (Wrenn, 1962). This challenge, voiced in the 1960s by C. Gilbert Wrenn, is even more important today as we close the first decade of the new millennium. School counselors of the twenty-first century must be multitalented individuals, culturally competent and responsive, and able to take advantage of the many resources and technological advances that help them perform a set of complex and complicated tasks. With the evolution of federal legislation (e.g., No Child Left Behind), school counselors, along with all educators in public schools, are confronted with issues of accountability and the need for data-based decision making regarding student learning and achievement. With this enhanced need for accountability, counselors are faced with the ongoing need to strike a balance in their work–between efforts to encourage student progress in the areas of academics (e.g., reading and math) with the "survival needs" of students and their families in the areas of personal growth and safety.

BRIEF HISTORY AND DEVELOPMENT

A brief history of school counseling and guidance begins with the initial emphasis on vocational guidance in the 1920s. In the early 1900s, many individuals in the United States had the opportunity (or were forced) to move from rural to more industrialized work settings. Along with this movement came the idea that public schools could provide students with assistance in matching their abilities, interests, and personalities to certain jobs. This "best fit" approach became known as the Trait-Factor Theory, attributed to Frank Parsons (1909), the "father of guidance." The basic assumptions of this theory were that counselors (or teachers at this time) could help students: (1) examine their individual "traits;" (2) explore the "factors" in the environment; and (3) make a rational decision as to what job would represent the best fit between the person and the environment. Even today, this popular approach continues to influence the area of career choice and the field of career development.

As the position of guidance officer or counselor emerged in the 1920s and 1930s, the role changed from an emphasis on vocational education and guidance to a broader range of pupil personnel services which involved orientation, appraisal, counseling, information, placement, and follow-up. This change reinforced the position of guidance counselor as a provider of many important services available to students in schools.

By the mid-1940s and 1950s, the definition of school counseling was expanded to include helping students with personal problems. It was at that time that Carl Rogers developed the nondirective approach to counseling, and the field's interest in counseling became greater than its interest in testing. Most counselors were trained in the Rogerian approach and believed that three conditions were necessary and sufficient for client change: (1) counselor genuineness; (2) accurate empathy; and (3) positive regard for the client. The assumption of this approach was that given the appropriate relationship with the counselor, clients would be capable of solving their own problems in a natural, progressive movement toward positive growth and development. The Rogerian approach is still taught today in most counselor education programs as part of the basic training necessary for counseling effectiveness.

With the passage of the National Defense Education Act in 1958, many individuals were trained to become school counselors. At that time, counselor education programs were preparing counselors in the "student-services model" that promoted personal counseling as a primary service. This model reached its peak popularity during the 1960s

and early 1970s. However, by the mid-1970s, it was thought by some education professionals that counselors were spending too much time on crisis-related and remedial problems (individual counseling) and not enough on education and development. With an early interest in wellness and holistic education, the elementary school counseling movement, which began in the early 1970s, contributed to the development of the role of the counselor as a prevention specialist. This role encouraged counselors to spend more time working with students in the classroom on basic developmentally appropriate issues, rather than just working with individuals and their problems in the counselor's office. It was believed that issues such as friendship, appreciating individual differences, cooperating with others, learning to solve problems, and decision-making were important to all students and that the counselor's time was better spent in the classroom teaching such skills to students. The percentage of time spent by the counselor in the classroom varies by grade level, but delivering an in-class counseling program continues to be an important part of school counseling curricula.

Throughout the later 1970s and 1980s the influence of "systems theory" brought about another important change in the role of the school counselor—the emergence of "human systems theory." Human systems theory assumes that individuals living or working in groups are influenced by each other (i.e., a change in one member produces changes in the entire system). Thus the counselor was identified as a key person or "agent of change" in a comprehensive network of related educational opportunities and services for students. While working with students directly through individual counseling, small group counseling, and in the classroom, counselors could increase their effectiveness and range of influence to help students through the use of indirect skills. These skills, along with counseling, became known as the "Four Cs for Counselors"–Counseling, Consulting, Collaborating, and Coordinating.

As the needs and demographics of students became more diverse in the 1990s and early 2000s, counselors began taking more of an advocacy role for students in order to assure that schools were places where all students could, and would want to, learn. It is this priority which counselors should have today as they look to the "comprehensive developmental counseling model" as a way of organizing their work. This approach, which has grown in interest at the local and state level, has developed into a nationwide model for schools around the country (ASCA, 2005). With 2010 and the next decade approaching, school counselors will be required to adjust and adapt even more to the "ever-changing world" described by Wrenn in 1962.

MISSION AND OBJECTIVES

The mission of school counseling has evolved over time to promote the idea that school counselors should become catalysts for educational change and assume greater leadership roles in education reform. Campbell and Dahir (1997) provided a definition of school counseling adopted by the American School Counselor Association (ASCA) Governing Board that helps to illustrate this challenge:

> Counseling is a process of helping people by assisting them in making decisions and changing behavior. School counselors work with all students, school staff, families, and members of the community as an integral part of the education program. School counseling programs promote success through a focus on academic achievement, prevention and intervention activities, ad-

vocacy, and social/emotional and career development. (p. 8)

ASCA developed the National Standards for School Counseling Programs that serve to identify specific student attitudes, knowledge, and skills that should be addressed by K–12 counselors (ASCA, 2004). These standards help counselors remain focused on student development, as well as to articulate a professional mission for current and future practice in their particular setting. While national standards are important, it is critical that counselors align their mission statement and program goals with their local school district's improvement plan. In this way, they are able to communicate to others the value of their program and how it helps advance the broader mission of the school and district (Green & Keys, 2001). One example of how the national standards are helpful and how they affect the entire climate of the school is in the area of personal-social development. For example, Standard A states, "Students will acquire the attitudes, knowledge, and interpersonal skills to help them understand and respect self and others." Counselors, with the help of classroom teachers and other professionals in the school, can develop appropriate curriculum-based activities that incorporate this standard as a learning objective. This standard, like others, can contribute to the primary mission of schools–the academic achievement of students (House & Martin, 1998). Students who understand and respect self and others are more likely to achieve and learn in school.

CONSUMER PROFILE

Types of Clients

Although school counselors may be certified to work at all grade levels (PreK–12), they typically work at the elementary, junior high, middle school, or high school levels. By specializing in students within certain grade levels, they can help both students and parents adjust to the age-specific problems typically encountered (e.g., ages 5–6: adjustment to school; ages 13–14: acceptance of peers; ages 16–18: decision-making and goal setting). While counselors tend to focus the majority of their attention on students, they also consult with administrators, teachers, parents, and other professionals to improve the learning environments that affect students and their achievement.

Typical Needs of Clients

The national standards developed by ASCA have provided goals and objectives for students in three important areas: (1) academic, (2) career, and (3) personal/social. Counselors base their intervention programs around these standards and use them as goals for classroom guidance activities as well as evaluation markers and measures for successful student development. Students who may be underperforming or have difficulties in any of these areas may need additional individual and/or small group counseling. At times, counselors may also work with students having situational or adjustment problems that can range in intensity from moving to a new school (loss of friends) to the death of a parent or close family member. If an event or loss is so severe that it impacts the entire school or district, a crisis response team, composed of counselors and other helping professionals, may be called in to help assist students and staff members deal with such events.

School counselors also play a major role in both organizing and coordinating school-wide programs to enhance student growth and development. Some of these programs include parent education, bullying and violence prevention, peer mediation, small group advisories for middle schools, community-based service projects, suicide awareness, and character education. (For more information on these programs see the Websites section at the end of this chapter.)

PHILOSOPHICAL ASSUMPTIONS AND THEORIES

There are at least four philosophical assumptions underlying the role and purpose of school counseling and a counseling program. The first assumption is that all students are capable of healthy cognitive, emotional, and social growth and development. This holistic viewpoint appreciates the interrelatedness of these three growth and development areas and their influence on student achievement. For example, a student who is upset because of a conflict or problem with a friend may have difficulty concentrating and staying on task in the classroom. Helping a student like this learn to cope successfully with the unpleasant emotions caused by conflict can promote positive adjustment when facing new situations and events that in the past may have thrown him or her off balance or out of focus.

The second assumption involves the belief that successful development means coping positively with the many external challenges students face today. A rapidly changing world that includes transitions in families due to job loss or career change, violence in homes, schools, and communities; divorce; teenage suicide; substance abuse; and sexual experimentation all serve to impact the lives of students today and will continue to influence them in the future (Gysbers, 2001). Students must be prepared and able to cope with uncertainty, be resilient in the face of loss and continue to take calculated risks that increase their opportunities, as well as make good decisions if they are to be successful in the future (Pelsma & Arnett, 2002).

The third assumption is that student growth and development are enhanced through personal contact and ongoing, consistent relationships with positive adults in their lives. Human attachment theory underscores the importance of students feeling connected to other people in their lives. As society and the structure of families change, schools have continued to provide a constant source of positive relationships for students. Through a positive relationship with the school counselor, a student's identity and sense of well-being can be greatly enhanced. Although this is often viewed as secondary to the actual mission of schools, positive relationships with adults can serve to validate and improve a student's quality of life— which is good for not only the individual but for society as well.

The fourth and final assumption is that a student's ethnic and cultural context plays a key role in their development, and thus in their relationship to school and learning. The counseling profession has been at the forefront in recognizing the importance of such contextual factors, which, in addition to culture and ethnicity, include gender, sexual orientation, and disability status. For school counselors to be effective, they must be well grounded in cross cultural theory in general and aware of the particular issues most common to the "individual" students they serve.

MAJOR COUNSELING THEORIES

School counselors generally employ several theories of counseling in their work with students. These theories reflect the counselor's personal belief system about students and the cause and nature of their problems

and how the counseling process helps change to take place. Counseling approaches are also somewhat dependent on the values and beliefs of the local community and the setting in which the counselor works (rural vs. urban). Ethical principles and standards of behavior (ASCA, 2004) require that counselors be able to articulate their theory of counseling, explaining not only what they are doing but also why they are doing it. It is also essential that counselors use evidence-based strategies that are shown to be effective through research and evaluation (Western Regional Center for the Application of Prevention Technologies, 2001).

Developmental Counseling

Developmental Counseling Theory assumes that, although there are some gender differences, all students will progress through normal stages and transitions. Understanding the changes, both physical and emotional, that are taking place in students of a particular age group allows counselors to encourage teachers and parents to anticipate some of these problems and to offer strategies to help students cope successfully. Counselors also base their curriculum on the Developmental Counseling model as they plan with teachers on age-appropriate classroom guidance activities.

Adlerian Counseling

A second theory that many counselors use in understanding student behavior is based on the work of Alfred Adler and is known as Adlerian counseling. This approach, popularized in the United States by Rudolf Dreikurs (Dreikurs & Soltz, 1964), assumes that (a) all behavior has a purpose; and (b) all individuals, having social interest, seek to contribute to and gain significance from the various groups to which they belong. Beginning at birth, children acquire a psychological "position" in the family based on the child's birth order (in relation to other siblings) and the expectations of parents. Adler described four basic positions: the oldest, the middle, the youngest, and the only child. The viewpoint or perception from each position, along with the reinforcement and encouragement provided by parents and others in the family, help determine the individual's understanding of themselves and what Adler called one's lifestyle. The youngest child or "baby" in the family may have the view that he or she should be protected and taken care of by others. The resulting actions and behaviors are understood as the individual's attempt to keep an established place in the group and to reinforce this lifestyle. As the "baby" joins other groups (kindergarten, for example) these behaviors will represent the student's best attempt to find a place within a new group. Unfortunately there may be five or six other "babies" who are also seeking to keep their "unique" positions. If positive methods are not successful, the student may become discouraged and use other behaviors such as attention getting, displays of power, revenge, or assumed disability to try to establish a unique place. The counselor can help students understand how to make a positive contribution to the group and avoid operating from a position of feeling dejected. Adlerian counseling is very useful in teacher and parent education as adults can learn to alter responses to students/children and avoid reinforcing negative behaviors.

Solution-Focused Counseling

The final counseling approach to be described in this section is a form of brief therapy known as solution-focused counseling. This theory, which evolved from family therapy, has been effectively used in various educational settings (Metcalf, 1995). It is ap-

plicable to working with students because it: (1) is brief and concentrates on small changes and solutions rather than on problems; (2) is positive and focuses on student competence and capabilities; and (3) lacks the emphasis on exploring the past and instead looks at solutions for the future (Goldenberg & Goldenberg, 2000). Knowing that school counselors often have only a short time to work with individual students, the solution-focused approach employs a series of questions (e.g., "What will you notice if you wake up one morning and the problem is gone?") as a part of the counseling process. Such questions serve to help examine exceptions to a problem or concern in order to uncover possible alternatives (new or old) that may work, define goals, notice small changes, and assess and determine student progress in counseling.

These three approaches have the common belief that students are competent and can learn to solve their own problems through techniques learned in individual, small group, and classroom activities. These theories also provide counselors with strategies when consulting with parents and teachers.

AREAS OF APPLICATION

As a helping professional working in an educational setting, school counselors are not trained (or expected) to do psychotherapy or in-depth counseling. Their primary focus is on developing and advancing student knowledge, skills, and abilities in three domains: (1) academic, (2) career, and (3) personal/social. Through the delivery of a comprehensive program, counselors help students acquire life-skills that encourage success in school and their personal lives. Working with people who are important in the lives of students, counselors can foster better communication between students, teachers, parents, and other adults who play important roles. While encouraging specific actions or interventions, the counselor is viewed as an advocate or "agent of change" bringing about necessary conditions for student success. In many cases, with the help of others in the school and community, a student's environment can be altered and adaptations made to better provide for individual needs and particular learning requirements.

PROFESSIONAL PREPARATION AND DEVELOPMENT

For admission into graduate study in school counseling, candidates generally must have at least a 2.5 grade-point average (GPA) in the last 60 hours of undergraduate study or an overall GPA of no less than 3.0. The application process usually requires scores on the Miller Analogy Test (MAT) or the Graduate Record Examination (GRE) where applicable. Acceptable scores on these exams vary with individual universities and programs. Candidates must complete a formal application that includes employment history and references. Personal interviews with members of the departmental faculty are typically required.

School counselors are certified by the Department of Education in the state in which they work. Most counselors have an undergraduate degree from a four- or five-year program, often in teacher education. In addition, some states require counselors to have one or two years of classroom teaching experience before they can become certified or licensed. Preparation for becoming a school counselor requires a master's degree in school counseling, which usually involves 40 to 48 hours of graduate coursework. During their training, counselors are required to complete several field experiences, including a practicum and an internship. These experiences are very important because they allow Counselors in Training (CITs) to practice counseling skills while receiving supervision from both on-site supervisors and university instructors. CITs are observed and "coached" in the effective use of counseling skills, as well as being provided mentoring and encouragement as they get ready to enter the profession of school counseling. After completing the master's degree, most counselors are eligible to apply for state certification or licensure allowing them to work in the public school system. They also are eligible to apply for state or national licensure as a professional counselor, though this designation may require some additional coursework and/or practicum experience. This designation also allows them to work in other mental health settings if they so desire. Candidates for a professional license in school counseling are required to pass a standardized test (Praxis-II) with passing scores varying from state to state. Like all counselors and others working in the helping professions, annual continuing education requirements must be completed and state certifications must be renewed on a regular basis.

WORK SETTINGS

School counselors typically work in an educational setting and are assigned to a particular building or location. They require offices that are used for confidential conferences with students and parents, and they spend a significant amount of time providing guidance lessons in regular classrooms. At times they may visit students' homes and may also visit local employers in connection with career development activities. In small school systems, they may be required to travel to more than one site.

PURPOSE OF COUNSELING

Types of Interventions

The primary goal of most interventions used by school counselors is to promote positive student growth and adjustment. Drawing from the theories described previously, interventions are designed to help students not only adjust to current concerns or problems, but to learn to cope in the future. In addition to the basic techniques of active listening (e.g., paraphrasing and reflection of feelings), counselors may use a wide range of counseling techniques in their work with students. Encouragement, an important technique in Adlerian counseling, is considered one of the most important elements in promoting change (Dinkmeyer, Dinkmeyer & Sperry, 1987). In working with children, Dreikurs and Soltz (1964) defined encouragement as a "continuous process aimed at giving the child a sense of self-respect and a sense of accomplishment" (p. 39). Encouragement is viewed as being different from praise in that it comments on the process or effort the student has made and not on any outcome or product. For example, a counselor may say to a student, "I appreciate how much work you put into your grades this semester." This response encourages the positive aspects of a student's performance even if the grade was not an "A."

Counselors may also use a form of questioning, which is the primary intervention for solution-focused counselors. Such questions may examine exceptions ("What is different about classes where you are doing better?"), promote goal setting and awareness of changes ("What would you notice first if a miracle happened and you no longer had the problem?"), and allow for the assessment of client progress ("When you first came in to counseling you were at a one, and now

where would you put yourself?"). An example of the use of questioning is as follows:

A ninth-grade student who is failing several classes is referred to the middle school counselor. After a short period of socialization and rapport building, the counselor asks questions of the student about the problem of failing. The counselor helps the student determine what may be different about some classes in which he or she is not failing. It is these exceptions that become important and the focus of inquiry. To the "exception" question, the student may reply, "I don't feel as embarrassed in biology class." This serves to open the door for possible reasons for this lack of embarrassment. Second, to the "miracle question," the student may respond by saying, "The teacher asks me a question in class and I give the right answer. I bet that would feel good." Finally, to the question that involves the use of scaling, the client may respond, "When I came in I was at a one or two with the problem and now, maybe a five or six." In this way, both the counselor and the student can appreciate the positive changes that have taken place.

Goals of Interventions

From an Adlerian perspective, each student must find or create a place of significance within the group. This means making a positive contribution and believing that they are appreciated and respected. If students are unable to create such a place, they may become discouraged and use more maladaptive methods for gaining importance (e.g., attention getting, revenge, power, or assumed disability). Counselors using this approach can help students understand their "faulty logic" and set goals for more effective means of finding their place and making a contribution to the group. If a child is an "only child" in the family of origin, for example, he or she may require special attention by others. At school, the counselor (possibly with the aid of the teacher) can help the child discover positive ways to gain recognition and to be special and unique.

The type or nature of the problem and the reasons for it are not necessarily important when using the solution-focused model. Counselors using this approach help students examine the current concern or problem and find new (or rediscover old) solutions. The primary goal is to help students to do "something different," making small changes that can result in positive consequences.

USE OF SERVICES

Clients

Students are typically referred to the counselor for individual counseling by classroom teachers, parents, or through self-referral. Counselors may have regularly scheduled appointments with some students and see them individually or in small groups. Otherwise, through the delivery of the comprehensive counseling program, students have contact with the counselor through regularly scheduled classroom guidance activities. Counselors also may be involved indirectly with students through resource teams that help plan academic programs or Individual Educational Plans (IEPs). These plans, especially at the elementary school level, serve to provide necessary services for students in order to assure academic success. Often teachers and administrators may ask the counselor to be involved in parent-teacher conferences where personal/social or emotional problems may be affecting the student's progress in learning. These activities can occur at any time throughout the year, although more often at the end of the quarter or semester. At the secondary levels, counselors are often consulted to help students determine appropriate courses and schedules for upcoming semesters or for the academic year.

Agencies/Businesses

If the student's individual problem or concern is considered chronic or severe, the counselor will encourage the referral of the student to other mental health or social services within the community. Most counselors have a list of resources and community agencies that are designed to help students and families. Counselors typically are asked to work with these professionals and agencies in monitoring student progress during the assistance or treatment.

Post High School Education and Training

Counselors frequently help students make plans for education and training beyond high school. This can include vocational training institutions, community colleges, or four-year colleges and universities. Counselors should understand the admission requirements for these educational opportunities and can help students and parents with the application process and with decisions about scholarships and financial aid.

PROFESSIONAL ORGANIZATIONS

The professional organization representing school counselors at the national level is the American School Counselor Association (ASCA), which is under the umbrella of the American Counseling Association (ACA), the group that represents the general counseling profession. Each state also has its own local branch of the ACA as well as regional affiliates.

CAREER ADVANCEMENT, OPPORTUNITIES, AND SALARY

Salary for school counselors is generally based on counselor's school district's teacher salary schedule and involves a base rate plus additional payment for advanced graduate hours and degrees, as well as for years of experience. Although most teachers work an average of nine months per contract year, counselors may get an extended contract providing them with additional pay. For example, some larger school districts employ a district-wide director of counseling programs who is responsible for developing and managing the district-wide comprehensive counseling program. This person is usually considered an administrator and is paid on a 12-month contract. The median income for school counselors in 2006 was approximately $48,000, with over half falling in the range of approximately $36,000 to $60,000 (Bureau of Labor Statistics, 2008).

OUTLOOK FOR THE FUTURE

In the past few years, increasing enrollments and expected retirements have created a high demand for teachers and counselors. It has been reported by the Bureau of Labor Statistics (2008) that employment of school counselors is expected to increase 13 percent or *about as fast as the average* for all occupations through the year 2016. Nonetheless, there are many factors that affect counselor supply and demand. Some states are increasing funding for school counseling through state mandates while others are attempting to reduce or eliminate funds for school counselors. Due to a national teacher shortage, many states have initiated alternative teaching licenses (e.g., a restricted lic-

ense) that allow noneducation professionals with advanced degrees the opportunity to work in schools as "resource specialists." Despite this movement, given the expanding responsibilities of school counselors and the increasing needs of students and their families, it is likely that school counseling positions (especially at the elementary level) will be available.

SUMMARY

Today, more than ever, choosing to work as a school counselor holds much promise for those individuals wanting to make a positive difference in the lives of children and adolescents. To make such a difference, school counselors must be adequately prepared and supported in their role as advocates for all students. Similar to other helping professionals, school counselors must serve as positive role models in both their school and community. It is often said that teachers influence or affect eternity through their day-to-day work with students. This statement could very well include school counselors. What better way could there be to make a contribution to future generations?

REFERENCES

American School Counseling Association (2004). *ASCA national standards for students.* Alexandria, VA: Author.

American School Counseling Association. (2004). *Ethical standards for school counselors.* Retrieved from www.schoolcounselor.org/content.asp? contentid=173.

American School Counseling Association. (2005). *The ASCA model: A framework for school counseling programs* (2nd ed.). Alexandria, VA: Author.

Bureau of Labor Statistics (2008). *Occupational outlook handbook (OOH)*, 2008–09 ed. Retrieved March 19, 2008, from www.bls.gov/oco.

Campbell, C. A., & Dahir, C. A. (1997). *The national standards for school counseling programs.* Alexandria, VA: American School Counselor Association.

Dinkmeyer, D., Dinkmeyer, D., Jr., & Sperry, L. (1987). *Adlerian counseling and psychotherapy* (2nd ed.). Columbus, OH: Merrill.

Dreikurs, R., & Soltz, V. (1964). *Children: The challenge.* New York: Penguin Books.

Goldenberg, I., & Goldenberg, H. (2000). *Family therapy: An overview* (5th ed.). Belmont, CA: Wadsworth/Thomson.

Green, A., & Keys, S. (2001). Expanding the developmental school counseling paradigm: Meeting the needs of the 21st century student. *Professional School Counseling, 5,* 84–95.

Gysbers, N. C. (2001). School guidance and counseling in the 21st century: Remember the past into the future. *Professional School Counseling, 5,* 96–105.

Gysbers, N. C., & Henderson, P. (2006). *Developing and managing your school guidance and counseling program* (4th ed.). Alexandria, VA: American Counseling Association.

House, R. M., & Martin, P. J. (1998). Advocating for better futures for all students: A new vision for school counselors. *Education, 119,* 284–291.

Metcalf, L. (1995). *Counseling toward solutions: A practical solution-focused program for working with students, teachers and parents.* West Nyack, NY: The Center for Applied Research in Education.

Parsons, F. (1909). *Choosing a vocation.* Boston: Houghton-Mifflin.

Pelsma, D., & Arnett, R. (2002). Helping clients cope with change in the 21st century: A balancing act. *Journal of Career Development, 28,* 169–179.

Western Regional Center for the Application of Prevention Technologies. (2001). *Program planning and best practices.* Reno, NV: Author.

Wrenn, C. G. (1962). *The counselor in a changing world.* Washington, DC: American Personnel and Guidance Association.

SUGGESTED RESOURCES

Campbell, C. A., & Dahir, C. A. (1997). *Sharing the vision: National standards for school counseling programs.* Alexandria, VA: American School Counselor Association.

Gysbers, N. C., & Henderson, P. (2006). *Developing and managing your school guidance and counseling program* (4th ed.). Alexandria, VA: American Counseling Association.

Metcalf, L. (1995). *Counseling toward solutions: A practical solution-focused program for working with students, teachers and parents.* West Nyack, NY: The Center for Applied Research in Education.

WEBSITES FOR SCHOOL COUNSELING

American Counseling Association (ACA)
www.counseling.org
American School Counselor Association (ASC)
www.schoolcounselor.org
Anti-Bullying Network
www.antibullying.net
CACREP Directory of Accredited Preparation Programs www.counseling.org/CACREP/directory/htm
Education World
www.educationworld.com/counseling
The Guidance Channel
www.guidancechannel.com
National Board for Certified Counselors (NBCC)
www.nbcc.org
National Career Development Association (NCDA) www.ncda.org
National Youth Leadership Council Website
www.nylc.org
School Counselor Standards
www.schoolcounselor.org/content.asp?contentid=173
Suicide Awareness Voices of Education
www.save.org

Chapter 17

SCHOOL PSYCHOLOGY

MICHAEL B. BROWN & PAUL S. TRIVETTE

School psychologists are professional psychologists who apply a psychological perspective to a variety of learning, emotional, or social problems experienced by children, adolescents, and young adults. School psychologists have training in both psychology and education and make a unique contribution toward the goal of fostering optimal social, emotional, and academic development. The majority of school psychologists work in the public schools, although many school psychologists also work in a variety of other settings providing services to children, adolescents, and adults. School psychologists must be licensed or certified in the state in which they work in order to practice inside or outside of a school system.

School psychology traces its roots to Lightner Wittmer and G. Stanley Hall around the turn of the twentieth century. Wittmer established the Psychological Clinic at the University of Pennsylvania and treated many children referred from schools in and around Philadelphia. Although Wittmer referred to this specialty as clinical psychology, he characterized the clinical psychologist as "a psychological expert who is capable of treating the many difficult cases that resist the ordinary methods of the schoolroom"

(Wittmer, 1897, p. 117). Around the same time, Hall was developing child study centers to provide services to children who had learning or behavior problems. In these early years of practice, persons functioning as school psychologists often were trained as clinical or educational psychologists as there were no school psychology training programs.

The establishment of compulsory public schooling along with the prevailing notion that education was the pathway to progressive change in America furthered the need for school psychologists. The first person with the title of school psychologist was Arnold Gesell, who worked for the Connecticut State Board of Education from 1915–1919 (Fagan & Wise, 2007). Gesell traveled around the state conducting diagnostic assessments and providing consultation to school staff about children with learning or behavior problems.

School psychology became a distinct field of psychology after World War II. Following the war, clinical psychology became more adult-oriented and focused on the treatment of mental illness. The Division of School Psychology was formed within the American Psychological Association in 1946. The 1954 national Thayer Conference defined modern school psychology by establishing uniform qualifications, training, and practice standards. As the practice of school psychology grew, the National Association of School Psychologists was formed in 1969, which solidified the nondoctoral degree as the entry level of training for the practice of school psychology. The establishment of special education programs through the passage of the Education for All Handicapped Children Act during the 1970s further defined the role of the school psychologist in diagnostic assessment for children with special needs. As the demand increased, the number of school psychology training programs and practitioners also grew rapidly in the 1970s and 1980s.

The school psychology Futures Conference in 2001 was held to map out the challenges and develop an agenda for the future of the profession (D'Amato, Sheridan, Phelps & Lopez, 2004). In the twenty-first century school psychology is moving toward a greater focus on prevention and intervention activities with a reduction in the traditional emphasis on psychological assessment. School psychologists are increasingly involved in all facets of providing behavioral health services to children and adolescents to reduce or remove barriers to student learning and development. For example, school psychologists have been influential in developing prereferral intervention programs to help reduce the need for special education and in developing school crisis intervention programs that help students and staff who have experienced a traumatic event.

PHILOSOPHICAL ASSUMPTIONS

The National Association of School Psychologists' *Professional Conduct Manual*

(2000a) establishes the philosophical underpinning for school psychology. A major philosophical principle underlying school psychology practice is that school psychologists act as advocates for their clients and "speak up for the needs and rights of their clients even at times when it may be difficult to do so" (NASP, 2000a, p. 13). School psychologists use their training and skills to partner with parents, educators, and other professionals to promote learning in a safe, healthy, and supportive environment. School psychologists also utilize their understanding of school systems, developmental psychology, and principles of effective teaching and learning to improve the educational and emotional environments for all children in the schools. Research-based interventions and program evaluation are used to assure that school psychologists are effectively meeting the needs of children.

A second philosophical assumption of school psychology is that an ecological view of factors that impact learning and behavior, rather than a deficit-oriented approach, will provide the maximum benefit for students. Rather than assuming that there is something "wrong" with the child if he or she has difficulty with learning or behavior, school psychologists are paying attention to identifying and removing factors that are barriers to learning (Adelman & Taylor, 1998). Significant barriers to learning include such things as lack of resources, poor study skills, and home environments that do not support learning, as well as learning disabilities and emotional problems. Psychologists collaborate with others in the school and community to identify barriers to learning and develop and advocate for interventions that remove or alter these barriers and facilitate optimal learning.

An appreciation for the diversity of values, interaction styles, and cultural expectations in the communities in which they work is another philosophical underpinning of school psychology. School psychologists have a critical role in providing culturally competent and responsive services for all students and their families and in assisting schools to become culturally sensitive environments (Ysseldyke et al., 2006). School psychologists must be able to recognize when issues of diversity are present and modify or adapt their services to better meet the needs of their clients. Prevention and intervention programs are also designed to fit the cognitive, behavioral and emotional developmental levels of the children they serve.

MAJOR THEORIES

School psychologists draw from the entire range of psychological theories in their work with children, families, and schools. The theoretical orientation that a school psychologist applies to a problem is determined by both the referral concern and the individual practitioner's training and skill. Practitioners use cognitive psychology, including information-processing theory, to explain and remediate the many problems that children have with learning. Principles of behavioral psychology are frequently used in developing interventions to alter maladaptive behavior or teach more appropriate behavior in the school setting. School psychologists often utilize behavioral principles through a consultation process with a teacher, parent, or school administrator. Systems theory contributes significantly to a better understanding of how schools work and how to develop interventions that attempt to change the larger school or community environment to prevent or resolve learning and behavior problems.

Knowledge of developmental psychology helps the school psychologist assist parents and teachers to understand children's behavior in the context of age and have appropriate expectations for future development. Behaviors and cognitive processes appropriate at one age may be an indication of a significant delay or impairment at later ages, and school psychologists must be aware of the typical behaviors and expectations of children with whom they work. For example, a two-and-one-half-year-old child who acts stubborn, defiant, and argumentative with parents is likely to be exhibiting developmentally appropriate behavior. An eight-year-old child with the same behavior is more likely to have oppositional defiant disorder because these behaviors become less developmentally appropriate past the third or fourth year of life.

Finally, school psychologists are increasingly adopting a public health/health promotion perspective in designing and delivering services to children and their families. A public health/health promotion approach to problems shifts the emphasis toward preventing problems rather than merely treating problems once they develop. For example, competency and skill-building programs are aimed at reaching children before they develop reading problems (Mather & Kauffman, 2006). As a student's difficulties become more severe, increasingly intense interventions are utilized. In the case of reading problems, a research-based instructional program typically would be used with a student who has poor reading skills. A more intensive intervention, such as special education, would be recommended only after the student had failed to improve his or her reading skills.

AREAS OF APPLICATION

The school psychologist is a member of a team that identifies the factors that hinder a student's learning and devises interventions to overcome the learning problems. The typical assessment process might include interviews with teacher and parents, observations in the classroom, and the administration of standardized assessment techniques. A school psychologist might administer cognitive ability or "IQ" tests, tests that measure academic achievement or tests that assess a variety of processing skills. The psychologist also might use behavior rating scales completed by parents to evaluate the behavioral, social-emotional, and developmental influences on learning. Learning problems can range from mild delays in reading, math, and writing to significant problems or deficits in cognitive processing. Students who have significant achievement problems and processing difficulties may be identified as having a specific learning disability, while some children may have difficulty in academics due to impaired cognitive ability. Students with educational disabilities are eligible for individualized educational programs and services.

Behavioral or emotional problems, such as school refusal, depression, attention disorders, and anxiety disorders, are a frequent cause of concern for children served by school psychologists. A variety of problems with interpersonal relationships may be a focus of assessment and treatment. Anger control problems, bullying, poor social skills, and discipline problems may be the focus of attention and intervention for some students. Students who have experienced abuse, neglect, or the death of a family member or close friend also may come to the attention of school psychologists. School psychologists are often members of the school's crisis intervention team, providing counseling and support following crises involving members of the school community.

School psychologists increasingly work with children with medical problems (Brown & Bolen, 2003). Advances in medical care have resulted in an increase in survival rates for those having serious medical problems; thus, understandably, an increasing number of students with medical problems attend school (Brown & DuPaul, 1999). Chronic and acute medical problems (such as asthma, diabetes, or traumatic brain injuries) often may affect a student's cognitive, emotional, and social development, which in turn negatively impact school performance. The psychologist, working with family members and other health professionals, identifies the immediate and long-term effects of medical problems on learning and development. An understanding of how specific symptoms manifest over time along with continuous monitoring are used to create interventions that maximize students' development.

PROFESSIONAL PREPARATION AND DEVELOPMENT

The entry-level training for school psychology practice in public schools is the *specialist-level*, which takes three years of full-time study past the baccalaureate degree and includes a minimum of 60 semester hours of graduate coursework. Both the master's degree (the M.A., M.S., or M.Ed.), the specialist degree (the C.A.S. [Certificate of Advanced Study]), and the Ed.S. (the Educational Specialist) degree are awarded by most training programs, although some schools grant only the master's degree. Training includes coursework in psychological foundations areas such as developmental psychology, educational psychology, and biological psychology, along with courses in educational foundations (special education, curriculum, and the organization and operation of schools). Courses covering ethics and professional practices, psychological assessment, and intervention (counseling, consultation, and prevention programming) provide the applied knowledge and skills for the school psychologist. Graduate students also take coursework in research methods, statistics, and measurement that round out their program of study. A comprehensive examination and/or a thesis (an original research study) or other project is required by some training programs to complete the degree.

School psychologists are health services providers–they apply their knowledge and skills to working directly with persons who have, or are at risk of, a variety of problems. School psychology training programs therefore include a heavy emphasis on practice skills. Students often have exposure to school or clinic settings in the first year, shadowing practicing school psychologists or even working part-time as teachers' aides. Formal practicum experiences in the schools introduce the student psychologist to the professional roles of school psychologists and include graduated practice under the supervision of a licensed school psychologist. Following completion of all coursework, students have a one-year, full-time internship in a school setting (for which they usually receive a stipend or salary). The internship is the capstone of the training experience, whereby the psychologist-in-training takes on increasing responsibility for professional practice while continuing to receive supervision from an experienced school psychologist.

Doctoral training in school psychology includes the academic and practice experiences of specialist level training with opportunities for more in-depth knowledge in one or more areas, such as counseling, consultation, or neuropsychology. Doctoral programs place a greater emphasis on research skills, and all require a dissertation or final project for graduation. Doctoral programs awarding the Doctor of Philosophy (Ph.D.) degree usually adopt the *scientist practitioner model* which promotes the development of both research and clinical skills. Doctoral

programs awarding the Doctor of Psychology (Psy.D.) or Doctor of Education (Ed.D.) degrees frequently adhere to the *practitioner model* of training, which emphasizes the development of practice skills along with the use of research skills for program implementation and evaluation. Students applying to graduate programs are wise to consider programs that have American Psychological Association or National Association of School Psychologists approval and/or accreditation.

Most students enrolled in school psychology graduate programs have an undergraduate degree in psychology, although applicants may have degrees in related fields such as child development, sociology, or education. Graduate programs usually require students accepted into their programs to have completed basic coursework in psychology (introductory psychology, statistics and research methods, and the psychological foundations area courses). Experience working with children and families is valuable preparation for graduate school, and it is recommended that students seeking entry to doctoral programs have some undergraduate research experience. This can be either as a research assistant for a faculty member or by completing independent research. An entrance examination, such as the *Graduate Record Examination* or the *Miller Analogy Test*, is usually required for admittance into these programs.

The most up-to-date list of school psychology training programs in print is available in the newest edition of *Best Practices in School Psychology* (Miller, 2008). This list provides a description of most of the master's, specialist, and doctoral-level school psychology programs in the United States. The American Psychological Association's Graduate Study in Psychology (APA, 2007, updated each year) provides information on graduate programs in all areas of psychology, but with an emphasis on doctoral programs. The

American Psychological Association and the National Association of School Psychologists maintain a list of approved training programs on their websites, as do other Internet resources listed in Appendix II.

WORK SETTINGS

The majority of school psychologists work in public schools, although others work in private schools or the Department of Defense Dependent Schools (overseas or in the U.S.). School psychologists with appropriate credentials are also involved in work settings outside of schools, such as vocational rehabilitation programs that provide opportunities for adolescents and adults with disabilities to develop skills for independent living (Pfieffer & Dean, 1988). School psychologists also work in college counseling centers or programs providing support services to adult learners with learning or adjustment issues. School psychologists work in medical settings such as hospitals, pediatric clinics, developmental evaluation centers, or school-based health centers. School psychologists also provide evaluation and treatment services for children and families in hospitals, community mental health centers, and in private practice.

School psychologists with doctoral level training can also become college or university professors–teaching classes, supervising field practice for psychologists in training, and conducting research in school psychology and related areas. They also frequently provide consultation and service to their universities, communities, and the profession. With the increasing emphasis on life-long learning, school psychologists even work in human resource development programs in business and industry.

HOW SERVICES ARE UTILIZED

School psychologists work with students, parents and professionals in education, mental health and medical fields. Services typically provided by school psychologists include: (a) assessment; (b) consultation; (c) direct interventions; (d) prevention; (e) education; (f) program evaluation; and (g) research.

School psychologists perform diagnostic evaluations for students who have learning or behavior problems. Students who are referred for special education services are required to have a psychological evaluation, which usually involves the administration of standardized tests of cognitive skills, achievement, social/emotional status, and adaptive behavior. The psychologist may also use informal behavioral or academic assessments to facilitate an understanding of a child's current status and to assist in developing interventions. Following the diagnostic assessment, the psychologist completes a report summarizing the results and makes recommendations for planning interventions that address the student's learning, behavior, or social difficulties.

Consultation is the intervention method most commonly used by school psychologists. Consultation involves working with a teacher, parent, or administrator to help the adult work more effectively with a student or a particular situation. For example, a student may need assistance to increase the amount of time that he or she spends working on academic tasks. Using a consultative approach, the school psychologist would help the teacher collect data about the problem and analyze the factors affecting the time spent on-task. The teacher and psychologist might determine that the student needs assistance with increasing motivation or that the work level is too difficult for the student. The psychologist and the teacher would then develop an intervention to remedy the identified problem. If motivation is a problem, the teacher might develop a reinforcement program for increased time on-task. For example, the student could earn extra free time on a computer when he or she completes increasing amounts of assigned work. The teacher then would keep track of progress in order to monitor how well the intervention is working. Furthermore, the psychologist would meet and talk with the teacher periodically to provide support and to help decide if adjustments to the intervention are necessary.

School psychologists also implement direct interventions such as group or individual counseling. The psychologist could work alone or as a coleader with another psychologist or school counselor. School psychologists often teach students behavioral or educational strategies to help them in a particular area. For example, students with anger problems are taught specific anger management skills that they practice in counseling sessions and are helped to apply such skills in "real life." Crisis situations, such as when there is a violent incident at school or someone in the school community dies, may require working with groups of students or adults in the school to help manage their reaction to the crisis and reduce future negative outcomes from the traumatic event.

Prevention programs are aimed at preventing or reducing the risk of negative outcomes for children and adolescents. These programs help children develop general competencies, strengthening social support for children and families at risk of a negative outcome or provide targeted interventions for children at-risk because of specific life events. School psychologists might develop and conduct a divorce support group for children who have recently experienced divorce. They could implement a drug abuse prevention program that helps students develop stress management and decision-making skills. School psychologists might also work with school administrators to restructure how the school is organized to reduce the impact of stressful events or situations (such as the move from elementary school to middle school).

In-service training programs enhance the knowledge and skill of teachers, staff, and parents (Brown, 2008). School psychologists provide training on a variety of topics, ranging from what teachers can do if they suspect that one of their students is depressed to helping teachers develop skills in curriculum-based assessment. A school's parent/teacher organization may request a training program for parents on effective parenting skills. School psychologists often use formal or informal needs assessments to identify the school community's training needs. Training for school staff can be an important part of a system's change process that modifies important aspects of the functioning of the school and/or school staff.

Finally, school psychologists have an important role in translating and distributing psychological research to nonpsychologists (parents and teachers). For example, they might help teachers understand how memory works in order to devise an effective intervention for a child who needs help in retaining academic material. The psychologist may use a form of research known as *single case design* research to monitor the effectiveness of interventions. Knowledge of effective program planning and evaluation also is necessary to help schools establish and maintain effective programs for students.

PROFESSIONAL ORGANIZATIONS

There are two national professional organizations representing school psychologists in the United States: The American Psychological Association (APA) and the National Association of School Psychologists (NASP). APA is the major scientific and professional organization representing psychology in the United States and is the largest association of psychologists in the world. The mission of the APA is to promote the science and practice of psychology, which is accomplished through the establishment of a code of ethics (APA, 2002) and standards for practice and training (e.g., APA, 1981), and accredits doctoral-level training programs in professional psychology, including school psychology. The Association encourages research and the dissemination of psychological information through conferences and the publication of books and scientific journals. There also are affiliated state psychological associations promoting the practice of psychology in their respective states.

APA has 54 divisions comprised of individuals who share interests in specific areas of psychology research and/or practice. Division 16 is the School Psychology Division and publishes the *School Psychology Quarterly*, a scientific journal in school psychology; develops other publications about school psychology; and sponsors programs at the APA Annual Meeting. The division has emphasized the role of school psychologists as health care providers. School psychologists without the doctoral degree can join the division as affiliate members.

NASP was formed in 1969 by a group of school psychologists who were concerned that the APA did not adequately represent the interests of school psychologists without a doctoral degree. NASP's mission is to promote educationally and psychologically healthy environments for children and youth through research and training in school psychology, advocacy, and leadership for the profession. NASP publishes the scientific journal *School Psychology Review* along with many books and other publications for practitioners. Affiliated state associations of school psychologists provide advocacy and service to school psychologists practicing within each state.

NASP has developed credentialing and practice standards (NASP, 2000b) and has a code of conduct for its members (NASP, 2000a). The National School Psychology Certification System was developed to help create a nationally recognized standard of training for school psychologists. Individuals who meet the educational and experience requirements can receive the National Certified School Psychologist credential, a measure of professionalism that is also used by 31 states as part of their standards for certification for practice in the public schools. NASP also provides program approval for specialist and doctoral-level school psychology training programs that meet the Association's training standards (NASP, 2000b).

CAREER ADVANCEMENT, OPPORTUNITIES, AND SALARY

School psychologists who practice fulltime in a school system are overwhelmingly satisfied with their jobs (Brown, Hohenshil & Brown, 1998; Worrell, Skaggs & Brown, 2006). School psychologists are most satisfied with the opportunity to provide service to others, to work independently and exercise professional judgment, and to work with congenial coworkers. The factor that school psychologists find most frustrating in their work is school system policies and procedures. Schools tend to be bureaucratic institutions that change slowly. Psychologists, as change agents, often find this frustrating, and these policies and procedures may restrain them from engaging in the types of activities that they believe are their "ideal" role.

The majority of school psychologists works in public schools and intends to remain in the profession of school psychology (Brown, Hohenshil & Brown, 1998; Worrell, Skaggs & Brown, 2006). Career advancement for school psychologists, as it is for public school personnel in general, is often into administrative positions that may not be directly related to school psychology (such as becoming a principal or the director of special education). Most school psychologists are employed in systems that have seven or fewer school psychologists in the district and therefore don't work in systems large enough to have the position of director of psychological services to which they can aspire.

Opportunities frequently exist for school psychologists to informally "specialize" in certain areas of practice based on their interests, training, and the needs of the school district. For example, a practitioner may become proficient in the assessment of children with autistic spectrum disorders or become behavior management specialists and work exclusively with children with emotional or behavioral problems. Some school psychologists (particularly those who hold doctoral degrees) become licensed for independent practice and have a part-time private practice and/or do consulting in addition to their school system employment.

School psychologists' salaries compare favorably with those of other types of psychologists. A number of factors impact salaries, such as the number of days that a psychologist works in a year, the number of years that a school psychologist has been practicing, the number of years in a particular school district, the type of school district (urban, rural, suburban), and the degree level all influence salary (Thomas, 2000a). In addition to salary, school psychologists usually have a state benefits program that includes a retirement plan, insurance of various types, and often assistance with continuing education and conference attendance. School psychologists working in the public schools usually work nine- or 10-month contracts (summers off!) and have a similar holiday schedule to other government employees. School psychology is often viewed as a "family friendly" occupation because parents who are school psychologists have a similar holiday and vacation schedule to their children who go to school in the district.

The national median salary of full time school psychologists in elementary or secondary schools (typically working on nine- or 10-month contracts) is $66,040 (Bureau of Labor Statistics, 2007a). The average salary varies significantly by state, with as much as a $22,000 difference between the highest and lowest paying states (Thomas, 2000b). The APA also conducts salary studies every few years, the last of which was in 2007 (Center for Psychology Workforce Analysis and Research, 2007a). The overall median 11–12-month salary for licensed, doctoral-level school psychologists providing school psychology services ranged from $92,000 to $101,000 per year depending on number of years of experience.

The salaries of school psychologists with doctoral degrees and who teach in college or university settings usually increase based on years of experience and rank (e.g., full professors make more than assistant professors). Faculty members at larger schools tend to make higher salaries than those at smaller schools. Although figures for school psychology faculty were not yet available in the newest salary survey, the median nine-month salary of respondents in the 2007 APA salary study who were professors of psychology ranged from $48,000 for assistant professors in four-year colleges to $95,000 for full professors in university psychology departments (Center for Psychology Workforce Analysis and Research, 2007b). Professors can also earn additional salary by teaching in the summer, obtaining grant funding, consulting and/or providing clinical services in an independent practice.

OUTLOOK

School psychology began in the early part of the twentieth century, and experienced its greatest growth in the 1970s and 1980s. Many currently practicing school psychologists who started in the field in the 1970s and 1980s are reaching retirement age. In fact, over 50 percent of currently practicing school psychologists in a number of states will be retiring within 10 years (Thomas, 2000c). The demand for psychological services in the schools is also expected to grow in the next few years. *The Occupational Outlook Handbook* (U.S. Bureau of Labor Statistics, 2007b) predicts that demand for all psychologists, including school psychologists, will grow faster than average (an increase of 10 to 20%) through 2010. School psychologists have some of the best job prospects of nondoctoral degree-level psychologists.

SUMMARY

School psychology is an attractive career field that offers a good salary and a bright employment outlook for the foreseeable future. School psychologists utilize some of the same skills that clinical psychologists use (diagnostic and intervention skills) along with knowledge of educational psychology, developmental psychology, and consultation skills. School psychologists are very satisfied with their jobs and like the opportunities to exercise independent judgment, help others, and work in congenial job settings (Brown, et al, 1998). The training for school psychology is made somewhat more affordable because entry-level training for school practice does not require the doctoral degree and students usually receive a stipend or salary on the required internship. Finally, school psychologists with appropriate training and credentials may have the option of working in a variety of nonschool settings or in private practice.

REFERENCES

Adelman, H.S., & Taylor, L. (1998). Mental health in schools: Moving forward. *School Psychology Review, 27*, 175–190.

American Psychological Association. (2007). *Graduate study in psychology.* Washington, DC: Author.

American Psychological Association. (2002). Ethical principles of psychologists and code of conduct. *American Psychologist, 57*, 1060–1073.

American Psychological Association. (1981). *Specialty guidelines for the delivery of services by school psychologists.* Washington, DC: Author.

Brown, M. B. (2008). Best practices in designing and delivering training programs. In A. Thomas & J. Grimes (Eds.), *Best practices in school psychology–V* (pp. 2029–2040). Washington, DC: National Association of School Psychologists.

Brown, M. B., & Bolen, L. M. (2003). Children with chronic health disorders in the classroom. In W. S. Thomson & C. M. Shea (Eds.), *Teacher's manual for North Carolina educators* pp. (464–487). Boston: McGraw-Hill.

Brown, M. B., Hohenshil, T. H., & Brown, D. T. (1998). Job satisfaction of school psychologists in the United States. *School Psychology International, 19*, 79–89.

Brown, R. T., & DuPaul, G. J. (1999). Introduction to the mini-series: Promoting school success in children with chronic medical conditions. *School Psychology Review, 28*, 175–181.

Bureau of Labor Statistics. (2007a). *Occupational Employment and Wages, May 2007.* Retrieved April 18, 2008, from http://www.bls.gov/oes/current/oes193031.htm.

Bureau of Labor Statistics. (2007b). Psychologists. *Occupational outlook handbook 2008-2009 Edition.* Retrieved April 18, 2008, from http://www.bls.gov/oco/ocos056.htm.

Center for Psychology Workforce Analysis and Research. (2007a). *Table 7: Direct human service positions (licensed only): School psychology– Doctoral-level, 11–12-month salaries for selected settings: 2007.* Retrieved May 14, 2008, from http://research.apa.org/t7salaries07.pdf.

Center for Psychology Workforce Analysis and Research. (2007b). *Table 1: Faculty positions–Doctoral-level, 9-10-month salaries for selected positions: 2007.* Retrieved May 14, 2008, from http://research.apa.org/t1salaries07.pdf.

D'Amato, R. C., Sheridan, S. M., Phelps, L., & Lopez, E. C. (2004). Psychology in the Schools, School Psychology Review, School Psychology Quarterly and Journal of Educational and Psychological Consultation editors collaborate to chart school psychology's past, present, and *"futures." Psychology in the Schools, 41,* 415–418.

Fagan, T., & Wise, P. (2007). *School psychology: Past, present and future.* Washington, DC: National Association of School Psychologists.

Mather, N., & Kaufmann, N. (2006). Introduction to the special issue, part one: It's about the *what,* the *how well,* and the *why. Psychology in the Schools, 43,* 747–752.

Miller, D. (2008). School psychology training programs. In A. Thomas & J. Grimes (Eds.), *Best practices in school psychology–V* (pp. clv-cxcviii). Washington, DC: National Association of School Psychologists.

National Association of School Psychologists. (2000a). *Professional conduct manual.* Washington, DC: Author.

National Association of School Psychologists. (2000b). *Standards for training and field placement programs in school psychology/Standards for the credentialing of school psychologists.* Washington, DC: Author.

Pfeiffer, S. I., & Dean, R. S. (1988). Special issue on school psychologist in non-traditional settings. *School Psychology Review, 17* (2).

Thomas, A. (2000a). School psychology 2000: Average salary data. *Communiqué, 28*(6), 28.

Thomas, A. (2000b). School psychology 2000: Salaries. *Communiqué, 28*(5), 32.

Thomas, A. (2000c). School psychology 2000: Personnel needs in the next millennium. *Communiqué, 28*(4), 10.

Wittmer, L. (1897). The organization of practical work in psychology. *Psychological Review, 4,* 116–117.

Worrell, T. G., Scaggs, G. E., & Brown, M. B. (2006). School psychologists' job satisfaction: A twenty-two year perspective in the USA. *School Psychology International, 27,* 131–145.

Ysseldyke, J., Morrison, D., Burns, M., Otiz, S., Dawson, P., Rosenfeld, S., Kelly, B., & Telzro, C. (2006). *School psychology: A blueprint for training and practice III.* Bethesda, MD: National Association of School Psychologists.

SUGGESTED PRINT RESOURCES

Barringer, M., & Saenz, A. (2006). Promoting positive school environments: A career in school psychology. In R. J. Sternberg (Ed.), *Career paths in psychology: Where your degree can take you* (pp 227–248). Washington, DC: American Psychological Association. This is a discussion of school psychology from the perspective of the practicing school psychologist. Includes a look into a typical day in the life of a school psychologist.

Fagan, T., & Wise, P. (2007). *School psychology: Past, present and future.* Washington, DC: National Association of School Psychologists. This is a classic introductory textbook on school psychology. This book does a nice job of covering the field with the perspective of future or current school psychology students in mind. It describes working conditions, training, and professional and practice issues.

Hoy, A. W. (1999). Psychology applied to education. In A. M. Stec & D. A. Bernstein (Eds.), *Psychology: Fields of application* (pp. 61-81). Boston: Houghton-Mifflin. This is a brief description of the field of educational psychology, which is the study of teaching and learning. Educational psychology is a distinct field from school psychology, although school psychologists utilize research findings from educational psychology in their practice.

Lee, S. W. (2005). *The encyclopedia of school psychology.* New York: Sage. This is a reference work in school psychology that provides wide-ranging coverage of the psychological and educational foundations of school psychology practice. Arranged A-Z, it contains more than 250 articles about school psychology from elementary school through university level. Each brief article provides a number of additional references and readings for further information on the subject area.

Merrill, K. W., Ervin, R. A., & Gimpel, G. (2006). *School psychology for the 21st century: Foundations and practices.* New York: Guilford Press. This is an excellent first textbook used in school psychology graduate programs. The book describes a comprehensive problem-solving approach to prevention and intervention in the schools. A good resource for students interested in a more academic approach to school psychology.

Thomas, A., & Grimes, J. (2008). *Best practices in school psychology–V.* Washington, DC: National Association of School Psychologists. This is a five volume book that provides a single source for information on the contemporary practice of school psychology. Its 141 chapters cover every conceivable topic area across the full range of activities of school psychologists. History, professional and ethical issues, assessment, prevention and intervention, and systems issues receive thorough coverage.

SUGGESTED INTERNET RESOURCES

The American Psychological Association. http://www.apa.org. APA is the largest organization of psychologists in the United States. This website has a lot of useful information on all areas of psychology. The section for students has useful career information (especially for students interested in doctoral-level training in psychology) and

the Education Directorate section provides good coverage of psychology in the schools. Salary data for various fields in psychology is also available here.

International School Psychology Association. http://www.ispaweb.org This group is devoted to promoting sound psychological practices in schools throughout the world. Its membership represents school psychologists from many countries. The site includes a number of informational resources about school psychology and psychologically related issues from an international perspective.

Intervention Central. http://www.interventioncentral.org. This site includes many free tools and resources for school psychologists and parents to promote positive behavior and foster effective learning for children. This is a nice example of the range of intervention strategies that school psychologists apply in the schools.

National Association of School Psychologists. http://www.nasponline.org. NASP is the primary organization for school psychologists who practice in the schools. This website is the single best source of information on school psychology as a career. A variety of informational resources for psychologists and educators is available, including information on certification and training, ethical standards, and career issues. The *About School Psychology* pages are especially useful for career information: http://www.nasponline.org/about_sp/index.aspx.

School Psychology Resources Online. http://www.schoolpsychology.net. A "portal" website that includes resources for school psychologists, educators and parents on a broad range of topics including special education, mental health issues, assessment, intervention, and educational disabilities. Very complete and often-referred to by practicing school psychologists, this site gives you a good idea of the complexity of issues and problems that school psychologists deal with each day. This site is created by Sandra

Steingart, a school psychologist in the Baltimore County (Maryland) Public Schools.

The School Psychology Program at the University of California, Berkeley. http://www-gse.berkeley.edu/program/SP/sp. html. This is an informative collection of resources about school psychology emphasizing information for prospective students. The Student section includes a great deal of information on careers in school psychology.

Chapter 18

SOCIAL WORK

SUSAN CRAFT VICKERSTAFF

Social work is the professional activity of providing "humane and effective social services to individuals, families, groups, communities, and society so that social functioning may be enhanced and the quality of life improved" (National Association of Social Workers [NASW] 1999, p. 1). Professional social workers assist individuals, groups or communities in efforts to restore or enhance their capacity for social functioning, while also working to ensure that the society in which they live is supportive of their goals (NASW, 2008a, p. 1). The practice of social work requires knowledge of human development and behavior; of social, economic, and cultural institutions, and of the interaction of all these factors. Perhaps even more important, social workers strive to make changes in social structures that would improve the individual's ability to function. In other words, social workers help people function to the best of their ability in their own social environment.

Social work is a values-based profession. At the core of social work's value system is *positive regard for every human being*. This means that all people who seek help from a social worker should receive the same respect and quality of service—regardless of age, race, gender, sexual orientation, mental or physical ability, or any other characteristic.

SOCIAL WORK'S HISTORY AND DEVELOPMENT

Although the social welfare needs of individuals have been addressed for centuries, social work is a relatively young profession. Historically, when people needed food, clothing, shelter, medical attention, or mental health services, their family, the church, or other nonprofessionals addressed such needs. The American social welfare system has its roots in England. The *Elizabethan Poor Law* of 1601 contained several important doctrines which influenced the formation of the social welfare system in the United States. First, the *Elizabethan Poor Law* formally shifted responsibility for the poor from churches to the government. Second, anyone capable of working was expected to work, and assistance could be sought only in the town or region from where an individual had originally come. This is the basis of "residency" requirements for assistance. Third, in order to qualify for help, individuals had to fall into certain categories: the elderly, children, or people who had mental or physical problems. Finally, The *Elizabethan Poor Law* required that families, when able, should assume responsibility for family members who could not take care of themselves. All of these principles are still represented in some form in the structure of agencies, services, and laws that make up our current social welfare system (Ferguson, 1969).

Social welfare agencies were first established in the United States in the early 1800s. Most of these agencies were affiliated with religious organizations–clergy and volunteers with no formal training in providing services. The focus was on meeting needs such as food, clothing, and shelter, and on dealing with mental or emotional problems with prayer and readings from the Bible. In the late 1800s, Charity Organization Societies (COS) were established in several large cities. Each COS was responsible for coordinating the services of agencies in an attempt to eliminate duplication. They investigated each applicant thoroughly to determine eligibility and to ensure applicants were not receiving assistance from more than one agency. The COSs also identified social problems, formed committees to explore them, and then planned solutions to address the problems. The executive secretaries of the COSs were the first paid social workers in the United States (Ferguson, 1969).

Another important movement in the late 1800s was the creation of settlement houses. The most famous of these was Hull House, opened by Jane Addams in Chicago. Settlement house workers lived in poor neighborhoods and helped residents determine ways to improve living conditions, health, education, and job opportunities. They focused on both individual and societal problems. This was the first time attempts were made to affect legislation and

social policy that would lead to better lives at the individual, community and society levels.

Many changes in social work began in the early 1900s. Colleges and universities began offering courses in how to provide social services. Social work was introduced into hospital settings in 1905 and soon emerged in many other types of organizations such as schools, clinics, and children's agencies. In 1917, Mary Richmond published the first textbook specifically for social workers. Titled *Social Diagnosis*, it was the first time a formal theory of social work was presented as the basis for assessing, diagnosing, and treating individuals. In the 1920s, Sigmund Freud's ideas were adopted by social workers and for the next 30 years, social workers focused on the intrapsychic functioning of the individual. It was not until the 1960s that attention returned to a psychosocial approach. Today, social workers work in many different settings and may focus on the individual at three levels: individual (micro), family or small group (mezzo), or community/ society (macro) (Zastrow, 2002).

SOCIAL WORK'S MISSION AND OBJECTIVES

According to *The NASW Code of Ethics* (1999), "the primary mission of the social work profession is to enhance human well-being and help meet the basic human needs of all people, with particular attention to the needs and empowerment of people who are vulnerable, oppressed, and living in poverty" (p. 1). Social workers work with people in all age groups, from all ethnic and cultural backgrounds, and in all socioeconomic classes. Historically, social work has been concerned with each person within his or her social environment. This concern has led social workers to focus not only on the individual but also on societal conditions impacting the individual's quality of life. Therefore, social workers must be concerned with social justice and social change in order to ensure that all individuals, families, small groups, and communities will have access to resources and the means to have their needs met.

Social workers work with people at three levels of intervention. First, at the micro level, social workers deal with an individual. Second, at the mezzo level, social workers work with families or groups of people. Third, at the macro level, social workers work with agencies, organizations, communities, and at the state or national level by advocating and making policy changes.

Social workers are trained to carry out tasks and functions appropriate at all three levels. At the micro level, social workers act as caseworkers and/or case managers. Social caseworkers provide numerous services such as counseling runaway youths, helping unemployed people secure training or employment, counseling someone who is suicidal, placing a homeless child in an adoptive or foster home, providing protective services to abused children and their families, finding nursing homes for people who have had strokes and no longer require hospitalization, counseling individuals with sexual dysfunctions, helping alcoholics to acknowledge that they have a drinking problem, counseling those with a terminal illness, serving as a probation or parole officer, providing services to single parents, and working in medical and mental hospitals as a member of a rehabilitation team (Zastrow, 2002).

Case managers provide services similar to those of caseworkers. The case manager's primary roles are to link clients to resources in the community and to advocate for their rights. The case manager also is instrumental in ensuring that the client does not get lost in what can be an overwhelming array of needs

and services (Hepworth & Larsen, 1993). An example of this is a high school student who is seriously injured in a car accident. Although his or her family may have health insurance, it typically will not cover costs for all of the services needed for his or her complete recovery. The social worker can assist in applying for additional benefits for this individual, help arrange transfer to a rehabilitation center, arrange for home health services, and assist the client and his or her family in coping with the injuries.

At the mezzo level, social workers work with families and groups. In addition to traditional group therapy in which people with similar social, emotional, or behavioral problems use the group process to deal with their issues, social workers also lead several other kinds of groups. A few examples of these include groups designed to improve socialization, to educate persons about certain illnesses or other topics, and to train people to become foster or adoptive parents. Social workers also work with entire families and groups of families to help them deal with problems or situations that are disrupting normal family functioning.

At the macro level, social workers attempt to initiate social change. This can be accomplished in several ways, most of which involve empowering the people directly affected. Examples of such activities include neighborhood organizing, community planning, and lobbying state and national legislatures to have laws and policies changed (Miley, O'Melia & DuBois, 2001).

CLIENT PROFILE

There is not a "typical" social work client. Social workers are employed in a wide variety of agencies and work with people from all age groups, races and income levels. One thing that social work clients do have in common is that they are experiencing some difficulty in their social functioning. Specific examples of clients include parents coping with the birth of a sick newborn; a child having problems in school; a teenager skipping school; a couple having marriage problems; a homeless man, woman, or family; an elderly man or woman facing nursing home placement; and many others. As stated in social work's mission, social workers are specifically mandated to pay "particular attention to the needs and empowerment of people who are vulnerable, oppressed, and living in poverty" (NASW, 1999, p.1).

PHILOSOPHICAL ASSUMPTIONS AND PREEMINENT THEORIES

The basic philosophies underlying the profession of social work are spelled out in *The National Association of Social Workers' Code of Ethics* (1999). The core values are service, social justice, dignity and worth of the person, importance of human relationships, integrity, and competence. Social workers use their knowledge and skills to help people in need while addressing the underlying social problems. Social workers respond to social injustice–particularly poverty, unemployment, and discrimination–by initiating social change, with special attention paid to vulnerable and historically oppressed populations. Social work professionals offer the highest-quality services to every client, not negating nor ignoring, but valuing individual and group diversity. Social workers believe in self-determination and strive to empower every individual they serve. Social workers help strengthen relationships between (and among) individuals, families, groups, communities, and society as a reflection of their belief that human relationships are powerful sources of change. Social workers are committed to their profession's Code of Ethics and structure their behavior according to its

guidelines. Finally, social workers continually upgrade their knowledge and skills, and practice to ensure that they remain competent.

Social work, a relatively young profession, has been able to utilize information from other disciplines, particularly biology, psychology, and sociology. Currently, in fact, one of the most influential theoretical approaches in Social Work is the *ecosystems perspective*, which contains aspects of all three. The ecosystems perspective, also referred to as person-in-environment (PIE), seeks to understand the interaction of individuals and groups within all elements of their environment and to use this understanding to determine what factors or conditions need to change and the best method to achieve that change (Miley, O'Melia & DuBois, 2001).

The psychosocial theory stresses the importance of and provides a base for studying human development. It links the individual's life stages–from birth to death–with cultural and societal expectations. Each life stage is described as having tasks that must be met in order to proceed to the next stage. The focus is on healthy development, and ways that disruption development may be addressed (Newman & Newman, 2005).

A third important approach in social work is the strengths-perspective in which the social worker's focus is not on the client's problems; instead, the social worker identifies the client's unique capabilities (Weick, Rapp, Sullivan & Kisthardt, 1989). This approach is consistent with the social worker's ethical responsibility to view every human being as having dignity and worth.

REAL WORLD APPLICATION AND SALARY INDICES

Social workers use their knowledge, skills, and values to help people across the entire lifespan in a wide variety of settings. Examples of such settings and the populations served include services to families and children, services to aging populations, substance abuse, health care, behavioral/mental health centers, schools, employment assistance programs (EAPs), corrections, disaster recovery, and the military. (These will be discussed later in the "Work Settings" section of this chapter.)

Opportunities for career advancement and salary ranges vary widely based on several factors. Obviously, a social worker with a graduate degree is going to earn more and be able to advance farther than someone with an undergraduate degree. Other factors may include the field within social work that an individual pursues and the geographic area where the individual resides and works. A study conducted by NASW (2008b) reported that the median income for their members was $44,400. Typically, an individual with a B.S.W. can expect to start at approximately $25,000 to $30,000 with beginning salaries for M.S.W.s at around $35,000.

PROFESSIONAL PREPARATION AND DEVELOPMENT

Preparation to work as a professional social worker occurs at several levels—bachelor's, master's, and doctoral. Undergraduate programs offer the Bachelor of Social Work (B.S.W.) or Bachelor of Science in Social Work (B.S.S.W.) degree. Graduate programs at the master's level offer the Master of Social Work (M.S.W.) or the Master of Science in Social Work (M.S.S.W.) degree. The Council on Social Work Education (CSWE) accredits bachelor's and master's level programs. CSWE requires that all programs provide education in the following areas: human diversity; human behavior and

the social environment; social policy; research; practice at the micro, mezzo, and macro levels; and field experience (internship).

CSWE requires that all bachelors' level students receive a "generalist" education, which prepares them to assess and intervene in problems faced by individuals, families, groups, agencies, and communities. Part of this education involves an internship–frequently called "field placement"–which allows students to put their education into practice in a supervised setting. In most cases, the internship will be the student's final semester and may involve 40 hours per week participation in an agency. An alternative in some institutions could be for the student to be placed in an agency part-time for two semesters while also taking coursework.

Like bachelor's level students, master's level students receive a generalist education but are also are usually required to select an area of specialization such as clinical or administrative. Students in the clinical specialization learn to provide direct services to clients in institutional and community-based settings and, in some cases, to progress into private practice. The administrative concentration prepares students for leadership roles in human service agencies. Full-time master's programs typically last two years (four semesters). Completion of the undergraduate program in social work is not always a prerequisite for entry into a master's program. However, many graduate programs in social work have an "advanced standing" program for individuals who have graduated from an accredited social work undergraduate program and whose grade-point average (GPA) meets the program's minimum requirement. These programs usually last one calendar year because they are able to give the student credit for the generalist portion of graduate study. In social work, the master's degree is considered the "terminal" practice degree, which means that a doctoral degree is not required for individuals who wish to have a private practice.

Doctoral programs offer the Doctor of Philosophy in Social Work (Ph.D.) or the Doctor of Social Work (D.S.W.) degree. Doctoral programs are not accredited by CSWE but are reviewed by The Group for the Advancement of Doctoral Education in Social Work (GADE). Doctoral programs in social work prepare individuals for careers in teaching, policy, and research. Entry into doctoral programs generally requires a master's degree in social work plus several years of practical experience after receiving the master's degree. Typically, doctoral programs require two years of coursework and two years or more to complete the dissertation (a major research project and paper). The doctorate in social work usually is obtained by individuals who plan to teach at the university level or want to do research.

Most states require social workers to be licensed in an effort to ensure that the professionals who work with the public have met certain minimum qualifications and standards. Requirements for licensure will vary from state to state. The Association of Social Work Boards (ASWB) provides information on licensing in all 50 states as well as Washington DC, Puerto Rico, and the Virgin Islands. Because licensure to practice as a social worker may be dependent on graduation from a CSWE accredited program, it is extremely important for prospective students to inquire about the accreditation status of a social work program. The websites for CSWE and ASWB where one can request information about this and other issues are provided in the list of references.

WORK SETTINGS

Social workers work with individuals, families, groups, and communities in a wide variety of settings. As mentioned earlier, at the bachelor's level, social workers are trained in knowledge and skills that can be used to help people learn to deal with issues or concerns that are causing them problems in living. In master's level education, social workers are trained in areas of specialization, such as clinical, administration or policy. The following describes many of the settings in which bachelor's and master's level social workers practice.

Services to Families and Children

When parents neglect or abuse their children, the state assumes responsibility for taking measures to ensure that the children are protected. It is typically social workers who investigate and assess what it will take to improve the family situation so that the children can remain with their family and also be safe. If this is not possible, the social worker is prepared to make other arrangements. One possible arrangement is for children to be placed with a foster family. Foster families are individuals or couples who have received special training from the state and are certified to take children into their homes on a temporary basis until the children can be returned to their home or until they are removed from their parents' custody and made eligible for adoption. Adoption is a legal process by which the courts mandate that a child becomes the responsibility of someone to whom he or she was not born. While foster care is temporary, adoption is permanent.

Services to Aging Populations

According to the United States Bureau of Labor Statistics (2008), the fastest growing segment of our population includes individuals over the age of 65. As people age, they frequently need more social services to help them maintain their quality of life. Social workers provide services to the elderly in many different settings such as the client's own home, hospitals, nursing homes, home health agencies, health departments, and mental health agencies. Unfortunately, there are many instances where older individuals are abused, neglected, or exploited. Similar to cases of child abuse or neglect, social workers assess the situation and make recommendations about what it will take to protect those persons and improve their situation.

Alcohol and Substance Abuse

Individuals who have problems related to substance abuse receive treatment in several different settings. First, inpatient treatment may be required–the person is admitted to a hospital for detoxification ("drying out" or "coming off of drugs"). Next, it is usually recommended that the person remain in an inpatient program for at least one month to learn–substance free–how to deal with his or her particular issues. After completing the inpatient program, a person may have no place to live if, for example, his or her family situation is not stable, and therefore a stay of up to one year in a halfway house may be beneficial. "Halfway" refers to a place where the person is between a hospital stay and living independently. Following inpatient detoxification or treatment, the person also will receive ongoing follow-up treatment on an outpatient basis, usually at a mental health center, clinics, and/or rehabilitation facilities.

Behavioral/Mental Health

Social workers assist people with behavioral and emotional problems in both inpatient and outpatient facilities. Examples of such facilities include community mental health centers, medical clinics, hospitals, homeless shelters, women's shelters, substance abuse programs, and employee assistance programs. In many settings, the social worker may also provide services to the families of people with these problems.

School Social Work

The school social worker helps children and teenagers who have problems or situations in their home environment that make it difficult for the student to do his or her best in school. For example, if a child comes to school every day hungry and dirty, there probably are issues occurring in the home that a social worker can address. In this situation, the social worker serves as a link between the school and the child's home environment.

Health Care

As was mentioned in the section on aging populations, social workers provide health-related services in varied settings. Examples of such include hospitals, nursing homes, home health agencies, family planning clinics, and rehabilitation centers. In these settings, social workers help the patient and family learn about and adjust to the illness or condition, make sure that the patient has an appropriate place to live after discharge, and link the patient and family to available community resources.

Employee Assistance Programs

Social workers also work in employee assistance programs (EAPs) which are clinics set up by employers so that their employees can receive help for problems that may be affecting their ability to do their jobs. Individuals may be self-referred or sent for assistance by their supervisors or human resource professionals.

Corrections

Correction facilities are another type of agency where social workers are often employed–usually as probation or parole officers. Probation officers work with juveniles or adults found guilty of a crime but whose sentence is put off as long as they comply with specific rules ordered by the court. Parole officers work with individuals who are being released early from jail or prison and have to report on their progress after release on a regular basis.

Disaster Relief

Social workers also help people in times of personal or large scale disasters. An example of a personal disaster is the loss of a home from a fire. Large scale disasters include the effects of hurricanes or earthquakes. Social workers help not only the individuals who have been personally affected but also the people who are helping them who may become stressed while dealing with the devastation.

PROFESSIONAL ORGANIZATIONS

There are many organizations a professional social worker may join. Several of these are very broad in nature and have members from different areas of social work practice. The National Association of Social Workers (NASW) is the largest association of professionals in the United States. It provides the Code of Ethics that is used by most social workers, social service agencies, and licensing boards. Two other general organizations are The North American Association of Christians in Social Work (NACSW) and The National Association of Black Social Workers (NABSW). Websites for these three organizations are included in the list of references.

There are also numerous national associations for social workers based on area of practice. A few examples are: The Association of Oncology Social Work, The American Network of Home Health Care Social Workers, The American Association of Marriage and Family Therapy, The Council of Nephrology Social Workers, The National Organization of Forensic Social Work, and The School Social Work Association of America. These websites also are included in the list of resources.

FUTURE OUTLOOK

The outlook for careers in Social Work is excellent. According to *The United States Bureau of Labor Statistics Occupational Outlook Handbook, 2008–2009 Edition,* job prospects for social workers will increase faster than most other occupations through 2016. The elderly population is increasing rapidly, creating greater demand for health and social services and resulting in particularly rapid job growth among gerontology social workers. Social workers also will be needed to help the large baby-boom generation deal with depression and mental health concerns stemming from mid-life, career, or other personal and professional difficulties. In addition, continuing concern about crime, juvenile delinquency, services for individuals with mental illness, mental retardation and physical disabilities, AIDS patients, and individuals and families in crisis will spur demand for social workers.

REFERENCES

Ferguson, E. (1969). *Social work: An introduction.* Philadelphia: Lippincott.

Hepworth, D. H., & Larsen, J. A. (1993). *Direct social work practice: Theory and skills.* Belmont, CA: Wadsworth.

Miley, K. K., O'Melia, M., & DuBois, B. (2001). *Generalist social work practice: An empowering approach.* Needham Heights, MA: Allyn and Bacon.

National Association of Social Workers. (1999). *Code of ethics of the National Association of Social Workers.* Washington, DC: Author.

National Association of Social Workers. (2008a). *Social work fact sheet. http://www.socialworkers. org/pressroom/features/general/profession.asp.*

National Association of Social Workers. (2008b). *Social work income, PRN 2:1, 2003.* Available at: www.socialworkers.org/naswprn/surveyTwo/ Datagram1.pdf.

Newman, B. M., & Newman, P. R. (2005). *Development through life: A psychosocial approach.* Belmont, CA: Thomson Wadsworth.

Richmond, M. (1917). *Social diagnosis.* New York: Russell Sage Foundation. United States Bureau of Labor Statistics. (2008). *Occupational outlook handbook, 2008–2009 Edition* (online). Available: http://www.bls.gov/oco/ocos060.htm.

Weick, A., Rapp, C., Sullivan, W. P., & Kisthardt, W. (1989). A strengths perspective for social work practice. *Social Work, 34,* 350–354.

Zastrow, C. (2002). *The practice of social work.* Pacific Grove, CA: Brooks/Cole.

SUGGESTED RESOURCES

Fiske-Rusciano, R., & Cyrus, V. (2000). *Experiencing race, class, and gender in the United States* (4th ed.). Hightstown, NJ: McGraw-Hill. First-hand reports from members of minority groups give the reader a bird's eye view into their lives.

Ginsberg, L. (2000). *Careers in social work.* Needham Heights, MA: Allyn and Bacon.

Grobman, L. M. (Ed.). (1999). *Days in the lives of social workers: 50 professionals tell "real-lift" stories from social work practice.* Washington DC: White Hat Communications. (The title says it all!)

Lieberman, A. (1998). *The social workout book: Strength-building exercises for the pre-professional.*

Thousand Oaks, CA: Pine Forge Press. This workbook provides a fun way for majors and non-majors to learn about social policy, contemporary issues, practice skills and theory.

Social Work is the primary journal published by the National Association of Social Workers. It addresses issues of general interest to social workers and provides results of up-to-date research.

Strom-Gottfried, K. (1999). *Social work practice: Cases, activities, and exercises.* Thousand Oaks, CA: Pine Forge Press. The exercises in this book will give the reader a look into what they might experience in a social work class.

The New Social Worker is a journal for social work students and recent graduates. It is available online. See below for website.

WEBSITES

The following websites will provide information on many different aspects of Social Work practice. At the time this chapter was written, they were all working. Hopefully they still are! If not, please use a search engine such as Google to look for your topic.

Association of Social Work Boards
www.aswb.org

Council on Social Work Education (CSWE):
www.cswe.org

Deaf, Hard of Hearing, and Hearing Social Workers http://academic.gallaudet.edu/prof/ dhhhswweb.nsf

National Association of Black Social Workers (NABSW) http://www.nabsw.org/mserver

National Association of Social Workers (NASW) www.socialworkers.org

National Organization of Forensic Social Work http://www.nofsw.org/

Nephrology (kidney) Social Workers http://www. kidney.org/professionals/CNSW

New Social Worker Magazine http://www.social-worker.com/home/index.php

North American Association of Christians in Social Work (NACSW) http://www.nacsw. org/2008/2008-index.shtml

Rural Social Work Caucus: http://www.marson-and-associates.com/rural

School Social Work Association of America
http://www.sswaa.org
Social Work Access Network http://www.social-workcafe.net
The Group for the Advancement of Doctoral Education in Social Work http://www.gade-phd.org

Chapter 19

SPECIAL EDUCATION

KAREN R. NICHOLAS & BRUCE M. MENCHETTI

Two roads diverged in a wood,
And I–I took the road less traveled,
And that has made all the difference.
–Robert Frost

The profession of special education is often seen as the "road less traveled" because professionals aspire to make a difference in the lives of children with special needs by designing individualized educational instruction that is not provided in general education classrooms. This chapter has three major purposes. First, it provides current information about the policies and practices that guide the profession of special education. Next, readers will find suggestions on how to prepare for a career in this exciting and challenging field. Finally, occupational information and professional resources are provided so that readers of this chapter may continue their exploration of careers in special education. (Appendix A presents several resources for exploring careers in special education.)

PROFESSIONAL REQUIREMENTS IN EDUCATION

Professionals in education are affected daily by two important legislative acts. These federal laws have significantly influenced instructional policies and practices at the state, local, and even the classroom level. The No Child Left Behind Act (NCLB) of 2001 and the Individuals with Disabilities Education Improvement Act (IDEA) of 2004 include principles that challenge American educators at all levels to meet the complex needs of an increasingly diverse student body. For the benefits of students with disabilities, NCLB and IDEA come together to place unique demands on special education professionals.

If you are considering a career in special education you must be aware of the core principles of both NCLB and IDEA. To a large extent, these principles will determine how you are prepared for your career, how you conduct your practice and how your performance is evaluated by other educators, parents, and society. By understanding the rules and regulations imposed on special educators, you will be better able to decide if this is the right career for you.

The next sections of this chapter will explain the principles of NCLB and IDEA. The core principles of each act will be described separately.

CORE PRINCIPLES OF NCLB

The No Child Left Behind Act (NCLB) of 2001 was enacted to improve education for all students, including those with disabilities (Turnbull, Turnbull & Wehmeyer, 2007). Cortiella (2006) suggested NCLB has four core principles: (a) professional accountability; (b) use of scientifically-based curricula and methods; (c) parental involvement; and, (d) local control and flexibility.

Professional Accountability

The most well-known requirement of NCLB has been the mandate that states create statewide standards in reading, language arts, math, and science. In addition, NCLB requires that all students, even those with disabilities, be tested to assess their performance on state mandated academic standards. Annual statewide tests of student progress combined with other indicators are used to determine if school districts achieve adequate yearly progress (AYP). All students, including students with disabilities, are required to participate in these assess-

ments. States must provide accommodations needed by students with disabilities for their participation in statewide assessments; this includes creating alternative assessments for students with more severe disabilities.

Use of Scientifically-Based Curricula and Methods

General and special education teachers must implement research-based curricular materials and instructional methods in their classrooms. The use of materials and methods supported by scientific educational research is an attempt to ensure that all children obtain a high quality education and reach proficiency on academic standards. Students with disabilities are also required to meet these standards; thus, it is imperative that special education teachers use empirically validated best practices.

Parental Involvement

NCLB recognizes the educational benefits of parental involvement. Under NCLB, all schools are required to report student outcomes, teacher qualifications, and safety procedures to parents of all students. As part of this requirement, schools must report on the achievement of specific subgroups of students; students with disabilities are part of these subgroups. Every year, each school in the United States must issue a report card to parents that details performance on AYP for the entire school and each subgroup of students.

Local Control and Flexibility

Decisions about what to include in state academic achievement standards and state assessments are left to individual states and districts. The outcome measures of students' performance are made at the state and local level. Decisions about accommodations for students with disabilities and the content of any alternative assessments are made by each student's individual educational planning team.

The core principles of The Individuals with Disabilities Education Improvement Act, or IDEA, work with these NCLB requirements: (a) to regulate the profession of special education, and (b) to provide both individualized instruction and school accountability for students with disabilities. Thus, the performance of students with disabilities becomes the shared responsibility of all educators. Now, let's review the core principles of the IDEA and how these bolster individualization and accountability.

IDEA PRINCIPLES AND PROCEDURES

IDEA requires that a free, appropriate public education be provided to every student with a disability regardless of the type or severity of his or her disability. This *right to education* is provided to every student with a disability, aged three to 21. First passed in 1975 as the Education for All Handicapped Children Act, or P.L. 94–142, the IDEA has articulated the procedures and safeguards for providing special education and related services (Culatta & Tompkins, 1999; Yell, 1998). The goal of the IDEA is "to assure that all children with disabilities have available to them a free appropriate public education which emphasizes special education and related services designed to meet their unique needs and prepare them for employment and independent living" (IDEA, 2004, Section 1400[d][1][A]). Related special services may include special transportation, speech pathology and audiology, physical and occupational therapy, as well as other services determined necessary through an "individualized education program" or IEP.

Turnbull, Turnbull, and Wehmeyer (2007) delineated six principles and procedures found in the Individuals with Disabilities Education Act since its inception in 1975. In essence, the IDEA mandates appropriate education for all children. This education must be provided at public expense, without cost to parents or guardians. The six core IDEA principles have been guiding the delivery of special education services since 1975. According to Turnbull et al. (2007) the six guiding principles of the IDEA are (a) zero reject; (b) nondiscriminatory evaluation; (c) free, appropriate, public education; (d) least restrictive environment; (e) due process; and, (f) parental participation. These six principles illustrate the challenges and demands that are faced on a daily basis by all special education teachers and any other professionals working with students with disabilities in America's schools.

Table 19-1 lists each of these six principles of the IDEA and describes its major requirements. For more information of regulatory requirements regarding the alignment of the IDEA and the NCLB on the field of special education, consult the U.S. Department of Education, Office of Special Education Program's (OSEP's) IDEA website located at http://idea.ed.gov/explore/home.

Table 19-1
The Six Guiding Principles of the Individuals with Disabilities
Education Improvement Act (IDEA) of 2004

Principle of IDEA	*Requirement*
Zero Reject Locate, identify, and provide services to all eligible students with disabilities	In summary, the zero reject principle is based upon the proposition that all children with disabilities can learn and benefit from an appropriate education. The right to education for children with disabilities means that every child in the United States now has an equal opportunity to realize the promise of becoming a large stream or a tall oak. At its core, the zero reject principle found in IDEA truly means that every child belongs in our nation's public schools.
Nondiscriminatory Evaluation Conduct an assessment to determine if a student has an IDEA related disability and if he/she needs special education services	IDEA evaluation methods must not discriminate on the basis of race, culture, or ethnicity and must be administered in the child's native language. To further safeguard against discrimination, no single instrument can be used to determine whether a child has a disability or what type special education services are needed. The purposes of the IDEA nondiscriminatory evaluation principle is to provide a safeguard against unfair classification or labeling of children and to assure that children who are found to have a disability can receive the services most suited to their needs.
Free Appropriate Public Education Develop and deliver an individualized education program of special education services that confers meaningful educational benefit	The content of the IEP must contain: (a) present levels of educational performance; (b) annual goals and short-term objectives; (c) description of special education and related services the student will receive including supplemental aids, modifications, and supports provided to school personnel; (d) a statement of the extent to which the student will participate in the general curriculum; (e) any modifications to state or district-wide assessments or a plan for an alternative assessment procedure; (f) timelines for the beginning and end of all services; and finally, (g) progress measurement strategies and how parents will be informed about the student's progress. Several professionals have suggested that the IEP represents the foundation for improving the performance and educational achievement of special education students.
Least Restrictive Environment Educate students with disabilities with non-disabled students to the maximum extent appropriate	The LRE principle has also been known as mainstreaming, integration, or inclusion (Turnbull et al., 2002). As articulated in IDEA, LRE requires that to the maximum extent possible, students with disabilities must be educated with their nondisabled peers at each level of the continuum of educational placements from the least restrictive to the most restrictive options available.
Procedural Safeguards Comply with the procedural requirements of the IDEA	Parents of students with disabilities must be notified prior to any change in the educational status of their child. This includes notice of initial evaluation and placement, as well as any changes in the educational program. Notice must be provided in a reasonable amount of

Table 19-1 (cont.)

	time. Parental consent must be obtained prior to any eligibility evaluation or the initial placement in special education. If the parents and the school system disagree about a child's special education evaluation, IDEA allows parents to obtain an independent evaluation at public expense
Parental Participation Collaborative topics between parents and school officials	These topics include: (a) sharing their family history, priorities, and concerns with educators; (b) clearly stating their child's expectations, preferences, and needs; (c) helping to administer informal assessments that inform the educational program; and, (d) sharing family resources with the school.

SUMMARY OF NCLB AND IDEA PRINCIPLES

Cortiella (2006) identified several ways that the NCLB and IDEA work together to ensure the educational performance of students with disabilities. First, all students must meet challenging academic and content standards. Students with disabilities must have access to this general core curriculum; any accommodations to this curriculum are determined by the students' individualized education plan.

The NCLB and IDEA require that all students participate in state and district-wide assessments. Students with disabilities can participate in these assessments through their regular education courses, with no changes to the assessment. Other students with disabilities can participate in alternative assessments that are determined by the student's IEP team and included in their educational plan. Such accommodations might include extended time, alternative settings, and the use of special lighting during tests. Even students with significant cognitive disabilities must participate using an alternative assessment based on standards established by their IEP.

Finally, both the NCLB and IDEA recognize that student performance is linked to effective teaching. Both laws require that teachers are "highly qualified." State and local districts establish professional requirements for their teachers. Each state department of education has its own standards and guidelines for certification of public school teachers.

STUDENT POPULATIONS

The U.S. Department of Education (2004), Office of Special Education Programs, defines several categories of disabilities that are eligible for special education services. These include students whose disabilities occur at higher proportions in the general population, as well as students whose disabilities occur at much lower proportions.

High Incidence Populations

According to the U.S. Department of Education (2004), Office of Special Education Programs, several categories of students with high incidence disabilities (i.e., specific learning disabilities, speech/language, mental retardation, and emotional disturbances) are eligible for special education services. Together, these disability areas make up about 78 percent of the total population of students ages six to 21 with disabilities served under the IDEA. Children with these disabilities are considered to be in the high incidence disability category. A child will *not* be determined to be a child with a disability if the basis of the child's problem is a lack of scientifically-based instruction in reading, lack of appropriate teaching in math or limited English proficiency.

Specific Learning Disabilities (SLD)

The category makes up about half of all students with disabilities (40.7%) and is now used as an umbrella term that refers to a group of students with average to above average intelligence who have difficulties with academic tasks in the areas of reading, writing, or mathematics in combination with limited language processing, spoken or written abilities. Specific learning disabilities are highly represented in general education classes (5.6%) and are the single largest disability area (U.S. Department of Education, 2008). When determining whether a child has a learning disability, a local education agency (LEA) shall not be required to take into consideration a discrepancy between ability and achievement. Rather, the LEA may use a process that determines if the child responds to research-based instruction (RTI).

Many students with learning disabilities experience difficulties in expressive and receptive language and are most commonly assisted using classroom adaptations such as structured daily routines, learning and study strategies, modified instruction and materials, peer-tutoring, and individualized goal-setting.

Speech/Language Impairments

Students classified with communication impairments constitute 21.9 percent of all students ages six to 21 served under the IDEA (U.S. Department f Education, 2008). Speech disorders may exist as voice, articulation, or fluency problems. Language disorders are problems in using or comprehending language, either expressive (using language) or receptive (understanding the language of others). Language disorders may involve difficulties with phonology, morphology, syntax, semantics, or pragmatics. Most students receiving speech and language therapy work individually or in small groups with a specialist in brief sessions several times a week and usually spend the rest of the day in general education classrooms. Some students may also have a primary disability, such as a learning disability, cerebral palsy, or traumatic brain injury, which would call for an alternative or augmentative communication device to assist in communication.

Mental Retardation (MR)

Individuals with mental retardation represent 8.3 percent of the students ages six to 21 served under the IDEA (U.S. Department f Education, 2008), or about 1.1 percent of the population in general. Mild mental retardation represents the upper range of intellectual functioning with IQ scores between 55 and 70. Scores between 35 and 54 are considered moderate MR, scores of 20 to 34 are severe, and scores less than 20 is considered profound mental retardation. Genetic disorders, brain factors, and environmental influences are some of the known causes of mental retardation. Students with mental retardation exhibit deficiencies in intellectual functioning and corresponding deficits in adaptive behavior. These students also may exhibit learning problems related to language, social behavior, attention, reasoning, and problem solving. Careful preparation can greatly enhance the successful inclusion of students with MR. For example, providing the same educational materials in the classroom, an open environment, daily routine, and placing an emphasis on strong peer relationships can all greatly influence their success in the general classroom.

Emotional Disturbance (ED)

Individuals classified as severely emotionally disturbed (or behaviorally disordered) represent 7.1 percent of all students ages six to 21 served under the IDEA (U.S. Department of Education, 2008). Emotional disturbance refers to a number of different but related social-emotional disabilities, such as schizophrenia, selective autism, and Tourette syndrome. Students with behavior disorders or severe emotional disturbance may exhibit problems in classroom behavior, social relations, or may exhibit disorders of affect, such as anxiety or depression.

Autism

Autism is a complex neurobiological disorder that typically lasts throughout a person's lifetime. It is part of a group of disorders known as autism spectrum disorders (ASD). Today, one in 150 individuals is diagnosed with autism, making it more common than pediatric cancer, diabetes, and AIDS combined. Children with autism make up about 3.3 percent of the students served under the IDEA (U.S. Department of Education, 2008). While it occurs in all racial, ethnic, and social groups, it is four times more likely to strike boys than girls. Autism impairs a person's ability to communicate and relate to others. It also is associated with rigid routines and repetitive behaviors, such as obsessively arranging objects or following very specific routines, and characterized by varying degrees of impairment in communication skills and social abilities. ASD can usually be reliably diagnosed by

age three, although new research is pushing back the age of diagnosis to as early as six months. Parents are usually the first to notice unusual behaviors in their child or their child's failure to reach appropriate developmental milestones. Some parents describe a child who seemed different from birth, while others describe a child who was developing normally and then lost skills. Pediatricians initially may dismiss signs of autism, thinking a child will "catch up" and may advise parents to "wait and see." Nonetheless, new research shows that when parents suspect something is wrong with their child, they are usually correct (Silverman & Brosco, 2007).

Multiple Disabilities

Individuals with multiple disabilities make up about 2.1 percent of the students served under the IDEA (U.S. Department of Education, 2008). Students with severe and multiple disabilities generally have cognitive and adaptive behavior difficulties and require instruction in self-help skills; communication skills; functional academic and daily living skills; community awareness; and recreation, social, and vocational education skills. The creation of peer support networks, friendship circles, and participation in after school activities can be great educational enhancements for these students. Paraprofessionals often assist teachers and their students with multiple disabilities in daily classroom activities (i.e., hands-on tasks, academic and communication skills, etc.) and adaptations (i.e., reading text aloud, assistance with small groups, fine and gross motor activities).

Hearing Impairments

Individuals with hearing impairments constitute about 1.2 percent of the students served under IDEA (U.S. Department of

Education, 2008). Hearing impairments range in severity from mild to moderate to severe and profound, with the greatest distinction being between hard of hearing and deaf. Students classified as hard of hearing can hear speech tones when wearing hearing aids, while persons who are deaf cannot hear any tones even with the help of assistive devices. Some teachers use "total communication," which includes using speech (lip reading), gestures, sign language, and both oral and written methods of communication in the classroom. Adaptive technology, visual language and learning cards, hand signals and sign language interpreters are commonly used to assist students with hearing impairments in general education classrooms.

Orthopedic Impairments

Individuals with physical disabilities and other health impairments make up about 1.1 percent of the students served under IDEA (U.S. Department of Education, 2008). Physical disabilities are often described as either orthopedic (damage to the skeleton) or neurological (damage to the nervous system). Some common physical or health-related disabilities include cerebral palsy, spina bifida, and muscular dystrophy. Traumatic brain injury (.25%) and epilepsy are common neurological disorders. Fetal alcohol syndrome and acquired immune deficiency syndrome are also health impairments that coexist with disabilities such as mental retardation and emotional disorders that are served under the IDEA. School personnel must be aware of medications, dietary needs, and adaptations for chronic conditions, and must receive special training in positioning and moving students with physical disabilities. Classrooms and instructional materials are often adapted using technology such as adaptive switches, touch screens, and special grips for pencils, paper, and utensils.

Visual Impairments

Individuals with visual impairments make up one of the smallest disability groups (about .4%) of the students served under IDEA (U.S. Department of Education, 2008). Visual impairments, such as glaucoma and cataracts, can be present at birth or acquired later in life. Educational definitions are based more on the method for learning to read. For example, students classified as legally blind may have some vision, but need enlarged print or a magnifying device to read printed materials. Other students may have such limited vision that they are considered totally blind and will learn to read using Braille text and/or audiotapes materials. Instructional adaptations include enlarged printed materials, bold-lined paper, converted texts to Braille format, oral output devices, and tactile three-dimensional devices—all of which are common strategies used to assist students with visual impairments.

PROFESSIONAL PREPARATION AND DEVELOPMENT

Special education teachers are required to have a minimum of a bachelor's degree. Often, teachers find that they are interested in the profession of teaching, yet do not know what specific age (elementary, secondary, etc.) or student population (SLD, MR, etc.) they want to teach. The National Clearinghouse for Professions in Special Education (NCPSE) (http://www.specialed-careers.org) provides useful information for anyone wishing to further explore careers in special education.

Scientifically-Based Methods of Teaching

Majors in education typically will be provided a broad range of subject area coursework, pedagogy, and introductions to several student populations commonly found in the general education classroom. To meet the NCLB definition of "scientifically based," research must (a) employ systematic, empirical methods that draw on observation or experiment; (b) involve rigorous data analyses that are adequate to test the stated hypotheses and justify the general conclusions; (c) rely on measurements or observational methods that provide valid data across evaluators and observers, and across multiple measurements and observations; and (d) be accepted by a peer-reviewed journal or approved by a panel of independent experts through a comparatively rigorous, objective, and scientific review.

Typically, the teaching methods to be used or the models to be emulated must represent the latest advances in teaching (e.g., dialogic reading, explicit phonic-based instruction, and learning strategies). Special education teachers who teach core academic subjects must be qualified in both the academic subject and special education methods. This provides students with disabilities access to instruction from teachers who are qualified. Specific subject area training may be offered within general education programs; however, special education teacher preparation typically is designed to cover unique special populations (e.g., learning disabilities, mental retardation, physical or visual impairments).

Field Experiences

Preparation for special education teachers often includes seminars, intensive observation and feedback strategies, peer coaching, and field experiences. Teachers are required to apply their theoretical and textbook knowledge to practical teaching experiences. Typically termed "field experiences" or "internships," these requirements intend to prepare teachers to deal effectively with the "real world" of schooling–the management of classes, the conduct of lessons, planning and collaborating with other teachers and administrators, and the performance of tasks such as hall monitoring and serving on various school committees.

Teachers in training are typically required to design structured assignments, write journals about their experiences, and discuss their progress with a supervisor on a regular basis. Field experiences are quite helpful to new teachers by providing them a wide range of student populations to teach and can often assist them in narrowing the choices between elementary, secondary, or adult special education settings upon graduation.

Student Teaching

By and large, the final component to formal teacher training at a university or college is student teaching. This professional prerequisite is designed to provide soon-to-be teachers with an experienced teacher role model who will assist them in preparing lessons, classroom management, and development of individual student goals and overall teaching requirements. While field experiences are similar, student teaching typically is at least one semester in length, and student teachers actually are in direct command of an entire classroom for longer lengths of time.

STATE AND NATIONAL CERTIFICATION REQUIREMENTS

In most instances, teachers are required to have successfully passed and been granted certification within the field of education to which they will be assigned a classroom of students. Teachers can be employed to teach "out-of-field," however, and certification is granted on a temporary basis until required coursework is completed for a particular subject area and/or student population. Professional development courses are often required to keep a professional certification current and up to date.

GRADUATE PROGRAMS/CONTINUING EDUCATION

Teachers are in the business of creating "lifelong learners." As such, teachers frequently find themselves returning to the classroom (as students themselves) to continue their education to learn more about a specific student population, age level and/or to obtain an advanced degree within the profession. Programs of study are commonly designed for teaching specific student populations and tailored to meet individual career objectives, and the number of required credits often depends upon previous training and professional aspirations.

WORK SETTINGS AND CONDITIONS

Special education teachers work in a variety of settings. The continuum of special education placements discussed earlier in this chapter (Deno, 1970) defines work settings for special educators. Special education work settings include the regular class, a resource room, separate classes for students with disabilities, separate schools, residential facilities, and homebound or hospital instruction.

Special education teachers work in regular elementary and secondary classrooms. Usually, special educators in theses settings work in collaboration with general educators in either a team or consultative role (Mastropieri & Scruggs, 2000). In other settings, such as the resource room or a separate class, the special education teacher is primarily responsible for the delivery of instruction. Nonetheless, it is important to understand that school districts vary in their use of these settings. Very often, this responsibility includes the supervision of paraprofessionals or teacher's aides. Figure 19-1 describes each of the settings from least restrictive to most restrictive in the continuum proposed by Deno (1970) and is still applied to special education program design today.

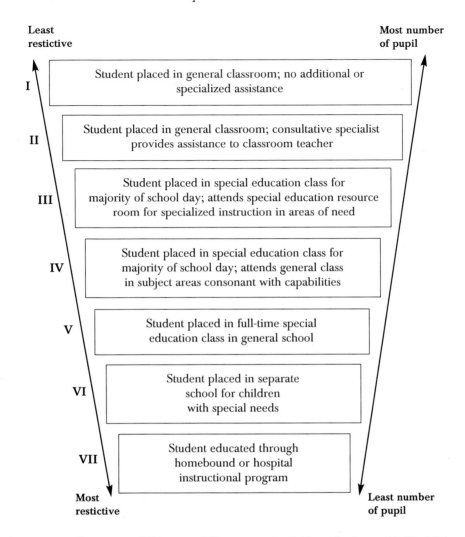

Figure 19–1. Continuum of Educational Placements Available to Students with Disabilities.
Note: Recreated by authors according to the model proposed by Deno (1970).

CONCLUDING COMMENTS

Large streams from little fountains flow,
Tall oaks from little acorns grow.
　　　　　–David Everett (1769-1813)
　　　　　Lines written for a School
　　　　　Declamation

These lines, written during a time when our nation was struggling to define its foundational principles and basic values, suggest a promising perspective on children and education. David Everett's simple, yet powerful ideals resonate today and should continue to guide educational policy and practice in the 21st century. Everett's perspective is particularly relevant to the profession of special education–special educators, like most dedicated teachers, believe that all children have potential to become large streams and tall oaks. Very often the children with whom special educators work are those whose growth requires the most nurturing. Perhaps because of the additional care required to nurture a child with special needs, others sometimes find it difficult to see the potential in such children. Special educators, however, know how to find the talents and abilities in all children and how to create the necessary conditions for children to flourish and grow.

REFERENCES

Cortiella, C. (2006). NCLB and IDEA: What parents of students with disabilities need to know and do. Minneapolis, MN: University of Minnesota, National Center for Educational Outcomes.

Culatta, R.A., & Tompkins, J.R. (1999). *Fundamentals of special education: What every teacher needs to know.* Upper Saddle River, NJ: Merrill/Prentice-Hall.

Deno, E. (1970). Special education as developmental capital. *Exceptional Children, 37*, 229–237.

Mastropieri, M.A., & Scruggs, T.E. (2000). *The inclusive classroom: Strategies for effective instruction.* Upper Saddle River, NJ: Merrill/Prentice-Hall.

No Child Left Behind (NCLB) Act of 2001, Pub. L. No. 107–110, § 115, Stat. 1425 (2004).

Silverman, C., & Brosco, J.P. (2007). Understanding autism: Parents and pediatricians in historical perspective. *Archives Pediatric Adolescent Medicine, 161*(4), 392–298.

Turnbull, A., Turnbull, R., & Wehmeyer, M. (2007). *Exceptional lives: Special education in today's schools* (4th ed.). Upper Saddle River, NJ: Merrill/Prentice Hall.

U.S. Department of Education (2004). *To assure a free and appropriate education for all children with disabilities: The twenty-sixth annual report to Congress on the mplementation of the Individuals with Disabilities Education Act (IDEA).* Washington, DC: U.S. Department of Education.

U.S. Department of Education, National Center for Education Statistics (2008). [On-line]. Available: http://nces.ed.gov/programs/digest/d07/tables/dt07_047.asp

Yell, M.L. (1998). *The law and special education.* Upper Saddle River, NJ: Merrill/Prentice Hall.

RESOURCES

National Organizations
Council for Exceptional Children
    http://www.cec.sped.org
US Department of Education
    http://www.ed.gov
Parent Organizations
Parent to Parent - National Parent to Parent Support and Information System
    http://www.nppsis.org
Kids Together, Inc.
    http://www.kidstogether.org/idea.html
Law and Advocacy
IDEA: The Individuals with Disabilities Education Act http://www.idea.ed.gov
NCLB and IDEA work together
    http://www.nea.org/specialed/ideanclbintersection.html
    http://www.ldonline.org/article/11846
NCLB: No Child Left Behind
    http://www.ed.gov/nclb
Clearinghouses
ERIC Clearinghouse on Disabilities and Gifted Education
    http://www.cec.sped.org/er-menu.htm
National Clearinghouse for Professions in Special Education (NCPSE)
    http://www.cec.sped.org/cl-menu.htm
National Information Center for Children and Youth with Handicaps
    http://www.aed.org/nichcy
Specific Populations
International Dyslexia Society
    http://www.interdys.org
National Center for Learning Disabilities
    http://www.ncld.org
The Association for the Severely Handicapped (TASH) http://www.tash.org
National Early Childhood Technical Assistance System (NECTAS) http://www.nectas.unc.edu
National Early Childhood Technical Assistance System (NECTAS) Coordinating Office
    http://www.nectas.unc.edu

National Association for Gifted Children
   (NAGC) http://nagc.org
Teacher Supports
LD Learning Disabilities Online
   http://www.ldonline.org
National Transition Network
   http://www.ici.coled.umn.edu/ntn

Part III

PROFESSIONAL HUMAN SERVICE OCCUPATIONS

Chapter 20

HUMAN SERVICE OCCUPATIONS: SELECTED EXAMPLES

Michael A. Richard & William G. Emener

As you may recall, Chapter 1 discussed the similarities and differences among a job, a career, an occupation, and a profession. Pointedly, a profession is an occupation, vocation, or career where specialized knowledge of a subject, field or science is applied. Furthermore, the term "profession" is usually applied to occupations that involve prolonged academic training and a formal qualification; fittingly, it is clear in that professional activity involves systematic knowledge and proficiency. As witnessed in the previous 19 chapters, professionals are usually regulated by professional bodies that may develop and administer examinations of competence, act as a licensing authority for practitioners and enforce adherence to an ethical code of practice.

An occupation, however, typically refers to a field of employment or work in which the jobs within them may or may not be performed by professionals. For example, some authorities consider police officers professionals; others do not, and some consider them semiprofessionals. By and large, such distinctions are predicated on the extent to which the individual workers are or are not in keeping with the Marks of a Profession as discussed in Chapter 1.

At times, people will enter a field of work in what is called an "entry-level position." For example, a person may complete an associate's of arts degree and begin working as a licensed practical nurse. While doing so, he or she may continue attending nursing school, graduate with a B.S.N. degree (bachelor's of science degree in nursing), become a registered nurse and a standing member of a professional nursing association, and thus then consider him or herself a professional.

There are hundreds of different kinds of semiprofessional jobs, paraprofessional jobs, and professional occupations in which thousands of individuals earn good incomes and enjoy high levels of job satisfaction. It may very well be possible that you, the reader, may already be in such a position or thinking of applying for one. Thus, while the following discussions of professional occupations—which fall into such classifications as semiprofessional, paraprofessional, and "entry-level"—are not designed to be inclusive in any way, they do offer an opportunity to further understand some selected examples of professional occupations within or closely related to human services. The following discussion also includes the kinds of information one may want to know when exploring a future career in a professional occupation.

SUPPORTING INFORMATION

In 2002 more than 70,000 individuals graduated with an undergraduate degree in psychology. The vast majority of these individuals joined the work force immediately instead of enrolling in graduate school. Some of these persons will earn a higher degree later, but others will not (Murray, 2002). These numbers do not include persons who graduate with other human service degrees such as social work, rehabilitation counseling, criminology, or education. Furthermore, there are many persons who graduate with Associate of Arts degrees from community colleges in a human service field who never obtain their bachelors degree (National Organization for Human Services, 2007). In addition, many students work in the human service occupations described in this chapter are simultaneously working on graduate degrees while accruing invaluable work experience along the way.

This chapter will look at examples of employment opportunities in five broad areas were these graduates often work: (1) Behavioral and Mental Health; (2) Human Resources; (3) Education; (4) Police and Public Safety; and (5) Leisure and Recreation. These broad areas as well as the examples given are only a sampling of possible jobs that can be obtained by an individual with an associates or bachelors degree in a human service field. In each of these areas salary ranges, employment availability projections and examples of specific jobs with general descriptions are be presented. Furthermore the reader is provided a list of websites that can be accessed to obtain more information about these and other jobs.

It first may be helpful to delineate the major generic knowledge, skills, and attitudes that are a part of all employment in human services and related occupations. These skill and knowledge areas are ingredients of most community college or undergraduate programs in human services. Nonetheless, the on-the-job training for workers utilizing this knowledge base will vary in each employment situation due to differences in clientele served, nature of the work and purpose of the job (National Organization for Human Services, 2007). These six broad knowledge and skill areas are as follows:

1. Preparation which helps a potential worker understand human development, group dynamics, organizational structure and community organization, and how social systems interact in producing human problems.
2. Preparation in understanding major models for promotion of healthy functioning and the treatment or rehabilitation of problems. Depending on the area of employment, it can include medically-oriented, socially-oriented, psychologically-behavioral-oriented, and educationally-oriented models.
3. Jobs in many of these areas require preparation in how to appropriately identify and select interventions which promote individual growth and goal attainment. An employee should be able to conduct an analysis of what the issues are and then select strategies, services, or interventions that help clients attain a desired outcome. Examples of interventions are assistance, referral, advocacy, and/or guidance.
4. An individual is expected to have skills in planning, implementing, and evaluating selected interventions. The worker should be able to design a plan of action for an identified problem and implement the plan in an effective manner. This involves some grasp of problem and decision analysis. This

ability can be useful in all organizations and modified for use with different consumers or organizations. In all human service and related areas, an ability to evaluate interventions is an important component of the service delivery process.

5. An individual is expected to be able to select interventions consistent with the values of clients and the purpose(s) of the organization. This requires recognition of one's own values as well as an appreciation and acceptance of the organization's values stated in the goal statements of the organization.

6. Individuals are needed who have "process" skills which are necessary to arrange and apply services. Employers will assume that the worker uses themselves as the primary instrument for responding to consumer needs. Therefore, a worker must be skilled in communication and relationship building. Other related personal skills, are also often desired such as writing skills, self-control and orderliness.

These jobs often expect employees to be self motivated and perform the primary functions the worker role requires (National Organization for Human Services, 2007).

Although this chapter explores jobs other than those performed in human services, a generic description of a "Human Service Worker" are provided as these skills and knowledge bases frequently are primary requirements of jobs outside of human services. Furthermore even in the context of human services, there are individuals who are employed in professional as well as semi or paraprofessional occupations that need these skills (National Organization for Human Services, 2007).

The specific areas explored in this chapter are those jobs in varied settings such as: group homes; correctional facilities; facilities for developmentally delayed individuals and community mental health centers; family, child, and youth service agencies; and others. Furthermore, persons having the training and skills in these described areas also are in demand in occupations other than human services such as schools, business, and law enforcement. Depending on the employment setting and the consumers of the service, job titles, duties, and salaries will vary. However, a major goal of human service workers, as well as those in other areas, is to assist the persons served to function as well as they can in the major domains of living. A desire to help others is of vital importance in all the areas and jobs described in this chapter. A person who can demonstrate composure, thoughtfulness, and appreciation in their relationships with others, is valued by employers in human services as well as in many other disciplines. Given this background information, let's look at the five prime areas and some examples of jobs where persons with such interests, knowledge, and an associate- or bachelor-level training are often employed (National Organization for Human Services, 2007; Murray, 2002).

The following presented and described human service occupations include specific jobs as described in the *Occupational Outlook Handbook* (Bureau of Labor Statistics, 2008-2009). Consequently, requirements, major duties, and salaries are similar. However specific duties may have some variation because of purpose, clientele, or job setting. Therefore, requirements, major duties, and salaries as presented may not apply to all jobs in the individual sections. Furthermore, variations related to experience or specialized training will be noted within the context of the description of a specific job.

I. BEHAVIORAL AND MENTAL HEALTH

Social and Human Service Assistants

In many mental health settings paraprofessionals with some level of training in social worker, health care, psychology, or other human service education are employed to provide services to people. The term *Social and Human Service Assistant* is a generic term used in the *Occupational Outlook Handbook* (Bureau of Labor Statistics, 2008–2009) to describe a group of workers with numerous and varied job titles such as human service worker, case management aide, social work assistant, community support worker, mental health aide, community outreach worker, life skills counselor, or gerontology aide. These individuals typically work under the supervision of professionals from a variety of disciplines, such as nursing, psychiatry, psychology, rehabilitation counseling, physical therapy, social work, and others. The duties performed and supervision given will have a great deal of variability. Some may work with only a small amount of immediate direction. An example being a job or life skills coach working "in the field" with a client who is geographically separated from the job coach's supervisor. Nonetheless, there are other jobs, such as a psychiatric technician, who may work under the close direction of a professional or professionals (Bureau of Labor Statistics, 2008-2009).

Job opportunities for social and human service workers are expected to grow. Growth should be excellent for persons having appropriate post high school education such as provided in most human service educational programs. Job openings are most likely to be the result of job growth and a continuing need to replace workers who advance into new positions, retire, or leave their jobs. Competition for jobs in urban areas will be greater than in rural locations; however, those qualified should have little difficulty finding employment.

Annual wages for social and human service assistants was $25,580 in May, 2006, with the average salary being between $20,350 and $32,440. The top 10 percent earned more than $40,780, while the lowest 10 percent earned less than $16,180 (Bureau of Labor Statistics, 2008-2009).

Job Coaches are specialists who use various structured intervention techniques to help a person learn and successfully perform job tasks that minimally meet an employer's job needs and task requirements. They also may assist individuals in acquiring necessary interpersonal skills so that they can be accepted by other workers at a job site as well as in their community contacts. In addition to job-site training, job coaching includes performance assessment; job development; and some degree of counseling or guidance, advocacy, travel training, and any services that are needed to successfully maintain an individual in competitive employment. Job coaches rely heavily on behavioral interventions to help their clients acquire requisite skills. However, supportive and empathetic measures are utilized to validate and motivate their clients. The clientele for job coaches are often persons with developmental disabilities, severe mental illness, or disabilities that severely impact a person's capability to perform a job (Bureau of Labor Statistics, 2008–2009; Jeschke, Rajecki & Johnson, n.d.).

Life Skill Trainers also provide individualized services to their clients. The goal, however, is to assess then remediate any barriers which may impede a person's successful assimilation into his/her community. Services provided may include training in how to get around their communities or in-home training for clients placed in independent living situations. These paraprofessionals work closely not only with the client but also with the family to establish target goals and how to determine success (Bureau of Labor Statistics, 2008–2009; Jeschke, Rajecki & Johnson, n.d.).

Child Protection Workers often have the job title of *Social Service Worker* and develop appropriate assistance plans in an effort to lessen the risk to an identified child. Their responsibilities also include the implementation of measures that assure the protection and safety to identified children at risk of abuse or further abuse. When necessary, workers in child protection evaluate then choose suitable alternate care for children needed to be placed outside their home. They will then routinely inspect prospective placements to ascertain that minimal physical, mental, educational, and developmental needs are met. Responsibilities also may include the interaction with the child's family of origin or family of residence to consult with them regarding treatment or prescribed care and to determine if there are negative impacts on the family or child–issues that need to be resolved. These workers often provide initial interventions once such concerns have been identified.

Substance Abuse Counselors work in facilities that meet the needs of individuals who have been diagnosed as having problems with the abuse of various substances and are attempting to end such use. Persons employed in such settings are required to evaluate a participant's level of need for the substance or substances. To accomplish this, they are often trained in the use of both manual and computerized assessment instruments. They also may complete family needs assessments and are required to be involved in the development of treatment and discharge plans. Person working in such agencies are expected to provide individual and group interventions, educational information to clients, and to have a deep understanding of Alcoholic's Anonymous and

other 12-step programs. Individuals who work in this area should be skilled or willing to learn more confrontational and assertive methods of interaction with clients (Bureau of Labor Statistics, 2008–2009; Jeschke, Rajecki, & Johnson, n.d.).

Residential Counselors provide direct daily supervision, social skills training, and structure to youth in residence. This includes varying levels of residence, from voluntary to involuntary. They can be employed at camps, colleges/universities, correctional facilities, group homes, etc. If employed in such jobs, it is vital that a worker be reliable, dependable, organized, and creative, and has good communication skills. Due to the inconsistent and unpredictable need for such services, persons who work in these settings must be willing and available to accept flexibility in scheduling (Bureau of Labor Statistics, 2008–2009; Jeschke, Rajecki, & Johnson, n.d.).

Nursing and Psychiatric Aides are employed to help meet the needs of the physically or mentally ill, injured, disabled, or infirmed individuals. Employment settings include hospitals, nursing care facilities, and mental health settings. The primary function of employees in these settings is to oversee the daily care and support of persons so placed. The specific care they give depends on their specialty and may include empathetic support, self-care assistance, and psychoeducational assistance, as well as a wide variety of individually specific needs (PsychologyMajors.com, 2008).

Home Health Care Aides have duties that are very similar, but they usually work in a client's home or in a residential care facility. Due to their role in working with patients who need long-term care, nursing aides or home health care aides are among the occupational titles commonly referred to as "direct care workers." Persons who work in these jobs are far more often required to attend to the self-care needs of consumers;

therefore, knowledge of or a willingness to learn primary physical care skills are more often required than not (Bureau of Labor Statistics, 2008-2009).

Volunteer Services Directors perform administrative work focused on directing a comprehensive volunteer services program for a major department or agency. Workers in these jobs are responsible for the planning, development, and implementation of volunteer services for a variety of departmental or organizational programs such as soliciting and developing interest of groups and individuals to serve in a volunteer capacity, monitoring the quality and effectiveness of volunteer programs, and recommending new initiatives or changes as needed. The direct supervision of a small staff engaged in volunteer program operations and the volunteers, as well as consistent contact with community action groups, are frequently required (Bureau of Labor Statistics, 2008–2009).

Other Jobs: Behavioral and Mental Health (Bureau of Labor Statistics, 2008-2009)

- **Counselor Aides** assist counselors or any other credentialed employee with tasks relating to an adult, student, or youth counseling and/or guidance services that involve educational and career planning, personal/social development, and follow-up activities. Settings may include mental health centers, substance abuse facilities, and schools, etc.
- **Mental Retardation Unit Managers** are employed to supervise and instruct unit staff in the care of developmentally de- layed residents. They are charged with the coordination and organizing of individual activity schedules, daily routines, and program plans for residents

in a facility housing such persons. They usually are required to assist and monitor the maintenance of all residents' records.

- **Occupational Therapist Assistants and Aides** work under the immediate direction of occupational therapists in order to provide rehabilitative services to persons having a mental, physical, emotional, or developmental impairment. The primary goals are to improve a person's ability to perform daily activities and ultimately their quality of life. For ex- ample, occupational therapist assistants help injured workers re-enter the labor force by teaching them how to compensate for lost motor skills or they may help individuals with developmental disabilities increase their functional independence.
- **Veteran's Psychology Aide/Technicians** perform much of the nonprofessional technical work required in connection with a program of veteran's social services. This may include provision of information, daily emotional support and technical support in one or more specialized areas.

II. HUMAN RESOURCES

In business and industry, there is a consistent need to attract and hire the most qualified employees for a wide range of jobs. Once these persons are employed and have demonstrated worth to the organization, there is a need to match them to other jobs and tasks for which they may be capable and to provide or arrange necessary training. Human resources, training, and labor relations managers and specialists are the professionals charged with this selection/training process. Some workers in human resources also are charges with a variety of administrative functions of an organization, such as handling employee benefits questions and assuring hiring practices are in accordance with policies and procedures established by top management (About. com:Human Resources, 2008).

Increasingly, human resources (HR) professionals are more involved working with the management of companies, suggesting and changing policies. Other duties performed by HR departments include efforts to improve worker morale and productivity, limit job turnover, increase the efficient use of employee skills, provide training and development opportunities to improve those skills, and increase employees' satisfaction with their jobs and working conditions. Some jobs in the human resources field require little direct contact with workers outside the HR workplace, "handling the varied needs of the people within the organization is the primary part of their job" (Armstrong, 2003, p. 3).

There are many jobs performed by HR departments and in small organizations where one or a few human resources professionals may be responsible for all HR functions. However, in larger organizations different aspects of the services provided by HR may be the responsibility of several professionals with specialized training and skills. General areas of employment in HR are presented below, with specific jobs described as performed by specialists. Although specialized on-the-job training is often required to master these jobs, a bachelor's degree in one of the helping professions is often acceptable for entry-level positions. Nonetheless, it is fast becoming a requirement that persons wanting to work in the HR field obtain specialized certification. Specific information about the two primary HR certifications can be obtained from the following two organizations' websites: (a) the International Foundation of Employee Benefit Plans which offer three certificates (www.ifebp. org/Resources/News/Information+Services

/default.htm); and (b) the American Society for Training and Development (ASTD) which offers 16 certificates (www.astd.org/ ASTD/aboutus/). These two professional organizations represent the two broad areas of HR specialties: employment and benefits (About.com:Human Resources, 2008; Bureau of Labor Statistics, 2008–2009).

Annual salary rates for human resources workers vary according to occupation, level of experience, training, location, and firm size. Therefore median salaries will be presented for each occupation presented below.

Of the jobs in all occupational areas in this category of Human Resources, managers and specialists are expected to grow faster than most occupations. College graduates who have earned certification in several HR areas should have the best job opportunities. Overall employment is projected to grow by 17% between 2006 and 2016 (Bureau of Labor Statistics, 2008-2009).

Employment Specialties

Employment and Placement Managers supervise the hiring and termination process for business and industry. In larger organizations they supervise specialists who perform duties such as recruitment, selection, and placement. The "manager" position is generally not an entry-level position and requires several years of HR experience. With experience in one or several of the areas presented below, an individual may be considered for such a promotion. The median annual earnings for human resources managers were $88,510 in May, 2006. The middle 50 percent of HR managers earned between $67,710 and $114,860 (Bureau of Labor Statistics, 2008–2009). The job titles and duties performed by these specialists follow:

Employment, Recruitment and Placement Specialists recruit and place workers. Each of these is a separate specialty. However, persons employed in one of these areas may move from one to the other or may work concurrently in all three (About.com: Human Resources, 2008). The median annual earnings for all positions as employment, recruitment, and placement specialists were $42,420 in May, 2006. The middle 50 percent of individuals in these occupations earned between $32,770 and $58,320.

Recruiters develop and maintain contacts within the community and may travel extensively and often. They often visit college campuses to seek out promising students and persuade them to apply for open positions within their company or organization. Recruiters screen, interview, and on occasion test individuals who apply for positions. They may also be responsible for checking applicants' references and offer them jobs. These professionals must be very knowledgeable about their organization and its human resources policies. This is necessary so they can discuss with potential hires salary, work environments and milieu, and opportunities for advancement within the organization. They must also be (a) informed about equal employment opportunity (EEO) and affirmative action guidelines and laws, such as the Americans with Disabilities Act, and be (b) aware of any new developments in these areas (About.com:Human Resources, 2008; (Armstrong, 2003 p. 4).

Employment Interviewers are also known by many other job titles such as human resources consultants, human resources development specialists, and human resources coordinators. These specialists frequently are employed by governmental agencies, but many opportunities exist in companies that provide this service in the private-for-profit sector. These workers help match employers with persons seeking employment who are appropriately qualified for a job opening. These specialists are sometimes charged with employer relations and asked to maintain working relationships with local employers, as well as to promote the use of public or private employment programs and services (About.com:Human Resources, 2008; Armstrong, 2003 p. 6).

Benefit Specialties

Employee Benefits Managers administer companies' employee benefits programs. Benefits include importantly health insurance and pension plans. These professionals must have acquired proficiency in the design and administration of all benefits programs. These positions are of great importance–as benefit plans grow in number and become more complicated, employer-provided benefits account for an increasing part of compensation costs. For example, pension benefits might include a 401K or thrift savings, profit-sharing, and stock ownership plans; health benefits might include long-term catastrophic illness insurance and dental insurance. Knowledge of all employee benefits is required of employee benefits managers. These professionals also supervise the work of Compensation and Benefit specialists. This position in not an entry-level position but may be open to Benefits specialists who have several years of experience (About. com:Human Resources, 2008).

The median salary for compensation and benefits managers was $74,750 in May, 2006. The middle 50 percent of these professionals earned between $55,370 and $99,690 (Bureau of Labor Statistics, 2008-2009).

Compensation, Benefit, and Job Analysis Specialists perform duties required to manage the compensation and benefit programs for employers and may specialize in specific areas such as pensions or position classifications. These are the individuals who meet with workers in order to enroll in or start receiving such benefits. This specialist must be aware of different plans, costs, exceptions, and employee and employer responsibilities regarding all benefits for which employees are eligible (About.com: Human Resources, 2008). The median annual earnings for all occupations classified as compensation, benefits, and job analysis specialists were $50,230 in May 2006. The middle 50 percent of this cohort earned between $39,400 and $63,800 (Bureau of Labor Statistics, 2008–2009).

Job Analysts or Position Classifiers collect and examine detailed information about job duties in order to prepare job descriptions. These descriptions explain the duties, training, and skills necessary to perform a job. This data is collected through a variety of methods such as observation, structured interview, and review of existing job descriptions from places where the job may already exist. Whenever large organizations introduce a new job or update an existing job, they uses a specialist skilled in job analysis (Bureau of Labor Statistics, 2008–2009).

Other Human Resource Occupations

Training and Development Specialists conduct ongoing training and development programs for employees. Such activities are designed to help employees develop skills in order to improve productivity and quality of work, and to develop employee loyalty. Most importantly, their purpose is to improve individual as well as organizational functioning so as to better achieve business results. Training has increasingly become seen as a necessary and valuable employee benefit. Furthermore, it is seen as a way to improve employee skills and morale (About.com:Human Resources, 2008).

The median annual earnings for individuals working as training and development specialists were $47,830 in May, 2006. The middle 50 percent of these persons earned between $35,980 and $63,200 (Bureau of Labor Statistics, 2008–2009).

Equal Employment Opportunity (EEO) Officers or EEO Representatives (also referred to as *Affirmative Action Coordinators*) handle matter related to EEO matters in large organizations. In general, they may consider any company practices that may be in possible breach of EEO standards, as well as examine and attempt to settle EEO grievances. Furthermore, they are responsible for collecting, writing, and submitting EEO statistical reports. Knowledge of EEO standards and sensitivity to the needs of minorities and women is generally required (Bureau of Labor Statistics, 2008–2009).

The median annual earnings for persons working in this area of HR were $47,830 in May, 2006. The middle 50 percent of these specialists earned between $35,980 and $63,200 (Bureau of Labor Statistics, 2008–2009).

III. EDUCATION

If one is interested in a career in education as a public school teacher, he or she will need to obtain a bachelor's degree and certification in the state in which he or she want to teach. However, there are other jobs in public elementary and secondary education that do not require teacher certification. Many of such jobs are filled with persons having no undergraduate or graduate degree in education but by persons with just a high school diploma and others with associate or bachelor's degrees in one of the human services. When looking for employment in one of the positions presented below, it is recommended that one look for specific information about the position in the school district where one wishes to work as each district's job requirements will likely have some variation (Smith, 2007).

Behavior Interventionists or Specialists work in the classroom with students having emotional, academic, developmental, and/or behavioral issues. These para-professionals work one on one, or with small groups, in a school setting. They often work as a member of a team to develop and then implement behavior plans which are designed to help individual students in a specific area of need (e.g., academic, anger management, concentration). As such, they are often responsible for observing and collecting behavior data in the provision of therapeutic support and intervention, including physical support when necessary. The ability to form strong individual relationships with students is a necessity as this relationship is often the basis for problem solving and gaining insight and behavior skill acquisition. Usually, a bachelor's degree in human services or an education related field is the minimal requirement (Bureau of Labor Statistics, 2008–2009; Gaither & Butler, 2005).

The annual salary for behavioral interventionist or specialist was $25,580 in May 2006. The average salary for persons working in these jobs was between $20,350 and $32,440 (Bureau of Labor Statistics, 2008–2009).

Teacher Assistants (TAs) may also have titles such as teacher aide or instructional aide, and also are referred to as paraeducators or paraprofessionals. They are responsible for providing instructional and clerical support for classroom teachers; moreover, they support and aid children in learning class material using the teachers' lesson plans. A primary role is to provide students having academic difficulties with individual attention. They may also be in charge of the entire classes' supervision while in the cafeteria, schoolyard, hallways, or when on field trips. Specific clerical duties may include recording grades, setting up equipment, and helping the teacher develop and set up instructional materials. Some teacher assistants perform exclusively non-instructional tasks; however, most TAs will carry out a combi-

nation of instructional and clerical duties. They may work with students individually or in small groups and listen while a student reads, review an instructional lesson, or help a student find information. TAs work at both the elementary and secondary levels. At the secondary level, they may be required to have special knowledge in certain areas such as math or science. More and more, nonetheless, there often will be a TA assigned to work with students in computer laboratories, helping them to use computers and educational software programs. Knowledge of information technology and computers typically is a secondary requirement in these labs (Lou, Bellows & Grady, 2000; Smith, 2007).

The median annual earnings for teacher assistants in May, 2006 were $20,740. The middle 50 percent of TAs earned between $16,430 and $26,160 (Bureau of Labor Statistics, 2008–2009).

After-School Program Supervisors and Aides work in schools that receive funding for "after-school programs" for children. These programs usually consist of a supervisor, often a teacher, and several aides. In some instances, the district may hire someone from the outside to run these programs, and in such circumstance the supervisors typically must have minimally an associate's degree, but most districts prefer someone with a bachelor's degree and an individual with a degree in some area of the human services field. Also, they often require some experience working with children. Supervisors direct the entire program including staffing, activity planning, and overall administration. After-school aides are responsible for the direct supervision of student activities and at minimum are usually required to have a high school diploma and some work experience. The aide position is a wonderful entry-level position for someone looking to get the experience required to become a supervisor in this area.

To work in this area, an individual must enjoy working with children and have the ability to physically manage them when necessary. It should be noted, however, that these positions are almost always part-time.

A search of job postings in this area revealed entry level salaries of aides to be in the range of $9.00 to $13.00 per hour. The salary range for supervisors was $14.00 to $19.00 per hour (Bureau of Labor Statistics, 2008–2009; Smith, 2007).

Adult Literacy and Remedial Education Teachers instruct adults and out-of-school youths in reading, writing, math, and at times learning to speak English. Most adult education programs require teachers to have at least a bachelor's degree. The reader should also be advised that in many states, a public school teaching license is also required; thus, these positions may not be available to persons having nonteaching degrees. They can, however, assist individuals in areas such as reading, basic math, and other skills that will provide them minimal skills to solve problems well enough to become active participants in our society, find a job, achieve a promotion on a job, or continue their education. The instruction provided by these teachers is typically divided into three areas: (a) *remedial* or *adult basic education (ABE)*, which focuses on adults whose skill levels in math, reading, and/or writing are at or below an eighth-grade level; (b) *adult secondary education (ASE)*, which generally targets individuals who are studying to obtain their General Educational Development (GED) certificate or a high school equivalency credential; and (c) *English literacy*–the primarily instruction that assists adults with limited English proficiency improve their English language skills (Bureau of Labor Statistics, 2008–2009; Prickel & Wolff, 2002 p.20).

The median earnings of adult literacy and remedial education teachers were $43,910 in May, 2006. The middle 50 percent of teachers in this area earned between $32,660 and $57,310 (Bureau of Labor Statistics, 2008–2009).

Health Educators work to help individuals and groups to develop healthy lifestyles and wellness. They provide information to individuals, groups, and communities about behaviors that advance healthy living, prevent diseases, and dealing with other health-related issues. They need to be knowledgeable about health-related topics such as proper diet and the significance of exercise in promoting health and well-being. They frequently will be responsible for conducting workshops or information sessions on a variety of topics, such as how to avoid sexually transmitted diseases, and lifestyle promotion that will assist persons in avoiding illness or injury. They will often need to be able to assess the needs of their communities in order to determine what topic needs to be covered. Further, they also must be able to determine what information may be needed by a specific audience. For example, they may hold programs on sexually transmitted disease for high school students or for persons in a substance abuse facility. Specific information and depth of information may vary because of the needs of these different groups. A bachelor's degree is the minimum requirement for entry-level jobs in this area, but be aware that many employers now prefer individuals with a master's degree (Bureau of Labor Statistics, 2008-2009).

The median annual earnings of health educators were reported to be $41,330 in May, 2006. The middle 50 percent of these individuals earned between $31,300 and $56,580 (Bureau of Labor Statistics, 2008–2009).

IV. POLICE AND PUBLIC SAFETY

In spite of a decade of declining crime rates, the law enforcement field is growing. The fact that crime rates now are reported to be on the rise, coupled with numerous post-September 11 events, as well as heightened media attention to crime and an emphasis on homeland security, collectively have contributed to a rising demand for persons in the field of law enforcement.

Individuals who work in this area interact with people from all walks of life that are often very stressful. Experts indicate that people interested in law enforcement careers should have a number of personal qualities to be successful. First, one must have real a sense of compassion and a need for adventure–working situations for law enforcement professionals can be extremely volatile and emotional. A high standard of personal morality plus humility are needed as police officers are given tremendous power. Because of this power, people choosing to work in this area must realize that they will be under a great deal of scrutiny. Fittingly, they must be prepared and willing to be an open book in both their personal and professional lives. The careers in law enforcement in this section provide a review of several that are in demand in today's security-conscious society. It is important to note, however, that for each of the jobs presented, specific training above and beyond a bachelor's or associate degree will be required (Baker, 2006; Bureau of Labor Statistics, 2008–2009).

Persons employed in any of the four jobs below will likely be required to have a bachelor's degree. The preferred degree may be in criminology, although many professionals in these positions have degrees in other human service areas. The jobs presented below do not include jobs in the law enforcement careers. (Persons interested in such jobs should refer to Chapter 8 on Criminal Justice.)

The median annual earnings of probation officers, parole officers, pretrial service officers, and correctional treatment specialists in May, 2006 were $42,500. The middle 50 percent of persons employed in these jobs earned between $33,880 and $56,280 (Bureau of Labor Statistics, 2008–2009).

Probation Officers are called Community Supervision Officers in some states. They are responsible for the supervision of people who have been placed on probation. There are several variations of this entry-level job, based on the location of an individual in the corrections system (Bureau of Labor Statistics, 2008-2009; Burton & Latessa, 1992).

Correctional Treatment Specialists are similar to case managers; they offer guidance to offenders and create postrelease plans for them to follow when they are released from prison and/or are placed on parole (Bureau of Labor Statistics, 2008–2009; Burton, Latessa & Barker, 1992).

Parole Officers have very similar job descriptions and perform many of the same duties probation officers perform. The distinction being that parole officers supervise persons who have been released from prison, whereas probation officers work with those who are sentenced to probation instead of prison by the courts (Bureau of Labor Statistics, 2008–2009; Burton & Latessa, 1992).

Pretrial Services Officers are responsible for conducting pretrial investigations; such findings are used by the courts to help make decisions such as whether a person and society would best be served by sending the person to prison or being placed on probation. Also they make recommendations based on their investigation if a person should be released before their trial (Bureau of Labor Statistics, 2008–2009).

Other Law Enforcement Jobs *(Bureau of Labor Statistics, 2008-2009)*

- **Fish and Game Wardens** are responsible for the enforcement of fishing, hunting, and boating laws. They monitor areas where people hunt and fish.

As part of their job, they conduct search and rescue operations, investigate complaints and accidents, and may be called upon to investigate some cases and aid in prosecuting cases. Good interpersonal and communication skills are necessary as well as a knowledge of the fish and game laws of the area where employed.

- **The Department of Homeland Security** is fast becoming a primary employer of law enforcement and security officers at multiple levels. Further, a person can find employment within many different governmental agencies, such as Customs and Border Protection, Immigration and Customs Enforcement, and the United States Secret Service.

V. LEISURE AND RECREATION

Individuals employed in recreation and leisure professions work with individuals involved in organized recreation to promote personal growth, fitness, wellness, creativity, healthy leisure choices, and overall good quality of life. These professionals must have knowledge and skills in recreation program planning, group dynamics, facilitation techniques, cultural competence, supervision, and administration. Frequently, a major in Recreation Management is required, although students may find opportunities if they have degrees in other areas such as psychology, sociology, health, coaching, or nutrition (Bureau of Labor Statistics, 2008–2009; Ross, Beggs & Young, 2006).

Recreation workers hold a variety of positions in many different areas and at varying levels of responsibility. Individuals work in the following settings: general recreation, outdoor recreation, youth services, travel and tourism, college campuses, and many others. Workers may provide instruction and coaching in art, music, drama, swimming, tennis, or other activities. Persons interested in this field should note that employment frequently typically is seasonal (Ross, Beggs & Young, 2006; SUNY- Cortland, n.d).

In May, 2006, median annual earnings of recreation workers able to find full-time employment were $20,470. The middle 50 percent of those employed full-time earned between $16,360 and $27,050. The *Occupational Handbook* reports that directors and supervisors earn "substantially more" but gave no specific salary range. A brief search for salaries on line revealed a range of $50,000 to $60,000 per year for directors (Bureau of Labor Statistics, 2008–2009). Examples of careers in this area follow.

Camp Counselors lead and instruct children and teenagers in outdoor recreation activities, such as swimming, hiking, horseback riding, and camping. In addition, camp counselors may provide instruction in special areas such as archery, boating, music, drama, gymnastics, tennis, and computers; skills and knowledge in these areas are required. In residential settings, they also provide guidance and support, and may supervise daily living and socialization. Persons workings in these positions frequently do not have a college degree nor are students. These positions are generally seasonal or part-time and staffed by students (Bureau of Labor Statistics, 2008–2009).

Camp Directors supervise camp counselors and are responsible for the overall planning and implementation of camp activities and/or programs. They also are responsible for performing the various administrative functions required for the camp to function. More often than not, camp directors have a bachelor's degree in Recreation Management or another related degree in the human service field (Bureau of Labor Statistics, 2008–2009).

Recreation Leaders are often in charge of a recreation program's daily operation. These programs can be at resorts, cruise ships, camps, colleges/universities, or agencies such as the YMCA. They principally are responsible for organizing and directing participants, and frequently need to lead and give instruction in a variety of areas including dance, drama, crafts, games, and sports. It is necessary for persons working in this job to be organized as they schedule the use of facilities, keep records of equipment use, and ensure that facilities and equipment are used properly by participants (Bureau of Labor Statistics, 2008–2009).

Recreation Supervisors oversee recreation leaders, and do the overall planning, organizing, and managing of recreational activities designed to meet the needs of many different populations in a variety of settings. Again, these programs can be at resorts, cruise ships, camps, colleges/universities, or agencies such as the YMCA. Furthermore, they frequently serve as liaisons between the director of recreation and recreation leaders. Recreation supervisors having some specialized skills may be responsible for directing activities or events in these areas or oversee major activities such as aquatics, gymnastics, or performing arts (Bureau of Labor Statistics, 2008–2009; Ross, Beggs, & Young, 2006).

Recreational Therapists, also referred to as **Therapeutic Recreation Specialists**, provide treatment services and recreation activities for persons with disabilities or illnesses. A wide range of techniques, including arts and crafts, animals, sports, games, dance and movement, drama, music, and community outings are utilized. The goal of such techniques is to improve and maintain the physical, mental, and emotional well-being of participants. Recreational therapists are different from recreation workers. Recreation workers work in settings such as camps, resorts, etc. and organize activities

for the enjoyment of the participants. Recreation therapists work at facilities with the mission of serving persons with disabilities and the purpose of enhancing the quality of life for these individuals. A bachelor's degree in recreation therapy or in a human service field with specialized training is required, but more often a master's degree is becoming the minimum degree accepted.

Median annual earnings of recreational therapists were $34,990 in May, 2006. The middle 50 percent earned between $26,780 and $44,850 (Bureau of Labor Statistics, 2008–2009).

SUMMARY

The wonderful thing about having a bachelor's or associate's degree in a human service field is that the training and education will provide an individual with a great deal of flexibility–more than most any other degree. In other words, one will have multiple career options, as witnessed by the occupations presented in this chapter. No matter what career path one chooses, he or she will likely be working with people. They may be clients, patients, customers, coworkers, employees, and/or bosses. To wit, a quality education in a human service field will prepare one to be a critical thinker, and the skills and knowledge acquired through coursework and out-of-class experiences will make one marketable in many employment settings. Even though a bachelor's or associate's degree in human services will not be considered a "professional" degree, one will be a well-educated and compassionate person, and career options will abound. Remember, if one chooses to pursue an advanced degree, the experience one might obtain working in any of these occupations will be invaluable.

REFERENCES

About.com:Human Resources. (2008).Success in career and personal development and management Retrieved June 21, 2008 from www.humanresources.about.com/od/careerplanningandadvice1/Success in education program design today.

Appleby, D.C. (n.d.). Descriptions of occupations of interest to psychology majors from the Dictionary of Occupational Titles. Retrieved June 21, 2008 from www.uni.edu/walsh/DOTdescrips.htm.

Armstrong, M. (2003). *A handbook of human resource management practice* (9th ed.). London: Kogan Page.

Baker, B. M. (2006). *Becoming a police officer: An insider's guide to a career in law enforcement.* Bloomington, IN: iUniverse, Inc. p1–2.

Bureau of Labor Statistics, U.S. Department of Labor. (12/18/07). *Occupational outlook handbook, 2008–09 Edition.* Retrieved June 18, 2008 from www.bls.gov.

Burton, V.S., Edward, J., Latessa, E.J., & Barker, T. (1992). The role of probation officers: An examination of statutory requirements. *Journal of Contemporary Criminal Justice, 8*(4), 273–282.

Gaither, G. A., & Butler, D. L. (2005). Skill development in the psychology major: What do undergraduate students expect? *College Student Journal, 9*(3), 540.

Jeschke, M. P., Rajecki, D. W., & Johnson, K. E. (n.d.). *Life beyond the bachelor's degree: A primer for psychology majors.* Retrieved June 21, 2008 from www.psynt.iupui.edu/Users/kjohnson/bulletin/primer.htm.

Lou, J., Bellows, L., & Grady, M. (2000). Classroom management issues for teaching assistants. *Research in Higher Education, 41*(3), 353–383.

Murray, B. (2002). Good news for bachelor's grads.: Psychology training opens doors for recent graduates. *Monitor on Psychology, 33*(6) retrieved June 21, 2008 from www.apa.org/monitor/jun02/goodnews.html.

National Organization for Human Services. (2007). *The human service worker.* Retrieved June 21, 2008 from www.nationalhumanservices.org/public-resources/about-human-services.

Prickel, D., & Wolff, S. (2002). Adult education and career and technical education. In M. A. Richard, & W.G. Emener (Eds.), *I'm a people person: A guide to human service occupations.* Springfield, IL. Charles C Thomas.

PsychologyMajors.com. (2008). Undergraduate psychology degree: Psychology career options. Retrieved June 21, 2008 from www.psychologymajors.com/what-can-i-do-with-my-undergraduate-psychology- degree.

Ross, C. M., Beggs, B. A., & Young, S. J. (2006). *Mastering the job search process in recreation and leisure services.* Sudbury, MA: Jones and Bartlett.

Smith, D. D. (2007). Non-teaching careers in education: Information on para-professional and support positions. Suite101.com. Retrieved June 20, 2008 from www.suite101.com/about/.

SUNY–Cortland Recreation and Leisure Studies Department. (n.d.). Careers in general recreation. Retrieved June 18, 2008 from www.cortland.edu/rec/career/general.htm.

WEBSITES

Academy of Leisure Sciences
www.academyofleisuresciences.org/

American Association for Leisure and Recreation (AALR) www.member.aahperd.org/sandbox/generationXXX/aalr/template.cfm?template=main.html

American Probation & Parole Association (APPA)
http://www.appa-net.org

American Society for Training & Development
www.astd.org/ASTD/aboutus/

International Foundation of Employee Benefit Plans (IFEBP) www.ifebp.org/Resources/News/Information+Services/default.htm

Occupational Outlook Handbook
www.bls.gov/OCO/

National Recreation and Park Association (NRPA) www.nrpa.org/

Society for Human Resource Management (SHRM) www.shrm.org/about/

SELECTED JOB DESCRIPTIONS FROM DICTIONARY OF OCCUPATIONAL TITLES

Academic Counselor
www.occupationalinfo.org/04/045107010.htm

Advertising Sales Representative
www.occupationalinfo.org/25/254357014.html

Alumni Director
www.occupationalinfo.org/09/090117014.html

Animal Trainer
www.occupationalinfo.org/15/159224010.html

Career Information Specialist
www.occupationalinfo.org/24/249367014.html

Caseworker
www.occupationalinfo.org/19/195107010.html

Child Development Specialist
www.occupationalinfo.org/19/195227018.html

Child Welfare/Placement Caseworker
www.occupationalinfo.org/19/195107014.html

Claims Supervisor
www.occupationalinfo.org/24/241137018.html

Coach
www.occupationalinfo.org/15/153227010.html

Community Organization Worker
www.occupationalinfo.org/19/195167010.html

Community Worker
www.occupationalinfo.org/19/195367018.html

Conservation Officer
www.occupationalinfo.org/37/379167010.html

Correctional Treatment Specialist
www.occupationalinfo.org/19/195107042.html

Corrections Officer
www.occupationalinfo.org/37/372667018.html

Customer Service Representative Supervisor
www.occupationalinfo.org/23/239137014.html

Department Manager
www.occupationalinfo.org/29/299137010.html

Dietician
www.occupationalinfo.org/07/077117010.html

Employee Relations Specialist
www.occupationalinfo.org/16/166267042.html

Employment Counselor
www.occupationalinfo.org/16/166257010.html

Employment Interviewer
www.occupationalinfo.org/16/166267010.html

Financial Aid Counselor
www.occupationalinfo.org/16/169267018.html

Fund Raiser I
www.occupationalinfo.org/29/293157010.html

Guidance Counselor
www.occupationalinfo.org/04/045107010.html

Human Resource Advisor
www.occupationalinfo.org/16/166267046.html

Information Specialist
www.occupationalinfo.org/10/109067010.html

Job Analyst
www.occupationalinfo.org/16/166267018.html

Loan Officer
www.occupationalinfo.org/18/186267018.html

Mental Retardation Aide
www.occupationalinfo.org/35/355377018.html

Minister, Priest, Rabbi, Chaplain, etc.
www.occupationalinfo.org/12/120107010.html

Nurse
www.occupationalinfo.org/07/075364010.html

Patient Resources and Reimbursement Agent
www.occupationalinfo.org/19/195267018.html

Personnel Recruiter
www.occupationalinfo.org/16/166267038.html

Police Officer
www.occupationalinfo.org/37/375263014.html

Polygraph Examiner
www.occupationalinfo.org/19/199267026.html

Preschool Teacher
www.occupationalinfo.org/09/092227018.html

Probation/Parole Officer
www.occupationalinfo.org/19/195107046.html

Psychiatric Aide/Attendant
www.occupationalinfo.org/35/355377014.html

Psychiatric Technician
www.occupationalinfo.org/07/079374026.html

Public Relations Representative
www.occupationalinfo.org/16/165167014.html

Real Estate Agent
www.occupationalinfo.org/25/250357018.html

Recreation Leader
www.occupationalinfo.org/19/195227014.html

Retail Salesperson
www.occupationalinfo.org/27/279357054.html

Social Services Aide
www.occupationalinfo.org/19/195367034.html

Substance Abuse Counselor
www.occupationalinfo.org/04/045107058.html

Veterans Contact Representative
www.occupationalinfo.org/18/187167198.html

Vocational Training Teacher
www.occupationalinfo.org/09/097221010.html

Volunteer Coordinator
www.occupationalinfo.org/18/187167022.html

Writer
www.occupationalinfo.org/13/131067046.html

Part IV

ETHICS AND PROFESSIONALISM

Chapter 21

PROFESSIONAL ETHICS AND PROFESSIONALISM

WILLIAM G. EMENER, MICHAEL A. RICHARD & JOHN J. BOSWORTH

The difference in success or failure can be doing something nearly right . . .
or doing it exactly right.

–Henry Ford

As we discussed in Chapter 1, underlying the 18 chapters in Part II of this book is the implicit assumption that you not only want to work with people, but you want to do so as a professional. And while Part III addresses nonprofessional occupations you may consider that are available in human services or related fields, they also require you to act in an ethical manner. If this is true, then it behooves you (1) to be knowledgeable and appreciative of what a profession is, (2) to remain aware of the essential role of ethics in professionalism, and (3) what ever you do–at least do it right.

PROFESSIONALISM IN HUMAN SERVICES

Critical to the provision of human services is the continuing assurance of consumer protection. Two generic attributes of human service consumers are that they most often are: (1) hurting, in trouble, and/or vulnerable; and (2) ignorant, unknowing, and/or helpless in terms of helping themselves. For example, few people see a medical doctor because they are feeling good and not worried about some aspect of their health. Typically, people are hurting or worried about some condition or situation they do not understand. In addition, they do not know what to do about their conditions or situations (otherwise, they would fix it themselves). Interestingly, it has been suggested that the two most powerful professions in American society are medicine and law (Emener, 1987). Most people who go to see a doctor or a lawyer are either hurting and/or in trouble and don't know what to do. Also, most people do not even know what knowledge and skills are minimally necessary for the professional assisting them. Thus, most societies have established, maintain, and publicize *regulatory mechanisms* to set, monitor, and enforce standards and requirements so when a "hurting, in trouble, vulnerable, unknowing, and uninformed" citizen goes to a professional for help, he or she can trust and have confidence in the assistance and help provided.

HUMAN SERVICE REGULATORY MECHANISMS

There are four regulatory mechanisms pertinent to human service professions: (1) certification; (2) licensure; (3) registration; and (4) accreditation.

Certification

If a professional is "certified," then the public can feel assured that he or she has met minimum published standards of competency in his or her discipline as evidenced by formal education, experience, supervisory evaluation, and, typically, the passing of a state or nationally standardized examination. Thus, for example, if a rehabilitation counselor has "CRC" after his or her name, it means that he or she is a "Certified Rehabilitation Counselor."

Licensure

Licensure to practice a profession or trade is regulated by state legislation, and typically is operationalized under the auspices of a state board of professional regulation. Some licensure boards also regulate nonprofessional occupations as well (e.g., plumbers, electricians). Importantly, if a professional is "licensed," he or she is able to: (1) go into private practice; (2) function autonomously (i.e., without required, direct supervision); and (3) qualify for "third-party funding" (i.e., he or she not only can charge and get paid by clients directly, but also can charge for services to be paid for by a third-party, such as an insurance company). Penalties associated with licensure typically are severe and restrictive (e.g., in most states, a person cannot even refer to himself or herself as a "psychologist" unless he or she is licensed as a psychologist in that state). Thus, for exam-

ple, if a professional has "LMHC" or "LPC" after his or her name, it means that he or she is a "Licensed Mental Health Counselor" or a "Licensed Professional Counselor" and is so licensed by a state regulatory body.

Registration

Most states have a list, or "registry," of certified and/or licensed professionals who have met state and/or national requirements to practice their respective profession. For example, nurses may have "R.N." after their names, signifying that they are "registered nurses."

Accreditation

In the human services arena, accreditation includes two main areas: (1) the accreditation of organizations, service agencies, facilities, and institutions; and (2) the accreditation of professional preparation programs. Regarding the former, if a rehabilitation facility such as a sheltered workshop is "CARF Accredited," it means that that facility has demonstrated high quality service-delivery standards and practices to the Commission on Accreditation or Rehabilitation Facilities. A person could have trust and confidence in the services provided at a CARF-Accredited facility. Regarding the latter, if a doctoral program in clinical psychology at a university is "APA Approved," it means that academic program has met the quality standards set by the American Psychological Association. Likewise, if you earn a Ph.D. degree from an APA Approved psychology program, you can trust you have received a high quality education; furthermore, prospective employers would have confidence in your knowledge, skills, and expertise.

AUTONOMY AND PROFESSIONAL BEHAVIOR

It is of conscientious importance to underscore the critical nature of "autonomous functioning" and "professional behavior" on behalf of a professional.

A few years ago, this chapter's first coauthor, Dr. Emener, received a phone call from another licensed psychologist asking if she could refer a client to him. Further discussion revealed that the referring psychologist had completed two sessions with a male client who was in recovery from alcoholism, and she realized that: (1) the client closely resembled the man from whom she was recently divorced; and (2) at this particular time in her life due to the recency of her emotionally challenging and difficult divorce, she was unable to be totally objective and "professional" with her client. Two of the critical "autonomous functioning" attributes in this example are (a) she was aware of her own issues and recognized her lack of objectivity, and (b) she did the right thing and referred the client to another psychologist who could be objective and professional.

The second coauthor of this chapter, recently was attending a picnic, and during a conversation with a small group of attendees was asked, "Dr. Richard, I would appreciate it if you would talk with me for a few minutes and tell me if you think I am depressed." With genuine warmth, care, and professionalism, he replied, "It sounds like you are concerned about feeling down and depressed. Here is one of my business cards, and if you would call me at my office, we could arrange an appointment at my office to evaluate you for depression. I'm sure you would agree this is not the time or place to do that." She smiled and acknowledged her agreement with his well-made point.

This chapter's third co-author, Mr. Bosworth, has had numerous examples of chronic pain patients who, in their best efforts, attempt to persuade him to sign off on disability applications due to lack of functioning and severity of their condition. However, he usually requires a thorough assessment and evaluation in order to rule out malingering, substance dependence/addiction issues, and other maladaptive behavior patterns often seen among people with chronic pain conditions. Recognition of these maladaptive behaviors is crucial in order to prevent enabling maladaptive coping responses, but also to make sure that those with legitimate conditions receive the proper care and support.

It is important to note that in all three of these situations, the professional was aware of what was going on, knew what to do, and did what was needed with class, concern, and consideration for the client (or potential client). Among other things, it is this self-awareness, self-monitoring, and self-direction that undergirds the public's confidence and trust in professionals.

PROFESSIONALS' CODES OF ETHICS

Among the attributes of any professional is the fact that his or her behavior is guided by a code of ethics (Corey, Corey & Callahan, 1988). As illustrated in all of the chapters in Part II of this book, every profession has its own code of ethics. Furthermore, each profession's code of ethics is known, endorsed, and practiced by its members.

Ethical codes are not designed to tell respective professionals what is right or wrong, or what to do or not do, in a given situation. They are not rules or laws; rather, they are philosophical principles designed to guide the professional in making the best decision for each individual client and/or each individual situation. Like every human being, every situation is different, unique, and requires a decision befitting the individual circumstance. Fittingly, inherent to any code of ethics are five guiding philosophical principles.

1. *Autonomy* . . . . . I will act in a manner that respects and facilitates my client's freedom of choice.
2. *Beneficence* . . . . I will act in a manner that promotes the growth and well-being of my client.
3. *Fidelity* . . . . . . I will act in a manner that keeps promises and commitments to clients, colleagues, and agencies, both stated and implied.
4. *Justice* . . . . I will act in a manner that will treat clients fairly.
5. *Nonmalfeasance* I will act in a manner that does not cause harm to clients and prevents harm to clients.

It is interesting to note that these principles are intentionally competing. For example, facilitating a client's "freedom of choice" may not guarantee that the client will act in a manner that will assure his or her "growth and well-being." But, as previously stated, every client with whom a professional works and every situation in which they find themselves is unique and different. By design every client and every situation calls for a unique decision. Codes of ethics do not provide the answers—they provide the professional with philosophical guidelines and principles with which to make the best possible decision.

THE ROLE(S) OF KNOWLEDGE IN A PROFESSIONAL'S DECISION-MAKING

Human service professionals constantly make decisions and assist others in making decisions. Usually, "good decisions" are not made by data or information alone; nonetheless, "poor decisions" usually are made in the absence of data and information. Having accurate, complete, and pertinent information is critical in good decision-making. For the human service professional, knowing what information he or she has, as well as the source and validity of the information, are important.

There are many sources of knowledge, such as: (a) tradition; (b) expert opinion; (c) documentation; (d) individuals in position of authority; (e) common sense; (f) faith; (g) intuition; (h) logical reasoning; (i) personal experience; and (j) habit. Do not assume that any of these or any other sources of knowledge are more important, pertinent or meaningful than the others. What is important is to know the source(s) of all information you have. Do not suffer from the transgression of *secondary ignorance.* Or as expressed in an informal way, "Primary ignorance is when you don't know nothin'; secondary ignorance is when you don't even know that you don't know nothin'." In your role as a human service professional there are four crucial things you need to know about "your" knowledge:

1. *Know What You Know.* Knowledge is critical in decision-making—you should know what you know.
2. *Know What You Don't Know.* This refers to the "secondary ignorance" notion—knowing what you don't know is an important piece of information.

3. *Know the Source of What You Know.* Be critical of your knowledge and it's source. A "They say. . . ." source of information is contingent upon who *they* are. Another illustration of this postulate is the light-hearted expression Dr. Emener uses in lectures on professional decision-making: "All Indians walk in single file–at least the one I saw did."

4. *Know How What You Know Affects What You Do.* Our knowledge affects and influences most aspects of our lives, our feelings, attitudes, perceptions, decisions, and especially behavior. Appreciating how knowledge (and lack of knowledge) affects us is very important.

PROFESSIONALS' "ULTIMATE" DECISIONS

Pertinent to professionals' decision-making, Saad Nagi (1977) suggested three "ultimate" decisions that professionals make (if they truly are professionals). The following will briefly discuss these "ultimate decisions" with representative illustrations.

1. *Who Do I Serve?* Professionals ultimately decide who they serve and who they do not serve. For example, if you look closely at courses listed in college and university catalogues, the term "Instructor's consent required" explicitly means that professor has the right (and responsibility) to determine who will and who will not be allowed to take his or her course. If a floor nurse in a hospital were to discover that a family member was a patient on his or her floor, he or she would have the right (and the responsibility) to request another nurse attend to the family member.

2. *How Do I Serve?* For a professor, this refers to the issue of "academic freedom"; no administrator at a college or university will dictate or tell a professor how to teach a course. Likewise, an agency may establish goals for clients receiving services but should not dictate to the professionals employed by the agency (e.g., counselors, social workers) how to best serve the clients on their caseload.

3. *When Do I Terminate Services?* When students complete a degree in higher education and attend their graduation ceremony, the appropriate academic officer, such as a dean, will introduce the graduating students by name and then say, "Mr. (or Madam) President, *based on the recommendation of the faculty*, I request that these students receive their aforementioned degrees." It is the faculty who decides when students have completed degree requirements, not the Dean, etc. Likewise, the only person other than yourself who can sign you out of a hospital is your attending physician. Thus, as a professional, you will be the person with the authority and responsibility of determining when a client has completed his or her program with you (e.g., counseling, treatment plan).

For almost a decade, numerous professionals (e.g., Janes & Emener, 1999) have suggested that the rise in the managed care model of human service delivery has eroded some of these areas of professionals' ultimate decision-making. Fittingly, it behooves professionals to work hard to preserve their capacity to make such decisions–the decisions that define their professionalism.

YOUR "PROFESSIONAL SELF-CONCEPT"

The phenomenon of self-concept could be expanded to include a person's concept of himself or herself in more than a general or overall sense. For example, a person could think about his or her "self" as a parent, an athlete, and/or as a professional–his or her *professional self-concept*. How an individual's professional self-concept significantly interfaces with an employer or a job, ultimately offers an insight into their primary source of identification–as an employee or as a professional. Consider, for example, the following illustration:

Lois has a master's degree in Rehabilitation Counseling from an accredited master's degree program, is a Certified Rehabilitation Counselor (CRC) and a member of the National Rehabilitation Counseling Association. She is employed by a state vocational rehabilitation agency and has the job title "Rehabilitation Counselor." Her professional self-concept, however, can be interestingly analyzed by finding out her primary source of professional versus employer affiliation. From an analytical perspective: does Lois think to herself: "I am an employee of the state, and I am working as a rehabilitation counselor." OR does Lois think: "I am a professional rehabilitation counselor, and I am employed by the state."

Central to Lois' or anyone's way of thinking about them self, is whether their primary sense of affiliation and identification is with their employer or with their profession.

CONCLUDING COMMENT

Winston Churchill said, "The best indication of the civilness of any society is in the way it treats its vulnerable citizens." This tradition primarily has included children, the elderly, and individuals with disabilities. It could be argued when working as a professional that caring for and helping vulnerable individuals (who also may be hurting, in trouble and/or uninformed, and unable to meaningfully help themselves), that you have a professional obligation to offer them the best help and assistance available. We suggest that this is not just a professional obligation; you also have a moral obligation to do so. If you believe in this challenge (to offer your clients the best help and assistance available), then you are obligated to be the best you can be. And ala Henry Ford, "Do it right." If you don't believe in this challenge, maybe being a human service professional is not for you. Hopefully it is (and maybe that's why you're reading this book and are now reading this chapter). Go for it! You owe it to people who will need you, and you owe it to yourself.

REFERENCES

Corey, G., Corey, M.S., & Callahan, P. (1988). *Issues and ethics in the helping professions* (3rd ed.). Pacific Grove, CA: Brooks/Cole.

Emener, W.G. (1987). Ethical standards for rehabilitation counseling: A brief review of critical historical developments. *Journal of Applied Rehabilitation Counseling, 18*(4), 5–8.

Janes, M.W., & Emener, W.G. (1999). The human side of health care in the new millennium. In C.G. Dixon & W.G. Emener (Eds.), *Professional counseling: Transitioning into the next millennium.* Springfield, IL: Charles C. Thomas.

Nagi, S. (1977). Disability concepts and implications to the structure of services. An address to the American Rehabilitation Counseling Association, Dallas, TX.

ABOUT THE EDITORS

William G. Emener, Ph.D., CRC, is a Distinguished Research Professor in, and the former Chair of, the Department of Rehabilitation and Mental Health Counseling, and a former Associate Dean at the University of South Florida, Tampa. Additionally, he has worked as a rehabilitation counselor and supervisor as well as a rehabilitation counselor educator and program director at Murray State University, Florida State University, and the University of Kentucky. Dr. Emener's publications and writings include seven research monographs, 23 books, numerous book chapters in 22 different books, over 50 nonpublished professional papers, over 100 authored/coauthored articles in 17 different professional refereed journals, and over 100 professional papers presented at professional association meetings. He also has been an editor/coeditor of over 20 special publications (including the *American Rehabilitation Counseling Association Newsletter*) and was Coeditor of the *Journal of Applied Rehabilitation Counseling* from 1978–1982. While many of his books have been textbooks and professional readings, his more recent books are pop-psych books, self-help books, and contemporary romance novels.

Dr. Emener's recognitions include being a recipient of the *1980 American Rehabilitation Counseling Association Research Award,* a recipient of the National Rehabilitation Administration Association's *1982 The Advancement of Research in Rehabilitation Administration Award,* and in 1988 was honored with the title of Fellow by the American Psychological Association. He was the 1983–1984 President of the National Rehabilitation Administration Association and the 1989–1990 President of the National Council on Rehabilitation Education.

For 33 years, Dr. Emener also had a part-time private practice as a licensed psychologist in Florida and Kentucky, with specializations in employee assistance programs, marriage/couples counseling, and addictions/substance abuse counseling. A former college basketball player, Bill's hobbies and interests now include playing his guitar and piano, fishing, boating, scuba diving, motorcycle riding, slow pitch softball, reading contemporary novels, playing golf, and occasionally walking a sandy beach with a six-pack.

Michael A. Richard, Ph.D., CRC, is an Associate Professor in the Department of Rehabilitation and Mental Health Counseling at the University of South Florida–Sarasota/Manatee. He serves on several university and departmental committees and provides ongoing advising and counseling services at the University Counseling Center in Sarasota. He has worked as a vocational evaluator, rehabilitation counselor, and behavioral program supervisor in the private sector for over 12 years prior to obtaining his doctorate, and also has taught graduate and undergraduate courses in rehabilitation counseling as well as providing undergraduate student advising at Emporia State University for three years. He received his B.S. degree from Athens College, his M.Ed. from Auburn University, and his Ph.D. from The Florida State University. He is a Certified Rehabilitation Counselor and worked for more than ten years in the field as a Rehabilitation and Mental Health Professional. His research interests include consumer satisfaction assessment of counseling services and diversity training for counselors. Dr. Richard also has coedited two books, and published six articles in peer reviewed journals and five book chapters.

John J. Bosworth, M.A., is a Licensed Mental Health Counselor in private practice (www.bozcounseling.com) and a member of the adjunct faculty of the Department of Rehabilitation and Mental Health Counseling at the University of South Florida, Tampa. There, he also serves as a member of the External Advisory Committee providing on-going consultation between academic endeavors and requirements and the practical application of student resources toward careers and employment in private settings. John received a B.S. in Psychology from Florida State University and a M.A. in Rehabilitation and Mental Health Counseling at the University of South Florida. He was trained in depth in Rational-Emotive Behavior Therapy at the former Albert Ellis Institute and The Rational Living Foundation/Center for Rational Living in Tampa. His areas of specialization in private practice include anxiety, depression, substance abuse, family and adolescent issues, and stress and pain management (he also is a member of the staff at Gulf Coast Pain Management in Palm Harbor, Florida–www.gulfcoastpain.com).

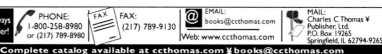

Reference Book - Room Use Only